Sport in the Global Village

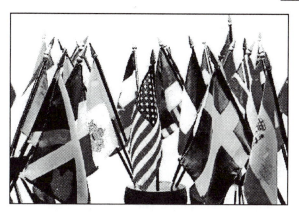

Ralph C. Wilcox

Editor

Fitness Information Technology, Inc.
P.O. Box 4425, University Avenue
Morgantown, WV 26504

Library of Congress Catalog Card Number: 94-70170

ISBN 0-9627926-4-0

Cover Design: Augusta Group
Production Editor: Greg Carte
Printed by: BookCrafters

Printed in the United States of America
10 9 8 7 6 5 4 3

Fitness Information Technology, Inc.
P.O. Box 4425, University Avenue
Morgantown, WV 26504 USA
(800) 477-4FIT (4348)
(304) 599-3482

Contents

Part 3: Professional Sport in Global Perspective

Part 4: Sport and the South African Question

Part 5:   Sport in the New Europe

Part 6:   International Sport

Part 7: Sport in the Global Village: Comparative Perspectives

Part 8: Theoretical and Methodological Considerations in the Cross-Cultural Study of Sport

Notes on Contributors

John Baxter is Head of Sports Administration at the University of the Witwatersrand, South Africa. He is a Trustee on the Board of the South African Soccer Academy and Honorary Treasurer of the South African Sports Sponsors Association. Since 1986 he has been a facilitator, advisor and consultant for the National Sports Congress, white establishment sports organizations, and foreign embassies and their government representatives. He is a committee member of the body coordinating the five commissions preparing a macro structure for non-racial sport in South Africa.

David Black is an Assistant Professor of Political Science at Dalhousie University, Canada. He has authored articles on Canadian foreign policy, Canadian policy towards South Africa, Canadian diplomacy and the Edmonton Commonwealth Games, and the political economy and foreign policy of Namibia and Botswana. His current research interests include sport in inter- and transnational politics, and Canada-Africa relations in the post-Cold War era.

Paul F. Blair is with the Department of Physical Education and Athletics at Mayville State University, North Dakota. His research interests are in the cross-cultural dimensions of sport.

Wolf-Dietrich Brettschneider is Director of Sport Pedagogy at the Institut für Sportwissenschaft at the Freie University of Berlin. His research interests are in sport and youth.

Asa Briggs was Provost of Worcester College, Oxford, from 1976 to 1991. He is the author of many books on social and cultural history, including five volumes on the history of the British Broadcasting Corporation.

Eric F. Broom is affiliated with the University of British Columbia, Canada, and served as President of the International Society for Comparative Physical Education and Sport, from 1988 to 1992. His research interests focus on comparisons of national, regional, and local sport and recreation systems, including policies, agencies, programs, funding, facilities provision, design and management, and coach education and employment.

Roy A. Clumpner is Chair of the Department of Physical Education, Health, and Recreation at Western Washington University. He has published and presented papers on American government involvement in sport,

Canadian/American cross-cultural studies in physical education and sport, pedagogy of physical education, and elite sport systems for international success. His current research interests in the sociocultural area relate to the historical development of inactivity in physical education.

Peter G. Craig is a Senior Lecturer in the Department of Physical Education, Sport and Leisure at Bedford College of Higher Education, England where he teaches in the sociology of sport and leisure. His research interests are in the cultural analysis of physical education, sport and leisure; sport and leisure in conflict societies; postmodernism; together with self and identity theory.

Jean Craven has competed, officiated and administered sport to the international level in three countries. Her current research interests focus on cross-cultural impacts on effectiveness in sport and she has worked as a consultant to Sport Canada, the Coaching Association of Canada, Alberta Ministry of Recreation and parks, the British Olympic Association; and the British Institute of Sports Coaches.

Scott A. G. M. Crawford is a Professor in the College of Education and Professional Studies at Eastern Illinois University where he also serves as Graduate Coordinator in the Department of Physical Education. He is on the editorial board of the *ICHPER Journal* and is a book review editor for the *International Journal of the History of Sport.*

Braham Dabscheck is an Associate Professor in the School of Industrial Relations at the University of New South Wales, Australia. He is editor of *The Journal of Industrial Relations* and the *Australian Society for Sports History Bulletin*. He has published widely on Australian industrial relations as well as economic and industrial relations aspects of professional team sports. His most recent book is the co-edited *Contemporary Australian Industrial Relations: Readings* (Melbourne: Longman Cheshire, 1992). He is currently working on unionism in Australian Rugby league, and a book on recent developments in Australian industrial relations.

Soeren Damkjaer is a Senior Lecturer at the Center for Sports Sciences at the University of Copenhagen. His research interests are in the sociology and history of sport; the sociology of the body; the aesthetics of dance and performance; and sport and cultural change in Eastern Europe.

Karen P. DePauw is the Associate Dean of the Graduate School and Professor in the Department of Physical Education, Sport and Leisure Studies at

Washington State University. She teaches and conducts research in the area of physical activity and sport for individuals with disabilities.

Ted Fay is an adjunct faculty member at the University of Massachusetts-Amherst, teaching courses in international sport and event management. He serves as Nordic chairperson and a member of the Sports Council Executive Committee for the International Paralympic Committee. His research interests are inclusion and equity for athletes based on race, gender, and disability.

Frank H. Fu is Reader and Head of the Department of Physical Education at Hong Kong Baptist College. He is an International Fellow of the American Academy of Kinesiology and Physical Education and has held faculty appointments Springfield College, USA, the China National Research Institute of Sports Science, and Guangzhou Institute of Physical Culture, China. His research interests are in sports physiology and psychology, and comparative physical education and sport.

Siegfried Gehrmann is affiliated with the Department of History at the University of Essen, Germany. He is the author of *Fußball—Vereine—Politik. Zur Sportgeschichte des Reviers 1900-1940*. Essen: Hobbing, 1988, and is presently at work on a book on Max Schmeling and the history of professional boxing in Germany.

Grace Goc Karp is an Assistant Professor in the Department of Physical education at the University of Idaho. She teaches and conducts research in the area of sport pedagogy, specifically in teacher behavior and curriculum development.

Herbert Haag is a Professor of Sport Pedagogy, and Director of the Institute for Sport and Sport Sciences at the University of Kiel, and is Director of the German Olympic Institute in Berlin. He serves as editor of the *International Journal of Physical Education* and the book series, *Texts on the Theory of Sport Disciplines*. His research interests include curriculum and instruction in sport; evaluation of teaching and learning processes in sport; comparative sport pedagogy, and scientific foundations of sport science.

Ken Hardman is a Lecturer in Physical Education at the University of Manchester, England. He is President of the International Society for Comparative Physical Education and Sport and serves as Editor of the *Physical Education Review*. His current research interests include the identification and development of young sporting talent, and the status of physical education worldwide.

Ilse Hartmann-Tews is a Senior Lecturer at the Institute of Sport Sociology, German Sport University, Cologne. Her research interests include the processes of social differentiation in sport from a comparative perspective; women's studies in sport sociology; sport and environment (green policy of sport governing bodies). Her most recent publication (with P. Gieß-Stüber) is *Frauen und Sport in Europa*, (Skt. Augustin: Academia Verlag, 1993).

Denver J. Hendricks is Deputy Dean in the Faculty of Arts at the University of the Western Cape. His most recent publication is "Physical Education as Power in South Africa: A Figurational Perspective," in Jonathan Jansen (ed.), *Knowledge and Power in South Africa: Critical Perspectives Across the Disciplines*. His current research interests focus on the role of sport in South African society. He is presently involved in composing a new "sports model" for the post-apartheid South Africa.

Roman Holcek is affiliated with Comenius University and the Slovak Union of Physical Culture.

Reet Howell died, in Australia, of cancer on June 10, 1993, only 48 years of age. She authored 18 books (including *Her Story in Sport, The History of Sport in Canada, The Genesis of Sport in Queensland, The Sporting Image, Aussie Gold, Foundations of Physical Education, Concepts of Physical Education,* and *The Greatest Game Under the Sun*), and had over 100 research publications. She presented papers in more than 20 countries. Born in a refugee camp in Sweden, of Estonian parents, she was renowned as a Baltic scholar and was an authority on sport in the ancient world, women in sport, and indigenous games.

Robin Jones is a Lecturer in the Department of Physical Education, Sports Science, and Recreation Management at Loughborough University. His current research interests embrace the topics of sport and physical education in China; the effect of economic reforms on sport; and the integration of sport into Chinese culture.

Clark C. Jwo is in the Department of Physical Education at the National Taiwan Normal University, Republic of China. His research interests are in the psychosocial dimensions of sport; and wellness and fitness management.

Hiroshi Komuku is a sport sociologist in the Department of Physical Education at Tenri University, Japan. His research interests lay with sport in culture, and sport and the body.

March Krotee is affiliated with the School of Kinesiology and Leisure Studies at the University of Minnesota. He is past President of the International Relations Council of the American Alliance for Health, Physical Education, Recreation and Dance. His research interests are in the psychosocial, comparative, and international dimensions of sport, and in the organization and management of sport.

Ming Li is an Assistant Professor in the Department of Sport Science and Physical Education at Georgia Southern University where he teaches in the area of sport management. His research interests include the administration of intercollegiate athletics, and the financing of sports organizations.

Rotislav Matousek is affiliated with Comenius University and the Slovak Union of Physical Culture.

Kazunori Matsumura is a sport sociologist with the Institute of Health and Sports Sciences at Tsukuba University, Japan. His research interests are in sport and the rural community.

Richard V. McGehee is Professor of Kinesiology at Southeastern Louisiana University, where he teaches history of physical education and sport. His current research interests include the development of modern sport and sport festivals in Middle America, and the history of the New Orleans Athletic Club.

Oleg Milshtein is affiliated with the Central Institute of Physical Education, Russia.

Roman Moravec is affiliated with Comenius University and the Slovak Union of Physical Culture.

Roland Naul is with the Department of Sportpadagogik at the University of Essen, Germany.

John Nauright is a Lecturer in the socio-cultural aspects of human movement at the University of Queensland, Australia. He is co-author (with Tim Chandler) of an upcoming book on Rugby and masculine identity and of another, co-authored with Dave Black, on New Zealand-South African Rugby relations. He is also working on the history of sport and female identity.

Werner Neuhaus is with the Department of Sportpadagogik at the University of Essen, Germany.

Jacob Nteere is Chair of the Department of Physical Education at the University of Kenyatta, Kenya. His research interests are in the politics of physical education and sport.

Pirkko Numminen is in the Department of Physical Education at the University of Jyväskylä, Finland. Her research interests lay in the areas of motor development and learning.

Catherine "Kitty" O'Brien is Program Director for Human Movement and Health Education at the University of Sydney, Australia. She teaches undergraduate and graduate courses in comparative physical education and sport. Her current research examines the sociocultural factors affecting women's participation in sport in Southeast Asia.

Lisa L. Pike is an Assistant Professor of Sport Law in the Sport Management program at the University of Massachusetts-Amherst, where she teaches courses in Amateur and Professional Sport Law, as well as Labor Relations in Professional Sport. Her primary areas of research are in sport law and international sport management. She is a member of the Massachusetts bar and counsel to Sport Ventures International, an athlete management firm.

John C. Pooley is a Professor in the Department of Exercise Science and Movement Studies at East Stroudsburg University. He has taught and coached in six countries across three continents, and has studied sport in 15 other countries throughout Europe, Asia, and North America. His research relating to cross-national issues, with particular reference to youth sport and physical education programs, has been published in national journals in Australia, Canada, Portugal, the United Kingdom, and the United States. A Founder Member of the International Society for Comparative Physical Education and Sport, he has served two terms as President.

C. Roger Rees is a Professor in the Department of Physical Education and Human Performance Science at Adelphi University, where he teaches courses in the sociology and social psychology of sport and physical education. He is interested in how sport is used as a cultural symbol, and has lectured on this topic in several countries (including South Africa). He is the co-author (with Andrew Miracle) of a forthcoming book entitled *Lessons of the Locker Room: Myth and Ritual in High School Sport*, to be published by Prometheus Press.

Antonin Rychtecky is affiliated with Charles University, Czech Republic.

George H. Sage is a Professor of Kinesiology and Sociology at the University of Northern Colorado. Among his recent publications are *Power and Ideology in American Sport: A Critical Perspective, Sociology of North American Sport* (co-authored with D. Stanley Eitzen), "The Golf Boom in South Korea: Serving Hegemonic Interests," *Sociology of Sport Journal* (1992), and "Sport and Physical Education and the New World Order: Dare We Be Agents of Social Change? *Quest* (1993). His current research interests include the political economy of sport and globalization.

Jaromir Sedlacek is affiliated with Comenius University and the Slovak Union of Physical Culture.

Darwin M. Semotiuk is a Professor of Kinesiology at The University of Western Ontario, Canada. He is a member of the Executive Board of ISCPES and serves as Co-Editor of the *Journal of Comparative Physical Education and Sport. Cross Cultural and International Studies.* He was recently elected as an International Fellow of the American Academy of Kinesiology and Physical Education. His research interests are in sport and politics, East Bloc sport, and Canadian public sports policy.

Barbara A. Smith is currently a doctoral student in sport pedagogy at the University of Idaho. She served as the graduate assistant for Professors DePauw and Goc Karp on their grant for internationalizing the physical education curriculum at Washington State University funded by the WSU International Program Development Office.

Joy Standeven is affiliated with the Chelsea School of Physical Education, Sport Science, Dance and Leisure at the University of Brighton, England. Her research interests are in sport and tourism—interdependency and infrastructures, market profiles, environmental and economic impacts; and leisure preferences and patterns on the basis of gender and age.

Brian Stoddart is Dean of the Faculty of Communication at the University of Canberra, Australia, where he was a founding member of the Centre for Sports Studies. One of Australia's leading authorities on sport and culture, he has been a keynote speaker at several international conferences and a commentator on sports issues for a wide range of media outlets. He has written several books, including *Saturday Afternoon Fever: Sport in the Australian Culture*, as well as a large number of articles in leading scholarly journals.

C. Lynn Vendien is Professor Emeritus with the University of Massachusetts at Amherst and former President of the International Society for Comparative Physical Education and Sport.

Michael J. Vitelli completed his graduate work, in the area of comparative and international sport and physical education, at The University of Western Ontario, after having graduated from The University of Toronto. In 1992, he was named recipient of the ISCPES's prestigious C. Lynn Vendien Award.

Ralph C. Wilcox is Professor and Chair, Department of Human Movement Sciences and Education at The University of Memphis. He served as Director of "Sport in the Global Village: Comparative Perspectives", the 8th Biennial Conference of the International Society for Comparative Physical Education and Sport. His current research interests include American sport and cultural imperialism in contemporary Europe, and the commodification of sport in Eastern Europe.

Victor Zilberman is a physical education teacher at Vanier College in Montreal, Canada. Born in the former Soviet Union, he was educated in the USSR, Canada, and Israel. His research interests include international sport systems; and high performance sport and physical education in East European countries, Germany, and China.

Preface

*T*he timeliness and global significance of the publication of *Sport in the Global Village* is quite apparent for much has changed in the world throughout the past few years. A dynamic, geo-political metamorphosis has seemingly spanned the globe, characterized by social dislocation, tension and realignment in Eastern Europe; preliminary settlements in the Middle East; optimistic shifts in South Africa; the tentative consolidation of a new European Community; and talk of a New World Order. While the problem and significance of sport may pale in comparison with concerns for overpopulation and world hunger, environmental disasters, health epidemics, and the wanton denial of basic human rights, this book has a very important role to play in the academic arena of international studies.

As technological advances and the ideological gravitation toward shared values, combine to draw the peoples of the world ever closer to the reality of a global village, it behooves us to maximize cross-cultural intercourse along the path to human betterment and improved global understanding. Whether out of raw curiosity or the desire to compare oneself with another, the chapters in this book will necessarily contribute to the enhancement of global awareness and cross-cultural literacy. As important is the examination of the nature and role of sport in contrasting cultures as well as the possibility of formulating reform measures in sport policy and practice around the world.

The chapters contained in this book represent a balanced collection of fine and relevant scholarly pieces that will fill a significant void in the literature. Including contributions from historians, political scientists, and sociologists, as well as by scholars in faculties of business, communication, and education, this is truly an international book reflecting authorship from four different continents. Throughout the editorial process, great sensitivity has been placed on preserving the unique cultural character of each contribution while at the same time striving for the highest standards of scholarship. What has emerged is a diverse account of the nature and role of sport in the world today. Replete with optimism yet tempered by domestic and global concerns, *Sport in the Global Village* represents a revealing and useful source for students and scholars within the broad field of international affairs.

Ralph C. Wilcox

Acknowledgments

This important collection of works by authors from 15 different countries is an outcome of *Sport in the Global Village: Comparative Perspectives*, the 8th Biennial Conference of the International Society for Comparative Physical Education and Sport (ISCPES), held at the University of Houston from June 12-18, 1992. I would like to take this opportunity to thank all delegates for their active participation in the conference. The quality of this work rests primarily with the authors.

The success of the meeting was due to the efforts of many. Above all, I wish to recognize the extensive and unselfish contributions of my personal friends and former colleagues at the University of Houston, James R. Morrow Jr. (University of North Texas, USA), and Shayne P. Quick (University of Western Sydney, Australia), who so readily accepted and ably fulfilled their respective roles as Associate Conference Director and Academic Program Coordinator. I also wish to extend my appreciation to members of the Program Committee who assisted in the formulation of the academic program, the selection of papers, the moderation of sessions, and the review of manuscripts. Noel D. Ryan maintained a sense of humor throughout, serving as Conference Administrator and ensuring that the frequently mundane, daily tasks of running an international conference were carefully attended to. Furthermore, the many and varied talents of Melba Morrow, particularly in editorial and registration matters, made my life as Conference Director so much easier.

The support of the ISCPES Executive Board, the University of Houston community, an Advisory Council of prominent figures in the international sports arena, together with keynote speakers Asa Briggs, Anita DeFrantz, Neal Gunn, Jack Kelly, Carl Lewis, Charles C. Ragin, and Brian Stoddart ensured that the conference was a major success. I am most grateful to the conference sponsors, including Continental Airlines; Houston Sports Association, Inc.; Mastercard International, Inc.; Mr. and Mrs. Roy H. Cullen; Rice University—Department of Human Performance and Health Sciences; Texas Association for Health, Physical Education, Recreation, and Dance; UNIGLOBE Dynamic Travel; and the University of Houston—Department of Health and Human Performance—College of Education—Office of the President. Moreover, the special contributions of students, whose names are too many to mention, their smiling faces, previously undiscovered talents, and genuine warmth remain among my most satisfying memories of *ISCPES '92*.

The people at Fitness Information Technology, Inc., most notably Andrew C. Ostrow, President, and Production Editor, Gregory A. Carte of Augusta Group, must be congratulated for their patience, so critical in the publication of international works, and the exceptional quality of the finished product. Finally, I would be remiss if I were not to recognize the people that through their sacrifice really allowed this work to come to fruition, my family—Barbara, Rachael, Rebecca, and Brian.

Ralph C. Wilcox
Memphis, 1994

Foreword

Eric F. Broom

Since the last conference of the International Society for Comparative Physical Education and Sport in 1990, the world of sport has undergone, and is undergoing, momentous change. The brochure for the 1992 conference *"Sport in the Global Village: Comparative Perspectives"* described the proposed academic program thus:

> Coming at a time of major political and economic change in the world, delegates will examine the nature and role of international sport in the emerging global village.

The brochure went on to identify thirteen thematic areas which focused upon many of the major issues confronting sport in the last decade of the twentieth century. These were the issues that were examined and debated throughout the conference, and I would congratulate the organizing committee on their vision and perspicacity in selecting the themes and I thank you for being here to present the fruits of your scholarly labor. The world of sport is in the process of unprecedented change and we are privileged to take part in the scholarly exchange that the conference program will provide. I look forward to the next five days with great anticipation. If you will permit me I would like to open the door ever so slightly and throw a chink of light on some of those themes, to whet our appetites so to speak.

There is no doubt that international sport has, in the past quarter century, become a multinational business in the global marketplace. The Summer Olympic Games in Montreal, in 1976, were a financial disaster with a deficit in excess of $1.0 billion, while the 1984 Los Angeles Games registered a surplus of $223 million, and the Seoul Games in 1988 a surplus of $497 million. Critics doubt that these latter Games actually generated a surplus because the balance sheet does not include an estimated $1.5 billion spent by the government on buildings and urban infrastructure. As in any business competition is fierce. While the Olympic Games do well financially the lower prestige sporting festivals, such as the Commonwealth Games and World Student Games, find it impossible to balance the bottom line as evidenced by Auckland in 1990 and Sheffield in 1991.

The Olympic Games and other major sport festivals are also in competition with two major sports, soccer and athletics (track and field), which have developed very successful World Cup competitions. A bitter protracted battle between the IOC and FIFA in 1989 resulted in the Olympic Games' soccer competition being limited to players 23 and younger. The IOC, which wants the best players in the world, irrespective of age, intends to re-open the struggle after 1992. In athletics the IAAF World Cup will now be held every two years, rather than every four years as it was prior to 1991. The Cup will be held in uneven years, thus avoiding a clash with the Olympic Games, but it will affect the smaller festivals such as the Pan American Games and a host of regional festivals.

In terms of salaries for professional players some sports are clearly in the big business league. The leading example must be baseball in the United States where, in 1992, 269 players will make at least $1.0 million in the year, up from 223 last year and 153 in 1990. In 1992, 28 players will each earn more than $3.0 million, 22 more than $4.0 million, 3 more than $5.0 million and 1 more than $6.0 million. Among major league players the average 1992 salary will be between $1.1 and $1.2 million, and 38% will earn $1.0 million or more.[1] These levels of salary owe much to the strength of player associations, or unions, and we shall hear several papers dealing with their development. At the other end of the scale in the traditionally amateur sport of Rugby football public attention, during the recent World Cup, was focused not only on the very high level of play but also on the question of remuneration of players to compensate for time off work for training and playing. Some countries have made 'under-the-counter' payments for many years; others still balk at the prospect. With the World Cup generating millions of dollars profit, change is inevitable. Somewhere in the middle of these two sports are previously amateur sports in which the top performers are able to command substantial fees. Athletics, or rather some of the events in athletics, is probably the best example. As far back as 1984 it was reported that Carl Lewis earned $783,000 in that year, and a further five athletes, two of whom were women, earned in excess of $350,000.[2]

As the Olympic Games in Barcelona draw near, the world anxiously awaits to see what the former Soviet Union can do in the arena in which it has performed with such success in the past four decades. Certainly, since the advent of perestroika, the Soviet sport system has undergone, and continues to undergo, major change. We at this conference anxiously await the insights which will be provided in presentations by sports scholars from within and without the boundaries of the former sport giant. In similar vein to the former Soviet Union the boundaries of many countries in Eastern Europe are being re drawn. We shall hear presentations from sports scholars on the developments in Estonia,

Slovenia, and the Baltic States. Sport in re-unified Germany is also of great interest to us, and to the sports world at large, and it has generated a number of papers. Papers by scholars from the former Federal Republic will be balanced by that of a scholar formerly from the Democratic Republic. What whets my appetite are those papers which focus upon unification but end with a question mark.

In many parts of the world countries are in the throes of either fragmentation or unification. Perhaps the most audacious example of the latter, as far as sport is concerned, are proposals by Jacques Delors, President of the European Commission. For $20 million the European Community (EC) purchased a political foothold in the form of a major presence in the opening ceremonies for both the Albertville and Barcelona Olympic Games. The EC's initial proposal that the Winter Games should be formally opened by Delors was rejected by the Albertville Committee. The proposals that the twelve EC nations should collectively march under the blue community flag and wear the EC symbol on all uniforms, were rejected by the European Association of National Olympic Committees. This latter body has since revealed that it was approached in 1986 by Delors who wanted the twelve nations to send one team to the Olympic Games in Seoul in 1988. It is interesting to note that the $20 million fee for involvement in the two 1992 ceremonies will go directly to the organizing committees of Albertville and Barcelona. Nothing will go to the IOC or National Olympic Committees.[3]

The ramifications of the Middle East crisis will be reported on in two papers. There has been voluminous material on the effects of the turmoil, both within the region and globally, but to my knowledge little or nothing has focused upon sport. I await these papers with great interest, as I do the paper on sport in Northern Ireland. It is my understanding that governments have made massive financial investments for the building of facilities in an attempt to alleviate social problems. How successful has this action been, I wonder?

Emerging and developing countries have long utilized sport to obtain international recognition and prestige, as well as to develop national pride and unity. Examples would be Pakistan, the German Democratic Republic, Cuba, and China. The conference will hear, at first hand, of sport development and its role in a number of East and West African countries, and also from a number of scholars on the situation in China. To learn of developments in Czechoslovakia, as it struggles to function under new governmental and social structures, will also be of great interest. The return of South Africa to Olympic competition after a hiatus of 32 years and its emergence from the sporting wilderness in many non-Olympic sports after a slightly shorter absence is a major event in world sport. International sport has undergone much change in the last quarter century, and South Africa is currently experiencing dramatic social and political change. It would therefore be surprising if the changes in sport, both internally and internationally, occurred without the odd hiccup. We welcome scholars from South Africa, who will provide commentary on developments in their country, and also scholars from other countries who will provide an international perspective.

Comparisons of the importance attached to and the methods of identifying and developing athletic talent in different countries are of widespread interest, and we have papers dealing with England, Germany, and China. I'm intrigued by the title "Selling international athletic talent to the global village's highest bidder." Does it deal, I wonder, with the sale of Russian and Czechoslovakian hockey players to National Hockey League teams in North America, or with players from the Yugoslavian soccer team Red Star, from Belgrade? This team, the European and World club champions in 1992, has been financially crippled by the United Nations' sanctions which ban Yugoslavian athletes from international competition and is being forced to sell its best players in order to survive.

The title also reminds me of an article I read recently on Mark McCormack in a newspaper series on the four most powerful people in world sport. The other three incidentally, whom McCormack far eclipsed, were Juan Samaranch, Joao Havelange of world soccer and Primo Nebiolo of world athletics. To quote from the article:

> ...the job of McCormack's more than 1,000 employees is to spot embryo talent, nurture it, massage its ego and then manage it to the point where no intrusive distraction from the real world disturbs the concentration of the talent that brings in the money,...[4]

Two recent additions to McCormack's International Management Group, which had a turnover in 1991 of over $1.0 billion, are Michael Schumacher, a 23-year-old German racing driver, and Anna Kournikova, a 10-year-old Russian tennis player. Miss Kournikova and her mother have already been shipped off to Nick Bollettieri's tennis ranch, which incidentally Mark McCormack owns.[5] Mark McCormack, and IMG, are at one extreme of the sport marketing consortium, and I imagine that Brian Stoddart's Keynote Address will focus in that area. Other sport management papers examine the status of the education process, with global implications.

A number of papers will examine the question "What will become of Physical Education?" The debate will focus primarily on England, Japan, and the State of Victoria in Australia. The potential role of the Olympic Movement in sport education will also be presented. Several papers will present comparisons of the extent of women's participation in sport, primarily in Asian and S.E. Asian countries. Provision for, and attitudes towards, sport for special populations are compared by a number of scholars.

The issue of deviant behavior—cheating, substance abuse, and violence—is one of sports' most pervasive problems. Since the Canadian Ben Johnson tested positive in Seoul, in 1988, Canadian sport has been required to bare its soul by the Dubin Inquiry. One conference paper examines the post-Dubin Report restructuring of Canada's national sport system. A small number of other countries have also been active in attempts to stem the use of illegal substance and practices. However, a recent publication suggests that much remains to be done. The Dubin Report should have revolutionized world sport. It has been ignored. The word 'Dubin' is seemingly blacklisted by the IOC Review and the IAAF Newsletter.[6] These authors plainly accuse the Olympic movement and its leaders of corruption, brought on by excessive commercialism. The charges range from the huge amounts of money now involved in cities bidding for the Games to the massive revenues from television rights.

The sums of money involved are immense. In its bid to secure the 1996 Summer Games the successful city—Atlanta, spent $7.0 million, while two unsuccessful cities, Toronto and Athens, respectively spent $14.0 million and $22.0 million. International sport and the mass media have developed a symbiotic relationship in the last quarter century. Each feeds on the other. For the US television rights to the 1992 Summer Olympic Games NBC paid $401 million, $101 million more than it paid for the rights to the Seoul Games in 1988. CBS paid $243 million for the US rights to the 1992 Albertville Winter Games and will pay $300 million for the 1994 Winter Games in Lillehammer. The average advertising rate for a 30-second unit during the Albertville Winter Games was $250,000 compared to $850,000 for the same time during the January 1992 American football Superbowl.[7] In 1991 US networks spent the following for the right to televise sport: National Football League: CBS (four years) $1.06 billion; ABC (four years) $925 million; NBC (four years) $752 million; ESPN (four years) $450 million; and Turner Network Television (four years) $450 million. Baseball, and to a lesser extent basketball, received comparable amounts. Notre Dame University alone received $30 million for football coverage.[8] In May 1992 the International Amateur Athletic Federation (IAAF) signed a massive television contract with the European Broadcasting Union amounting to $91 million for the next four years. The previous record, for the expiring four-year contract, was only $6 million.[9] With these levels of expenditures it would be surprising if television did not exert a great deal of influence on sport. Certainly commentators and color men have become the image makers and the shapers of public attitudes and values. I look forward to hearing the words of Lord Briggs and our other presenters on this topic.

A second recent British publication "More Than a Game," which is being broadcast in an eight-part television series by the BBC, has Sebastian Coe as one of its major contributors. If the first episode is anything to go by, the book and the television series lift the lid and reveal some very unsavory practices in sport.

All of us throughout this conference will be focusing on the future of sport, both international and recreational. In my very occasional low moments I sometimes say to myself, "It's not what it used to be;" but that is probably nothing more than a very early visit from Father Time. In sport, as in life, little if anything is as it was, and that is what makes both so fascinating. I firmly believe that sport, at all levels, is an excellent vehicle for human self-realization—discovery, expression, and development. That is not to say that all is well with sport. There is much that I would dearly like to change. Sport itself is fine, it is what people do to it that causes the problems. Sport has changed greatly in the past forty years. Some would say it has sold its soul to politicians, big business and television. As we go about our deliberations in the next few days we shall no doubt debate the extent to which that claim is correct.

Notes

[1]Hernandez, Martha P. Associated Press, New York, April 3, 1992.

[2]*Runner's World,* May 1985, p. 41.

[3]Miller, David. "Delors treads on dangerous games ground." *The Times* (London). February 4, 1992.

[4]Wooldridge, Ian. "The Power Brokers." *Daily Mail.* (London). May 9, 1992, p. 73.

[5]Wooldridge, p. 73.

[6]Simson, Vyv, and Andrew Jennings *The Lords of the Rings: Power, Money and Drugs in the Modern Olympics.* London: Simon and Schuster, 1992, p. 198.

[7]Associated Press, New York, February 26, 1992.

[8]Associated Press, New York, September 4, 1991.

[9]Miller, David. *The Times.* (London). May 27, 1992.

Part 1: Sport and Globalization

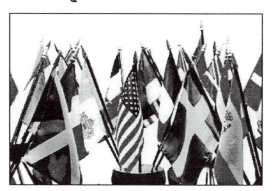

Chapter 1 *The Media and Sport in the Global Village*
Asa Briggs

Chapter 2 *Golf International: Considerations of
Sport in the Global Marketplace*
Brian Stoddart

Part 1: Sport and Globalization

The opening section of this book provides the reader with a fundamental philosophical platform upon which the remaining chapters build together with extensive and diverse evidence for the emerging internationalization of modern sport throughout the past one hundred years.

Asa Briggs, best known for his work in nineteenth-century British social and cultural history, and for his multi-volume history of broadcasting, presents a fascinating examination of the interdependence of culture, media, and sport in the global context. In his chapter (the text of his earlier keynote address), Briggs frames the topics for discussion developed further by subsequent contributors. With characteristic perception and incisiveness he raises a variety of questions concerned with sport as a signifying element of culture; the role of the media in the construction of popular sport; the political and economic control of sport and the media; and the impact of television on changing sport. Briggs' etymological diversion into the origin of key terms proves invaluable as does his account of Marshall McLuhan's conception of the "Global Village" in his 1968, co-authored book entitled, *War and Peace in the Global Village*. Aboveall, one is struck by the historian's contagious enthusiasm at witnessing such far-reaching global change for, as he wrote, "There is a new world around the corner and it will not be run by villagers."

Brian Stoddart's analysis of sport in the global marketplace follows the international fortunes of golf throughout the past century. Stoddart argues that the globalization of sport far-preceded modern technological development in the mass media and was the product of a variety of global events and patterns. The author furnishes an abundance of empirical evidence to support the global presence of golf today. Exploring the sport's diffusion from St. Andrews, in Scotland, during the late nineteenth century Stoddart attributes the contemporary, international popularity of golf to the early export of Scottish professionals to all corners of the globe; publication of golf manuals the world over; the establishment of international team competition; the emergence of globetrotting players drawn to international venues by appearance money; the global marketing of golf-related goods and services (including clubs, and course design); together with improved and instantaneous communication through both travel and the media. Recognizing the persistence of characteristic exclusive tradition, Stoddart recognizes the potential for demographic change as the process continues.

Chapter 1

The Media and Sport in the Global Village

Asa Briggs

Throughout this chapter, I am raising basic questions about the relationship between sport, itself a conglomerate term, and the media, an equally conglomerate term. For me it comprises print media, including literature, everything from diaries and autobiographies to novels and poetry, and I throw in music as well as electronic media. A contrast used to be drawn between the electronic and the rest. For technical and cultural reasons it no longer exists. It was never as sharp as it seemed, but while it continued to be drawn, it focused attention on 'standards,' however they were defined, on quality, not quantity, and on the differences between 'high culture' and 'popular culture.' For some, the advent of the electronic seemed a threat, as it did, of course, to many people involved in the management of sports who were afraid not only of its possible effects on the number of people passing through turnstiles but also of its impact on the distribution of leisure time.

Sports in the plural, for each has had its own distinctive history and orientation, figured relatively little in academic discussion of the age of the electronic media. Much has been made since of the way in which creative writers before the age of the electronic media dealt with sports in their writings, presenting them as mirrors of society. I am thinking, for example, of Allen Guttman's *A Whole New Ball Game*, "an interpretation of American sports."

As a historian of the nineteenth century I have often gone back to Mark Twain's lyrical proposition that baseball was "the outward expression of the drive and push and rush and struggle of the raging, tearing, booming nineteenth century," recognizing, of course, that like all statements about the nineteenth century—for that matter the twentieth also—it is highly selective. So, too, was T. S. Eliot when he put sport at the center of his list of what he called "the characteristic activities and interest of the English people"—what in his view made up their 'culture.' He was prudent enough to state in his title that the book constituted *Notes towards the Definition of Culture* rather than pretended to define it. More than half of the thirteen items in his list related to sports. Among them were Derby Day (horse racing), the Henley Regatta (rowing), the 12th of August (shooting), and the Cup Final (soccer). Of the four, the last three were 'popular culture,' the first three highly stratified class culture. Yet all four were great events in an annual calendar, two of which, Derby Day and the Cup Final, were presented to the public in words and in pictures by the media, a term not yet used in Britain in 1947.

Being Anglo-American, Eliot did not include cricket. There was no mention of a Test match. But then he did not mention Wimbledon either. Both of these were, of course, international events rather than national events. But then so too was the Henley Regatta. For that matter, as an Anglo-American he did not note the negative significance of the absence of baseball. Eliot did include in his list, however, three other English sporting activities which were activities, not events—'the dog races,' 'the pin table' and 'the dart board,' the last of these quintessentially English. Sports, therefore, were related to custom as well as to chronology or to literature—as an anthropologist would always relate them, and as I believe they always must be related. The pub comes into the picture as well as the stadium and/or in the United States, the park.

For those historians of sport who have not read Eliot and are curious about what nonsporting activities were in his list, a list that conjures up images and consti-tutes a picture, they included (and the first two come complete with smells as well as with pictures) "Wensleydale cheese, boiled cabbage cut into sections, beetroot in vinegar, Gothic churches, and the music of Elgar." It is a measure of the effects of the spread of television in Britain that dog races, the pin table and the dart board would now figure less prominently in anyone's list of sporting activities than snooker or golf, or even bowls and show jumping.

Television has had a different impact on different sports. Take snooker as a British example. "The shape of the snooker table, snugly fitting the screen, and the unit of competition, the frame, could have been custom built". There was the necessary tension and there was the necessary element of surprise. It required not just television, but color television, however, to convert snooker into entertainment. Thereafter, the story became complex. *Pot Black*, first intro-duced on BBC 2 in 1969, was a low budget program to begin with, one of the programs introduced mainly for that reason but also in a campaign to sell more color receivers. There was a problem, however, in introducing the championship element into the broadcasts since to become the snooker champion in 1969 you had to play no fewer than 73 frames. It took eleven months for Alex Higgins, a character made for television, but very different from Shaw's Professor Higgins—to win the championship title at his first attempt in 1972 on a road that led him from Ealing to Birmingham. That was too long a period, as would be the length of this chapter, for television. To continue to be televisually effective for what had now become a sizable television audience for snooker, most of whom had never played snooker in their lives, a different time scale had to be introduced into the game. It was so introduced. The 73-frame contest was cut down to 19 in the first round and best of 35 in the final—I love these strange numbers—and in 1977 the whole event was completed on two tables in two weeks. There was a new center, too, more adaptable for television, the Crucible Theater in Sheffield. We can now talk of theaters as well as stadiums, parks, grounds, and courts. In tournaments (a very old word) other than the championship (old too) where television cameras were not always present, winning on the basis of the best of 9 frames now became acceptable. So, too, did bigger prize money—and more tournaments in more places.

Such changes have accompanied the intervention of television into the history of different sports—for example, the advent of one-day cricket (although television did not end three-day or even longer cricket); the introduction of tie breakers into tennis (that stuck even in private games); or the shift in golf from match to medal or stroke play. Such changes left an impact, like changes in the lighting of snooker tables or, on this side of the Atlantic, the reduction by the National Football League (NFL) of the half-time intermission from 20 minutes to 15 minutes. The snooker change I know more about, as I know more about the role of sports in English, Scottish, Welsh or Irish culture than I do about their role in culture in the United States. What Eliot, had he known about snooker, would have called a 'traditional' trough shade, casting light over the snooker table, was replaced—if reluctantly—by television lighting. Television won, although not without occasional disasters, like bulbs exploding over the players' heads.

What I have said about these sports can easily be paralleled in the case of others. There have been multiple ramifications in most sports, with television being blamed and praised for what has happened—as in the case, too, with education and with politics. Yet television cannot be blamed for the fact that this year Wensleydale cheese, made 'traditionally' in the Yorkshire dales, not far from where I was born, has faced a crisis of its own with the decision of its now big-business owners—its production is part of a conglomerate—to cease producing it in Wensleydale and to transfer its production to a multi-product factory across the formidable local border in Lancashire. I should add that with no intervention from television—except for cookery programs, and these are part of television's staple fare—"boiled cabbage cut into sections" has virtually disappeared from English tables.

So many influences contribute to cultural change, which is at the very center of this chapter, that the exact role of the media, particularly the role of television, has been—and still is—highly controversial. Some acclaim, even defer; some complain, even resist. Eliot, however, was a man without doubts but with many anxieties. He was against television—and writing at the time when he did, before television had established itself, he saw it as a destroyer rather than as an entertainer. After a visit to the United States in 1950, he was sufficiently depressed to write to *The Times* in London questioning the wisdom of the BBC, which then had a broadcasting monopoly in Britain, spending £4 million on the development of British television over the next three years. Before, in his own words, "popularizing this pastime" in Britain, he urged people in Britain to consider the American experience very carefully. "The fears expressed by my American friends were not such as could be allayed by the provision of only superior and harmless programmes; they were concerned with television habit, whatever the programme might be."

A decade later, Newton Minow was to borrow an earlier Eliot metaphor and describe American television as a 'wasteland.' Eliot himself, however, stands out on the eve of the age of television in using those formidable words "whatever the programme might be." He would have been willing to add the words "wherever the programme may be." Already the medium was the message, although Eliot drew quite different conclusions from the proposition, which he never framed, than Marshall McLuhan was to do—also a decade later—when he claimed—and McLuhan's claim enters the title of this chapter and of the conference—first, that the content of the media is less influential than the media themselves, each of them with its own characteristics, and, second, that, in consequence of television taking over, the world was being turned into a 'global village.' Perceptions were changing and, in particular, perceptions of time and place, season and sequence. So, therefore, inevitably was culture, which was increasingly mediated through television rather than through books. It is necessary, therefore, according to McLuhan, to distinguish between a pre-television and a television age in all explorations of culture, including the cultures of sport, cultures about which he himself wrote very little. Already time has moved on, however, and in some respects at least we have moved or are moving into a post-television age, the age of the video, just as we are said to have moved into a postmodern age. Cultural characteristics are different as well as cultural attitudes.

McLuhan was little concerned with the question of who controlled the media, far less concerned, indeed, than Eliot was and far less concerned than sociologists or historians of the media, most of whom since 1966 have begun to write about Sport in the singular with a capital S. Nor did McLuhan ask questions about how and why forces other than television, notably mass tourism and concentrates of business power, including multinational companies dealing in marketable products, were themselves furthering 'globalization' during the 1960s. I cannot leave such forces out. Economics must be brought in, not least because television programs soon become marketable—or dumpable—products themselves.

As far as the cultures of sport are concerned, television has done much to turn sports into Sport—with the capital S. It figures prominently in television scheduling and in television budgeting. Expenditures on it are high when compared with, for example, Drama or Opera. Other reasons, however, why sports have become Sport are academic and political. Professors and ministers have influenced the story, even in Britain, as well as market forces. Sir Roger Bannister, of four-minute mile fame, was first Chairman of the Sports Council. Later we had a Minister of Sport, though his responsibilities are now subsumed in a Department called National Heritage.

A second obvious influence of television on sport is that sports, like food, are less seasonal than they used to be in many parts of the world—again not entirely because of television. And because of time differences in different parts of the world, 'globalizing,' a verb popularized by McLuhan, has had some curious effects on the starting times of sports as well as on the seasons. Let me give you one dramatic example. The boxing contest between Frank Bruno and Tim Witherspoon in 1986 was staged at Wembley Stadium in London after midnight to allow American viewers to see it live in the early evening. The signal to begin it was given not at Wembley but in New York. There are many less dramatic examples of Anglo-American cooperation, some of considerable social and cultural significance, like the switch of the last day's tennis at Wimbledon from Saturday to Sunday. At least one critic has taken such changes as examples of an adapted slogan, the medium is the massage.

Not everyone in the global audience has been massaged, however, and this remains the great strength of sport. I remember as a boy getting up in the early hours of winter darkness to listen to radio commentaries on cricket Test

Matches in Australia, and there fortunately are still people who live in their own time. Decades later in 1986, the year of the much publicized—hyped would be a better word—Bruno-Witherspoon contest, no fewer than 6 million British viewers stayed up for what for them was a very late-night show, the live television broadcast of the Super Bowl on Channel 4. Here the influence of television was quite direct. The size of this audience for the great American game at whatever time, day or night, that it was viewed would have been difficult to imagine when the first British televised sport was broadcast from Wimbledon in 1937 or, indeed, when Eliot wrote his *Notes on Culture* ten years later in 1947. The appeal of sports was becoming more international, although there had, of course, been a long history earlier of export and import, particularly, perhaps, in cricket. It was certainly surprising, more surprising than this year's general election result, when in 1990 a British Film Institute report suggested on the basis of research published in *Games and Sets* that in 1988 televised American football had overtaken soccer in popularity with 15- to 24-year olds, with 33 per cent saying that they lived to watch it compared with 32 per cent who preferred soccer. Soccer reversed the figure in 1989, however, but against a background of a slump in enjoyment of most sports on television, a social and cultural, not to say economic, phenomenon of considerable importance.

Super Bowl, which a latter-day Eliot would have had to include in any Notes towards a definition of American Culture, was not in the calendar, of course, in 1947. The game was old, but from the start, Super Bowl was a 'media event,' a term we cannot do without, a product of the new relationship between sport and television. For Ronald Cummings, writing ten years after Super Bowl, stated in a book significantly called *Mass Mediated Culture*, "the annual Super Bowl [might] not be culture with a capital C, but it was popular with a capital P, and it was surrounded by dollar signs and American flags."

For those, like ourselves, who are interested in comparative history, a necessary dimension of any global history, pre- and post-television, it is fascinating to compare Super Bowl with the English Football Association Cup Final, which celebrated its centenary in 1972, not least because the comparison must bring in other comparisons between media structures and policies as well as between sports and how they are played and watched, perceived and judged. We are not dealing simply with impact but with interaction. In the case of the Cup Final, of course, there was an earlier radio history. After it was transferred to newly built Wembley Stadium in 1923—very soon after the advent of radio—a commentary on it could not be broadcast until four years later because of opposition of the press, not opposition in soccer circles. It was first televised eleven years later to what was then a very small and well-off London audience, very different in size and in composition from the crowd at the stadium who were watching two teams from the North of England—Preston and Huddersfield. It is more memorable in history as a media event, a term that could not conceivably have been used in 1938, than as a football match, for the commentator, Thomas Woodroff, was made to eat his hat after foolishly saying "If Preston score now I'll eat my hat." Not every pledge made on radio and television has been so honored.

To recapture the mood of these early years, which seem like an age of innocence in the history both of television, then a small minority medium, and of sport, still with a strong amateur bias, I like to turn back to a letter from Gerald Cool, the BBC's first Director of Television, to Major Larcombe, the Secretary of the All England Tennis Club at Wimbledon in August 1936:

> Could we next June consider carrying out
> experimental transmissions... We would be
> tackling unknown quantities and as the
> apparatus has not yet been used over such a
> distance, we do not know whether we can
> achieve yet a satisfactory link between your
> good selves and Alexandra Palace.

The phrase "your good selves" stands out as sharply as "unknown quantities" in the history of the relationship between television and sport, but there have not always been "good selves."

Another point is important in relation to the title of this chapter. There was no sign, in 1937, that television would ever cross frontiers in the way that radio was already crossing them. Indeed, after the Second World War, when Arthur C. Clarke was already forecasting communications satellites, the head of the BBC's Light Programme and the future Head of Irish Radio, Maurice Gorham, wrote confidently in 1952 that:

> ...where television cannot replace sound
> radio is in long-distance transmission.
> Nobody has yet devised a way of making
> the waves used for television rebound from
> the upper atmosphere, regularly and reli-
> ably, as the waves used for sound broad-
> casting can be made to do.

Until Gorham's vision passed into history there could be no talk of a global village.

Live televised sport on a global basis—whatever the terms—has depended on the technological development of communications satellites, and that in turn has depended on a conquest of space which permitted us to see not only the dark side of the moon but also the face of our own globe from outer space. That was genuinely revolutionary. Yet it came after McLuhan had talked of a global village and at a time when there had already been proposed structural changes in the television business on both sides of the Atlantic and in the sporting world, which in some respects was more globally oriented than television when the 1970s began. There were certainly more intercontinental contacts in sport than in television—the World Cup in soccer, for example, and, of course, the Olympic Games, which had to be seen on newsreel in Britain—British Movietone News—before 1960.

There were important changes in television, however, pre-satellite, particularly the regional development of Eurovision and similar regional arrangements, and even before that films were being carried round the world as fast as possible to get them to viewers in other countries. Immediacy on the screen was not yet there in pictures, but the demand for immediacy already was. Within this context satellite technology was in some respects a response more than a cause. And the business backing for it was already there, even if as in cable television, more money was lost than was made during the critical stage of early development. In Britain there is still some resistance to paying for specialized immediate sports coverage on television. Even in 1992 the biggest British satellite company BSkyB, a company with a history as dramatic as that of any soap opera, had an audience figure of less than a million for its most popular program, not a sports programme but the American comedy series, *The Simpsons*. The highest BBC figures for international sporting events are something like ten times greater, while for ITV, the BBC's competition, the biggest soccer programme *Match of the Day* is seven times as great. There are big changes round the corner in relation to satellites and soccer—and indeed, to satellites and Test Match cricket, but they are just round the corner, not here. There are still far too few dishes and far too few cable viewers for a historian to rewrite the recent record. He must note, however, that the controllers of BSkyB, with Rupert Murdoch in charge, bear little resemblance to Gerald Cook, or for that matter, the controllers of Britain's planned new Premier Soccer League bear little resemblance to Major Larcombe. There is a new world around the corner and it will not be run by villagers.

In 1975 my Oxford colleague, Sir Roger Bannister, to whom I have already referred, wrote in a French publication *Sport et Societe 2000* that "sport [and he chose to use the word in the singular] is a natural, worthwhile and enjoyable form of human expression" and that he trusted that it would remain such beyond the year 2000. In fact, through concentrations of economic power spectator sport can be contrived and manipulative rather than natural and a form of escape rather than of expression. There is nothing new about this observation. Ethical questions always arise when we focus on money.

Memorable comments concerning money, free from jargon, public or private, revenue or capital, figure in every dictionary or anthology. "The root of all evil?" (the First Epistle of Paul to Timothy); "You pays your money and you takes you choice" (*Punch* 1847); "That's the way the money goes: Pop goes the weasel" (nineteenth-century ballad by W.R. Mandel); "Television is a license to print money" (Roy Thomson, Canadian born English newspaper proprietor and television magnate, 1955). And, applied not to sport, I emphasize, but to sex, a critic of an American novel of 1986, *Mayflower Madam* "Her book about the money in sex gives you the feeling of the sex in money."

I have reached the point in this chapter when I need both to recapitulate and to offer a longer list of themes that are relevant to my subject, the area where communication changes and changes in sport converge. Some themes are psychological as well as economic—the interpreting of habit and choice; the extent and use of leisure time; the measurement of time itself; the calendar of events and how and why it changes; annuals and perennials; rulemaking and rule breaking in sport; facilities and equipment; the relationship between performers and spectators; 'participation'; the relationship in sport and in television between women and men and between young, including children, and old; amateurism and professionalism, as prominent a theme in the history of communications as it is in the longer and more varied history of sport; values on the screen and in the stadium, on the field and on the terraces, including 'physical fitness,' 'sportsmanship,' recreation and 'competitiveness' and 'the will to win'; sport as faith and sport as fun; the role of government, which has usually had nothing to do with fun; violence, its causes and consequences and the extent to which the media have contributed to it; the relationship between seeing on the spot and seeing on the screen, which brings in comparisons with concert and theater; the relationship, an older one, between seeing for yourself and having what is seen reported through intermediaries; trappings, ephemera, publicity advertisement; the relationship between the local, which is where sport always began and begins, and the global, which brings in time as well as space since, as I have already stressed, many sports which were once seasonal are now in continuous operation all the year round.

I have used the word 'relationship' many times in compiling this list which is far longer than Eliot's but still incomplete. As long ago as 1977, the *Journal of Communication* in a number devoted largely to sport and the media used the word 'interdependence.' "Television and, significantly, the financial support it can offer have become so important to professional sports," Donald Parente wrote, "that they have moulded, adapted and changed their rules to meet the desires and needs of television." I prefer the word 'relationship,' however, because in dealing with interdependence we are dealing with individuals and institutions, not with anonymous forces. There has, indeed, been much interchange of individuals between the two sides. Sports commentators, for example, are often former active sportsmen, and even in ownership there are interlocking interests both in communications and in sport, some, it is true, extremely disturbing. I like a comment on soccer and television made by the journalist, David Lacey, in 1986, "A marriage guidance counselor," he wrote then, "would understand English football's uneven relationship with television—the awkward courtship, passionate honeymoon, years of bickering, and now it is obvious who wears the trousers."

If we revert back to the more neutral language of interdependence, Parente, writing on this side of the Atlantic nine years before Daley, and not about soccer but about spectator sports in general, agreed with Daley's conclusion when he claimed that in the patterns of interdependence television had called the tune. "It has been suggested," he went on, "that once a sport, league or team [these were the units] has had its 'product' bought by television for use as programming that entity can seldom exist thereafter, at least in the same style or manner, without the financial support of television."

If only because of slumps as well as booms, bankruptcies and fortunes—and we are now familiar with a wide range of economic situations—it is necessary, I believe, before passing such general judgments, to examine more closely the economic history of particular sports bargains and deals in the form of case studies, studies which take account of timing as well as terms. Just because television, even by 1977, as Parente recognized, had become "dependent upon sports to fulfill many of *its* programming needs" there was scope in circumstances that were favorable to a particular sporting interest for that interest to strike hard bargains, special bargains, that were advantageous to it. Moreover, specialist sports channels, particularly satellite channels—and these have been favored by the government in new broadcasting legislation—have brought in new levels of bargaining, which inevitably influence controllers of nonspecialist channels which cannot afford to leave sport out of their own mix. The changes have all been apparent in the most recent deal in Britain concerning television rights in soccer matches played by the teams in the new Premier League. I could devote a whole chapter to it, and I must be very selective indeed. After successful skyjacking, a £304 million deal has been carried through which gives television rights to show matches next year to Murdoch's BSkyB, with very limited rights left to the BBC (at significant cost) for what has become almost a 'traditional' soccer program, *Match of the Day*, a program which they lost to their ITV competitors two years ago. The highly controversial deal, which was opposed by six clubs in the new Premier League, including Liverpool, Manchester United, Arsenal and Leeds, went to the courts, but emerged unscathed, leaving ITV to pick up the remaining soccer clubs, including those in the new First Division. The viewing pattern for next year, therefore, will be completely different from last year or any previous year. The well-chosen title of an article about it in the *Sunday Times*, which is part of the Murdoch empire, was "Snatch of the Day." It had little to do with sport as Bannister had conceived it. The sub-heading ran "When BSkyB secured exclusive coverage of the English tour of the West Indies and the BBC was left with a paltry half-hour in the small hours while BSkyB provided coverage from mid afternoon to late evening."

I have deliberately introduced the topical because the relationship between sport and television is going through a new phase. Given the *furore* in Britain about the latest deal it would have been impossible to leave it out. I would like in conclusion, however, to look briefly at the range of issues that I listed in longer term historical perspective before ending by making a foray into language, I will look a little more closely at the terms of the title of my lecture—'media,' 'sport,' 'global,' 'village.' My main qualification for writing this keynote chapter, which is designed to offer a comprehensive overview, is that I am a social and cultural historian who began as an economic and political historian and who has always been interested in the history and in the practice of communications and sport.

Communications first. In researching and writing on the history of broadcasting in the United Kingdom I have deliberately tried in my various volumes—and it has been a hard task—not to keep looking round the corner to see what happened next after the end of the period that I was covering but to recapture the interests and language of the period with which I was specifically concerned. I realized that if I had been topical, I would have very quickly become out of date. I realized two other things also. First, that I had to be comparative. In particular, I would have to compare the contrasting broadcasting structures of Britain and the United States, asking myself how deep the contrasts were and whether or not the United States was setting the pace so that Britain would eventually, for good or ill, catch up. I also realized that I would have to be inter-disciplinary. Economics, psychology and sociology—not to speak of anthropol-ogy—introduce concepts and insights. All that I learned about the history of communications applies to the history of sport. It too must avoid hindsight, develop a comparative dimension and draw on a combination of insights and concepts from different disciplines. In both branches of history, however, I believe that we must always seek synthesis. I am an integrationist. I believe that we have to put together the four ingredients that are kept separate in *USA Today*—Newsline, Sports, Money, and Life.

I would like as a historian, however, to make two points about perspective which are very much historian's points. It has become common among social historians to draw a distinction between events and patterns. The latter may recur. Events, however, unfold. Many of them have an element of the unexpect-ed about them. In the present they constitute the newsline; and electronic media are concerned, above all else, with getting the news of events across as quickly as possible to as many places as possible, preferably instantaneously and uni-versally. Television, in particular, prides itself on being 'the universal eye.' Scoops are sought after. Because of the role of communications historians of sport have to look at the perception of events as well as at the events them-selves, and they have to take account of what Elihu Katz and others have identi-fied as one special category of events, 'media events.' It is not just that by con-verging on them the media make events different from what they would other-wise be. In certain circumstances they may influence their outcome. In other circumstances the media may invent events. What interests me most as a histori-an is how they deal within a framework not of their choosing with national and international events with a history, like, for example, Derby Day, the Cup Final, Wimbledon, and the cricket Test Matches to which I have already referred. Each country has its own list, and each event has its own historians, faithfully, often lovingly, recording what happens in terms of results, records, and memo-rabilia. Moreover, spectators' memories sustain such events as effectively as players' performances. The camera—and the people behind the camera—appre-ciate that no two occasions within the sequence of such events have ever been quite the same, and that has been part of their appeal—although Lester Piggott, who won the Derby nine times, must have felt that history repeated itself. So too must Helen Wills Moody or Ms. Navratilova at Wimbledon. How can tele-vision get at the essence of each occasion? Can it avoid stereotypes and formu-lae?

The question arises in relation to the best known—and oldest—of all events in sport, the Olympic Games, about which I have been able to write little in this chapter. This is an Olympic year—and the media have presented the Olympics in quite different ways at different stages in media history. At the same time, it is important to note that in considering both the facts and the perceptions of the Olympics since the advent of television, when the Olympics have become major 'media' events, the media are by no means the only agencies to take in to the reckoning. Athletics has gone through big changes too, by no means all of them 'caused' by media intervention.

So much for such events—and they do not lack historians—yet when the social historian turns from events to patterns—and they include both sequences and serials—he is seeking to identify stabilities as well as changes over spans of time. And this quest is followed both by the historian of sport and the historian of communication just as it is by the historian of religion. He or she wants to get at attitudes as well as activities and at *genres*, each of which has its own history. The electronic media, which have their own history, will be of help to historians who are not specialists in media studies, for they record as well as transmit. They add to the record evidence that was not previously there, and since it is such massive evidence, visual and verbal, they transform the historian's task.

The thrust of this chapter has been essentially historical, but in conclusion I would like to turn from both events and patterns to words and to metaphors. These are as revealing in the history of sport as in the history of everything else. Surprisingly the word 'global' in the title of this chapter, now so familiar, proves in some ways to be the most interesting of the three words when its history is traced. When the *Oxford Dictionary* first appeared in 1928—and according to its editors it was a dictionary devised on a historical basis—it described the adjective 'global' as rare. Indeed, it was not until the *Supplement* to the *Dictionary* appeared in 1972—more than a decade after Marshall McLuhan had coined the phrase 'the global village'—that the adjective 'global' was defined for the first time, as more recent dictionaries have defined it, "as relating to or involving the whole world," "worldwide." In the *Longman Dictionary of the English Language*, a synchronic not a historical dictionary, "global" has bracketed after it "warfare" and "communication" to describe the two main contexts in which it had been most frequently used. The *Longman Dictionary* was published in 1984, and while it includes an entry "global village," it appeared too early to include an entry 'global warming,' the context in which the adjective is now regularly used. 'Global village' is defined there in the dictionary, however, in non-McLuhanesque terms. There is no reference to 'tribalization.' Instead, the 'global village' is defined as "the world viewed as a totally integrated ecological, socio-economic and political system of which all the parts are dependent on one another."

The old *Oxford Dictionary*, which appeared in 1923, gave another older definition of the word 'global,' French in origin, which is now less common, although
it is very pertinent to this chapter. Before being used in a geographical sense the
adjective 'global' had been used in the late nineteenth century—in the best
nineteenth-century tradition—in a classificatory sense. It referred to "the totality
of a number of items, categories etc.; comprehensive, all inclusive, unified,
total." The first twentieth-century use of the word 'global' in a geographical
sense was not until 1927 when it was used in inverted commas in the periodical
the *Contemporary Review*: "the essence of the American proposal therefore was
its 'global' criterion." Significantly the United States was the source. The last
two examples of use are directly related to this chapter. In 1968 McLuhan and
Fiore published a book with the title *War and Peace in the Global Village* (note
again the use of the 'war' context), while in 1970 the *Scientific Journal* noted
that "the meteorological global telecommunications system required... an effective system of global numerical weather prediction." The entry ends, after dis-
posing of the adjective global, "Hence globalism, globalization, globalize." The
first use of the verb is traced back to 1962.

I have no time to deal adequately with the second word, 'village,' except to say
that McLuhan's choice of that unit to describe the world that was cohering
through the media is itself open to criticism. In talking of games at least—and
not least of the Olympic Games—cities, not villages, have been the centers of
action. They have been prominent both in pressing their claims as hosts, as
Barcelona was on this occasion, and in actually incurring sizable expenditures
to attract them. In the same number of *Sport et Société* where Roger Bannister
talked of sports as 'natural expressions' and where Lord Killannin discussed the
Olympic Games, Professor Haumont described how sport had already influenced the appearance and range of facilities offered by great cities. More recently, we have come to talk more of global communications in terms of networks
rather than in terms of coherence, a mechanical rather than an organic
metaphor.

Whether or not the use of the word 'village' when applied to the Olympics village is the right term is a different matter. Keeping more up-to-date than a dictionary, however, I noted in a cricket column in a recent London newspaper a
reference to real British villages as real as any that Eliot knew, and it touched
on a perennial sports theme:

> An outbreak of shamateurism in the
> Rothman's Village Cricket Championship
> has forced organizers to tighten up the rules

> forbidding player payment. The lure of a
> Lords' final [Lords is one of the two great
> London cricket centers] has been too much
> for some pot-hunting clubs who have cir-
> cumvented the regulations barring remuner-
> ation by arranging for payment from an out-
> side source.

The competition had been sponsored and organized for 21 years by *The Cricketer* magazine which hoped that its 'new get-tough policy' (a policy known far outside villages) would encourage renewed interest from villages "who have been steering clear of the event because of the professional faction."

I am back to the topical again. Let me end with the briefest of references to the last of the words in the title, 'sport.' It is a word which is often defined simply as Eliot defined it as a 'pastime,' but it is a word which has also come to carry with it all the heavy freight of rules and codes, not to mention the even heavier freight of betting and gambling. The statistics themselves constitute freight. Many languages have imported the word, but the *Oxford Dictionary* gives no specific language root. The word did not figure in the Gould and Kelb's *Dictionary of the Social Sciences* that appeared in 1964 or in the 1972 edition of the *Encyclopedia Britannica*, which does, however, include an entry on 'sporting records' covering 73 sports from archery to yachting, all of which have separate entries. There is also a brief entry on Sports (Articles on) which lists articles that include 'Games, Classical,' 'British Commonwealth Games,' 'Pan-American Games,' 'Highland Games,' Amateur (but not Professional), Gymnastics, and Physical Education. Clearly the then editors of the *Encyclopedia Britannica* had not thought of sport in the singular or of sport in the global village. Nor, indeed, have the editors of most other encyclopedias. Compilers of books of quotations sometimes have. I like a quotation from Jimmy Connors, as given in *Simpsons' Contemporary Quotations* (1988), that is, quotations of utterances since 1950, since the quote refers back to the development of the word 'global' and Connors is certainly a global character as well as celebrity. In Thomas Tutko and William Brun's *Winning is Everything and Other American Myths* Connors is quoted as saying, "People don't seem to understand that it's a damn war out there." I put that quote alongside some of the quotes given in James Michener's *Sports in America*, notably Vince Lombardi's "Winning isn't everything, it's the only thing," Leo Durocher's "Nice guys finish last," and, quote of quotes, Bill Musselman's "Defeat is worse than death because you have to live with defeat." War again provides the context as sport has become part of the 'leisure sector.'

Yet that is not its only context. 'Sport' can, of course, be used generically in questions like 'Do you like sport?,' and Shakespeare used it, as his fifteenth-century predecessors had done, to refer not to contesting but to mocking or deriding—"then make sport at me." There remains all the difference in the world between the two adjectives 'sporting' and 'sportive.' 'Sport' was used in 1593 to describe a theatrical performance — another of its contexts (Connors has also insisted that he is an entertainer)—and it can, of course, be used as a noun and applied to an individual. *Longman's Dictionary* describes as 'Australian' and 'New Zealand' the word 'sport' "used as a form of familiar address chiefly to men." The adjective 'old' in front of it—'old sport'—seems to me to make it sound more English, even if old-fashioned English, the English of P.G. Wodehouse.

I have tried to keep this chapter as 'global' and as little 'English' as possible. Yet I should emphasize at the end of it that even in an age of satellite and of multinational conglomerates as 'the media approach the millennium' the 'nation,' tribal or not, remains the main unit both in sport and in communications and that in each nation both are part of distinctive cultural complexes. This fact alone will keep historians busy as the millennia come and go.

Notes

---

[1]The text of this chapter was presented in the form of a keynote address at "Sport in the Global Village: Comparative Perspectives," the 8th Biennial Conference of the International Society for Comparative Physical Education and Sport, Houston, June 12-18, 1992.

Chapter 2

Golf International: Considerations of Sport in the Global Marketplace

Brian Stoddart

As we sit in our homes watching television bring us tennis from Wimbledon, soccer from Brazil, horseracing from Australia, the Olympics from several countries, and a myriad of other sports, it is easy to construct globalization as a modern phenomenon made possible by the technology of telecommunications. Moreover, if we think about it at any length, we become prey to the more simplistic interpretations of postmodernism. What we see in our sports is mere pastiche devoid of meaning and/or substance. At its extremes, the globalization of sport might in some minds be thought of as what David Harvey terms, "a condition of nihilism."[1] To take such a view would be to ignore several aspects of the globalization story. It includes the historical, spatial, intellectual, economic and cultural aspects of sport. Indeed, it might be argued that the spread of sport and its means towards the interpretation of cultures has been one of the most remarkable features of the twentieth-century experience.[2]

In order to demonstrate just a few corners of that experience, this chapter examines probably the most underinvestigated sport in academic literature, the game of golf. As a starting point, consider some of the following statistics. According to the National Golf Foundation, during 1987 at least 21.7 million Americans played at least one round of golf, with 15 million of those defined as core golfers. Those players spent approximately $20 billion on golf and golf-related services. At a calculated growth playing rate of 4% per year, that expenditure will rise to $40 billion by the year 2000.[3] In Australia, it is estimated that there were 1.2 million regular players during 1990, in a total population of 17 million, and that those players supported an industry worth $100 million.[4] In Japan during 1991, where the proportion of players is smaller (than in Australia and the United States), the government collected $723 million from its golf course users' tax, an 18.5% increase from the previous year.[5] One research report on Canada ranks the percentage of the population playing golf at a staggeringly high 18.4%, nearly four million players.[6] Statistics such as these suggest that golf is a "borderless industry," as declared by The National Golf Foundation President, Joseph Beditz.[7]

Golf is genuinely a global sport.[8] North Africa and the Middle East currently host events on the European professional tour. The Middle East tournament is played on a course constructed out of the desert in the United Arab Emirates. At the other extreme, games are played in the snow of Finland and at the heights of Gulmarg, in Kashmir. Traditional Scottish courses are carved out of seaside lands fertile for little else but grazing, while in other parts of the world fairways wind through beautiful lakelands and forests. Major world cities, like Buenos Aires and Johannesburg, boast elaborate golf complexes in close proximity to areas of dire poverty. In Japan, the cost is so high that most "players" experience little more than a multilevel driving range. Ocean-side resort courses in Hawaii and California are matched in their beauty only by those in the mountainous surroundings of Switzerland and Colorado. Australian courses boast kangaroos, while those in Florida are home to alligators.

The complexity of all this is framed by an analysis comparing the relationship of the course and nature, the sheer amount of land and associated natural resources consumed by this social passion, the relationship between course and host culture, and the concept of the course as a social space. As a starting point, the following questions should be considered:

> (i)   How did golf get to be this way?
> (ii) What are its recognized and emerging trends?
> (iii) What are some of its dimensions?
> (iv) Why is golf such a strong global subculture?

The points of emphasis are:

> (i)   Golf has been globalized since at least the later nineteenth century.
>
> (ii) The marketplace avenues offered by the game have increased exponentially during the past century.

(iii) What has changed and continues to
change in golf's globalism are the locations of influence and the sources of
power in terms of the market.

It was in Scotland, during the late nineteenth century, that the globalization of
the game began.[9] St. Andrews is the most famous golfing territory in the world,
home of the Royal and Ancient Golf Club which, along with the United States
Golf Association, governs the game worldwide. Scotland alone now has
approximately 600 courses ranging from humble nine-hole layouts to the great
names like Royal Troon (where Greg Norman lost to Mark Calcavecchia in
1989) and Turnberry (where Greg Norman won in 1986). These references to
Norman constitute an example not only of Australian chauvinism, but also of
subcultural jargon. "Winning," in Scotland, means inevitably to win the Open
Championship, first contested in 1860. These courses indicate the popularity of
the sport among numerous players. From the late nineteenth century onwards,
golf has been dominated by such leading players who have prospered from the
game. The only primary change over the past 100 years has been the variety of
available avenues for these leading players to use in order to capitalize financially upon their golfing skills.

The Triumvirate of Harry Vardon, James Braid, and James Taylor won the
Open Championship a combined total of 16 times between 1894 and 1914.
Additionally, Vardon won the United States Open, in 1890, at the Chicago Golf
Club. This win conquered Taylor who, at that time, was on tour promoting golf
clubs bearing his name and simultaneously writing for a magazine paying
$2,000 for his efforts. By the turn of the century, professional players were fre-
quent passengers on the transatlantic passenger liners as well as on ships going
all over the world. They capitalized upon their skills at what appeared to be a
mere game, but which was already an economic system.

Then, as now, tournament golf was the most obvious way to make money.
Employment with a club as a resident professional, teaching golf and selling
equipment provided a much more stable income. Furthermore, given the global
boom in golf between 1890 and 1910, there was a strong demand for good
teachers in the sport. In the years preceding and following 1900, for example,
the small Scottish town of Carnoustie exported at least 300 professionals to
clubs all over the world. Carnegie Clark arrived in Australia in 1894 to become
one of the country's most influential golfing figures. He began on a retainer of
50 pounds per annum at The Royal Sydney Golf Club, and his teaching fee was
2/6d per half hour.[10] Mac Smith journeyed to America in 1910 to join his broth-

ers where all became prominent players. Alex Duthie traveled to Portland, Oregon, in 1906 and then, in 1910, joined the Jericho Golf Club in Vancouver, Canada. He remained there, until his death, in 1947 having served, in many ways, as the city's founder of golfing practice.[11] Around the same time, other Carnoustie men traveled to countries such as South Africa, New Zealand, and Argentina. Therefore, by the end of the century, golf was already in a global mode.

This trend was confirmed between the wars with the Ryder Cup. This created great public speculation when the professionals of the United States and Great Britain met to match skills.[12] Global supremacy at the game was at stake here as the Americans sought to establish their own traditions, styles, and attitudes in distinction from those of Great Britain. Even at that point, the importance of cultural style was becoming apparent and had a considerable bearing upon the ways in which the golf industry developed moneymaking opportunities. This has continued into the 1990s with "Great Britain" transmogrified into "Europe" in the Ryder Cup to create better competition and more commercial interest.

The interrelationship between style and money was personified by Walter Hagen. The "Haig" was born in Rochester, New York, in 1893. He won the Open four times and the US Open twice. More significantly, he pioneered the "globe-trotting" ways of the modern professional by playing in tournaments, challenging local professionals and staging clinics for the public. His flamboyance attracted great crowds worldwide. In 1930 and 1937, accompanied by Joe Kirkwood, the first Australian player to venture to America, Hagen played before huge galleries worldwide. The "Haig" and Kirkwood were among the first to actually promote endorsed products. The humble tee, invented by an American dentist, was popularized by the pair, marking the beginnings of the diversified corporate push into golf.[13]

While there were many successful players like Ben Hogan and Byron Nelson in the 20 years after Hagen, his real successor was Arnold Palmer. From the late 1950s until the present he has created a vast financial empire. His golfing success is associated with a bewildering array of goods and services. Now well into his sixties, he is still generally considered the highest annual earner in sports by virtue of his golfing empire. Jack Nicklaus quickly followed, creating an enormous empire soon to eclipse Palmer's. Both men emulated Hagen by playing all over the world, attracting crowds, attention, and profit. Shrewd management teams perfected the ideas of appearance money to the point that these and many other prominent players demand and receive $200,000 and more simply to tee it up. Their corporate, if not championship successor, Greg Norman, has been nicknamed "Logo Man" by some critical American commentators.[14] Norman, now 37, has just two major titles to his name. However, he earns up to and beyond $10 million annually from endorsements and sponsorships. This phenomenon is not confined only to the United States and Europe. Some of the richest players in golf are people like Jumbo Ozaki whose victories in golf-crazed Japan ensure lucrative profits from equipment and clothing sales. Senior player Bob Charles won approximately $500,000 over several years on the regular US tour. However, in five years on the Seniors tour he has amassed over $3 million.

While the principle of globalism has existed for a long time, its scale has increased. Much of it is clearly marked by global change itself. Vardon, for example, sailed to America by ship while Palmer flew his personal jet to the Open Championship. The global marketplace for golf-related goods and services opened up concurrently. Media services are more instantaneous and heighten awareness faster than in previous years. Before the turn of the century it sometimes took weeks to learn the results of a major tournament. Now, Monday and Tuesday papers around the world relay the weekend's tournament results from Asia, America, Europe, and elsewhere. The game itself has become increasingly sophisticated, widening opportunities for maximized profit. Prominent players may now appear in Australia, Japan, America and Europe in successive weeks, simply because of this globalization.

The other existing dimension to the professional's income is that of the teacher. One of the main reasons so many Scottish players left home between 1890 and 1914 was the worldwide demand for knowledge as the game enjoyed its first great global boom. While teaching has always had a frustrating side, it has also provided a steady, often excellent income for the best proponents. The media also served as an aide, to these star teachers, as an alternative form of communication. James Braid, of the Triumvirate, was among the first to lend his name to a coaching manual.[15] Since then, many players have learned the game by following instructions in one of the many classics, *Modern Fundamentals* by Ben Hogan being one of the more favored.[16]

Dan Soutar, though not born in Carnoustie, grew up there from the age of five. One of his constant opponents was Carnegie Clark. In 1903 he emigrated to Australia, won several important titles, then turned professional. He was a prominent player, but his living was grounded in his teaching among the members of the clubs that he served. Among his protégés was Joe Kirkwood, who went on to partner Walter Hagen. In 1906, Soutar published *The Australian Golfer,* complete with diagrams and photographs of flat and upright swings, full and half shots, chips, putts and, of course, caution and advice.[17] The book was a tremendous success, modeling itself upon the principles established by Vardon and Taylor. Abe Mitchell was another English player whose *Essentials of Golf* became very popular between the wars. As a performer in the transatlantic Ryder Cup matches, Mitchell was able to use his profile to sell his book, thereby contributing to the further growth of the game.[18]

By this stage, however, the player-writers had become paralleled by professional teachers, like J. Victor East. Another Scot, East also emigrated to Australia, in 1901, and joined Carnegie Clark and Dan Soutar. Many years later, he wrote *Better Golf in Five Minutes* in which, along with the instructions, he recalled examples of his teaching at Royal Sydney and Royal Melbourne.[19] In 1921 he traveled to America as Joe Kirkwood's manager and remained based there until his death in 1969. During this period, he served as a teaching professional at many of the leading clubs. Never a great player, East's skills lay in analysis and imparting knowledge. In numerous ways, David Leadbetter is his natural successor. Born and raised in Zimbabwe, Leadbetter first appeared in Britain and Europe as a struggling tour player. He soon turned his attention to teaching, gaining a reputation as a swing doctor.[20] The big break came when leading English player Nick Faldo entrusted his career to Leadbetter. In 1987, Faldo won the Open, followed by two Masters titles. Other important victories included a second Open title, in 1990, and a third, in 1992. Leadbetter shifted to a lucrative post in Florida where, today, a variety of quality players from around the world come to seek everything, ranging from inspiration to the miracle cure, at approximately $200 per hour.

The Southern Hills Country Club in Tulsa, Oklahoma, seems an odd place to develop a summary of globalism in the teaching of golf. The key is a man named Richard Brain, who currently resides in Singapore, where he teaches golf to a range of students. Many of these travel from throughout Asia for their lessons. Brain estimates that he has traveled around the globe at least 26 times in search of the perfect golf swing. He has observed teachers at work on municipal driving ranges in Canada, courses in Taiwan and Indonesia, public links in Britain, and country clubs in America, including Southern Hills where he was the teaching professional for several years. Brain's most important contribution to this debate lies in his theory of "the tree of knowledge." This theory traces the heritage of most contemporary teaching back to the nineteenth century. So, who taught the teachers? In the answer lies the true globalism, the power of ideas, theories, and practices to override boundaries. Scottish migrants around the world developed local teachers, who influenced others to the point where there are no boundaries in the teaching of golf, especially with the proliferation of videos.[21]

Another important area of globalization, begun by the early masters, concerns the manufacturing of the playing instruments themselves.[22] Those dating back to the eighteenth century now bring $20,000 and more at an auction. With the late nineteenth-century golf boom, the demand for equipment became enormous and the old handcrafting developed into a rudimentary form of factory production, such as at Robert Forgan's in Scotland. The leading players lent their names to design and marketing processes, which dominated, until after the First World War. Wooden shafts and iron heads were the only materials involved, along with leather grips. The discovery that American persimmon trees made beautiful wooden golf heads stimulated both production and design, with the main break-through occurring in the 1920's creation of steel shafts. America became the main production site, shifting the seat of influence from Great Britain. This ties together the process in which Britain, the industrial entrepreneur at the end of the eighteenth century, was overtaken at the end of the nineteenth by the second gen-eration industrial powers. Men like Toney Penna were involved in the evolution. The son of an Italian migrant cabinetmaker, Penna won professional tournaments in the 1920s and 1930s before joining the McGregor company, where he revolu-tionized club making. His wooden clubs are now considered classics, and leading professionals scramble to purchase an old one, should it become available.[23]

In the last 20 years, the range of choice available to players has become bewil-dering. Embedded in that is the remarkable shifting of patterns in the global pro-duction market. I received one of my first clubs in New Zealand during the early 1960s. It was made in St. Andrews, around 1911, by Tom Stewart, one of the most famous handcrafters of his day. When I returned to the game, in the late 1980s, I discovered that one of my drivers was made of American persimmon, shaped in Australia, and fitted to an American steel shaft. Then I switched to a club made in Japan, but purchased in America, for use in Australia. It was made of graphite and metals originally gathered from various parts of the world. My current driver is designed to American specifications, but not necessarily made in America, as the 1990-91 Australian figures suggest.[24] Of all the fully assembled clubs sold in Australia during that period, almost 70% were manufactured in America. However, that section of the market is shrinking, as Australians resort increasingly to importing individual pieces of the club like the shaft, head, and grip because that incurs significantly lower tariff rates. Of the imported heads, 85% originate from Taiwan, which suggests that of the vast array of clubs now available to buyers, many of them come out of the same factories. Incidentally, an early Taiwanese practice was to "copy" famous American brand products, give them a different name, and then sell them below the standard price. While most shafts sold in Australia still come from America, other equipment comes from as many as 14 countries, including Namibia.

From the late nineteenth century, the global combination of demand and economics has shifted the forces of production from Great Britain to the United States, Japan, and Taiwan. Most other countries have had or continue to have their own manufacturers of clubs, but these have been the largest producers. In part, the global pattern of shifting influence has been dictated by the availability of raw material (the restrictive persimmon to the ubiquitous steel), the presence of skills (American shafts are still the weapon of choice), and the costs of production. The Mizuno Corporation is an instructive example here.[25] In 1906, Rihachi Mizuno began selling baseballs in Osaka, cashing in on the game's tremendous growth in Japan. Very quickly the company branched into sportswear and other equipment. In 1933 it produced its first golf clubs. By that time, golf was becoming very popular in Japan. The number of available courses for play had risen from 10 in 1922 to 35 in 1938, including one club for women only. The Mizuno group clearly saw the game promising a bright economic future. In 1939, the first offshore operation was established, in Shanghai. When the modern Japanese golf boom began, in the early 1960s, Mizuno sponsored its first tournament, and opened a new golf manufacturing plant. In 1979, the company sponsored its first golf tournament in Malaysia and established Mizuno America in Dallas. Three years later, the American and British Mizuno Golf Companies were founded, establishing a major foray into the international golf market. Its golf manufacturing subsequently developed in such diverse locations as Taiwan and Mexico. Among its myriad of contracted sports stars are golfers like Sandy Lyle, Nick Faldo, Jose Maria Olazabal, and many others. By the 1990s, Mizuno's annual golf equipment catalog consisted of hundreds of pages.

There are two noteworthy points to this story. First, it is too readily assumed that the globalization of sport is the prerogative of the West when, in fact, much of its past and present thrust has come from elsewhere. Second, Mizuno's globalization began very early and then mushroomed from the 1970s onward, a clear pointer to the need of understanding the prevailing context in which this globalization occurs. The inevitable trend, in all this process, is towards science. My clubs, mentioned earlier, range from something relatively simple to the highly complex. Tom Stewart's club, for example, was put together by instinct and experience. It does not look much different from the Henry Griffits, but the latter takes approximately 12 hours of fitting to develop the right lie angle, the right shaft, the right grip size, and every component weighed to keep absolute consistency through the set. Does the result matter? Fred Herd won the first four-round US Open, in 1898, with a total of 328. In 1906, Willie Smith won with 295, and in 1916, Chick Evans won with 286, a score not improved for 20 years. Ben Hogan broke 280, in the 1942 unofficial event, with a 271, a remarkable score rarely approached now.[26] In 1991, for example, Payne Stewart won a playoff after tying Scott Simpson at 282, just four shots better than Chick Evans 75 years earlier.

A global scientific search is now in progress to determine how to hit the ball further, make it spin more, maximize ball flight, eliminate deviation, overcome new architectural nightmares, look better, and feel lighter, stronger, and more responsive.[27] In some senses, looking at the historical scores, it is more a matter of marketing than of progress.

Golf provides many avenues for developing a business venture. Shoes are an extremely lucrative area for obvious reasons, and Footjoy, the American company, is an excellent example. The scientific push has become an important one, too, not to mention the sense of the aesthetic. Again, the available range is bewildering, with the options varying from the traditional to the high-tech.

Clothing offers even greater opportunities for producing capital. Ian Baker-Finch, 1991 Open champion, models for Lyle & Scot, one of the "big two" in Great Britain. The other, Pringle, has a great fan in Nick Faldo. Again, the tradition, the "look" of golf, is a major thread in the globalization of the game. This is greatly emphasized because of the class and/ or status images associated with the game. However, tradition can always be mixed with modernity.

Equipment is not the only important feature to consider. Golf's most conspicuous feature is its land hunger. In early days, golf courses "just happened." By the turn of the century, things began to change, and today, that is no longer the case. The influence of the architect is now a global phenomenon and contains potentially the greatest global impact as golf architecture, by definition, interacts with the earth itself.[28] There is enormous scope for the manifestations of local culture and landscape to be altered by the architect. Alternatively, it is also threatening for the architect to introduce completely foreign concepts into a local environment. One example was the recreation of Augusta National's famous 12th, the par 3, on-site in a Japanese exhibition so that, for three months or so, Japanese golfers could "play" the marvelous hole. Donald Ross was one of the first Scots to travel to America and specialize in design. His greatest accomplishments are the Pinehurst layouts, in North Carolina, which every year attract thousands of pilgrims. The equipment of early times had great limitations, thereby placing the emphasis of Ross and other pioneers on shotmaking, rather than on brute strength. Charles Blair MacDonald also had Scottish connections. He spent two years at the University of St. Andrews, became America's first national amateur champion, in 1897, and the country's first major course architect. He was the most instrumental in gaining American acceptance of the R & A rules, one of the major global influences on the game. In particular, The National Golf Links, which he designed on Long Island, were scrupulously based upon holes drawn from Scottish examples so setting the framework for the inevitable debate between traditionalists, modernists, and even postmodernists.[29]

Perhaps the first global architect was Dr. Alistair McKenzie, the Scottish medical practitioner whose work may now be seen all over the world, particularly at Augusta National and Royal Melbourne. McKenzie visited Australia, in the 1920s, at the invitation of Royal Melbourne. While there, he advised other clubs for £250 a time, a considerable amount of money in those days.[30] Royal Sydney was one of those advised and, for its £250, received five pages of typewritten notes, double spaced. McKenzie emphasized the natural, shifting very little dirt, planting few trees, but placing sandtraps with unerring accuracy.[31] Even now, with modern equipment, McKenzie traps undermine the confidence of the greatest players. At the 8th hole on the Royal Melbourne composite course, very few players tee off with a wood, even through the par 4 is driveable at just 279 meters. The yawning bunker on the left is almost 50 meters long and 4 meters deep. Despite the simplicity, a McKenzie course is distinctive, an important reason why Augusta National, home to The Masters, is so celebrated. While it would be false to suggest that the course is simple, it is certainly natural. The holes flow with the geography, difficulties created mostly by the placement of the water and sand to emphasize and reward shotmakers, especially those who move the ball right to left. Augusta National's subtlety is what most players emphasize, many needing a few years to come to terms with it.

In the context of this chapter, it is important to emphasize the symbolic nature of the club and what it represents globally. Augusta National is home to a mere 300 of the United States' richest and most influential men, with membership by invitation only. It is virtually impossible for anyone else to get on the course. Everywhere around the world, prestigious clubs represent a social oasis for these kinds of people. The exclusiveness and real estate value physically separate them from the rest of the community. As the expense of the architecture increases, so does the exclusivity. Classic courses, like Pebble Beach and Merion, are now replaced by spectacular constructions emphasizing either physical beauty or a demonstration of power over the landscape. In all this, the power of the machine has become paramount, but it is interesting to reflect that the most respected courses are those made by man, shovel, and horse, rather than by a Caterpillar D-8. Perhaps in an increasingly technological global sports world there is still a place for tradition, which is why designers like Robert Trent Jones Jr. and Pete Dye are so controversial.[32] Each of them has completed well over 100 courses worldwide and each charges around $1 million for a plan, the execution of which can cost many times that sum. Neither builds traditional courses, and with the possible exception of Japan, neither really relates to the local culture.

An important contributor to that dimension of golf's globalization is the relationship between course development and real estate investment. In some parts of the world, the rise of the golf club is an investment in its own right.[33] Private clubs have always implied distinction, as Pierre Bourdieu might put it. The wildly exotic Shiner clubhouse, at the Medinah Country Club, near Chicago perhaps says it all.[34] Real estate developments on and surrounding a course clearly increase the value of the investment exponentially. If land is scarce, as in some parts of Asia, the variation is to simply sell a membership. While there is insufficient space here to explore this aspect, it is important to note that this process is now highly globalized. Golf club memberships and/ or property is sought across national borders, in very high volume.

Perhaps predictably, another of the major global impacts of golf with a long history is that of tourism. Turnberry, for example, site for the 1977 epic Open contest between Tom Watson and Jack Nicklaus, was developed as a tourist resort, during the 1920s by British railway authorities. Remaining within golf's English classed image, rather than within its Scottish plebeian one, it was very upscale tourism as represented in the facade of the Turnberry Hotel. Its tourist role continues but now caters to a very different wealthy clientele, the Japanese traveling golfers. They are of very considerable number, and also now own interests in the hotel itself.[35] In Hawaii, the switch has been from the wealthy American golfing tourist to the Japanese one, with almost all resorts on Oahu being Japanese owned. Instead of inspiration coming from railway owners, it is from airline operators such as ANA which encompasses air travel, hotel accommodation and golf within its corporate structure. Golf made a substantial contribution to the company's profit margin.

Government agencies and private companies alike have long recognized the important spur to travel provided by golf. In the 1930s, despite the rise of Mussolini and the Fascists, golf provided an attraction to Italy for British upper classes, enjoying a twentieth-century version of the Grand Tour. Politically neutral Switzerland provided a more stable golfing environment. The variations in the European scene concern the mix of the limited upper market with the mass lower end. Switzerland continues to maintain an important attraction in golf. France has begun to develop several high quality locations, while in Spain, especially on the Costa del Sol, mass migration of winter golfers from Britain is highly significant in an economic sense. This trend is not confined only to Europe. Southeast Asian tourism is now highly geared towards golf, with "emerging economies" investing large sums of money in golf resorts in hope of attracting wealthy tourists from Japan and elsewhere.

An important feature of this tourism concerns women. Golf, in a global sense, is one sport in which women were treated more fairly. That is not to say that they were well-treated, but at least they were allowed to play. By the turn of the century, women's golf was well established on both sides of the Atlantic, as well as in British Imperial outposts, like Australia and New Zealand. There were very good women players, but many of their achievements were locked up in the social and/or fashion pages. In several cases, women became the golf widows who let their men go off to play. Much of that has now changed since the women's tours in Europe and the United States have progressed relatively well, stimulating interest in the game at local levels. By 1990, there were thought to be approximately 2.5 million women golfers over the age of 18 in the United States. At least half of these women resided in a household where the income was in excess of $50,000. They played at least 18% of all rounds of golf played in the United States during 1990.[36] Clearly, women provide a major economic dimension on the globalization of golf. Consequently, despite traditional views, women are more catered to today.

A major statistic from the 1990 National Golf Foundation's survey stated that 2.8% of blacks were golfers, compared to 9.6% of Hispanics, 15% of Asians, and 14.9% of whites. Similar figures are duplicated in many places around the globe. These statistics are now recognized as a major economic opportunity in the rapidly growing demographic sectors virtually untouched by the game. The point here, in relating to global sports, is that the marketplace is inevitably connected to cultural and socioeconomic structuring. This point has been ignored by many analysts and industry decision-makers, thus creating an important growth issue among minorities, since they have received poor service from golf manufacturers and suppliers. Therefore, the future involves niche marketing.

Golf is probably the best example of the inherent ironies in sports as a business. The game serves no essential social purpose, yet thrives by feeding on itself. If Marx and Engels had written a century later than they did, they might well have regarded golf as the purest form of capitalism.

Consumers of golf are indeed a very strange class. Like all sports subcultures, they have their own international language, customs, practices, and buying patterns. They are susceptible to the same forms of advertising as many other sports. Their passion for golf supports television coverage, creating multimillionaires of the game's great players. They also support a myriad of spin-off industries. One includes golf collectables, the most notable being golf art. There is a huge, long-term publishing industry. Consumers underpin clothing and equipment purchases and support tourist venues all over the world. The social significance of golf has long been recognized because of the economic opportunities offered by even the most tangential connection with the game.[37]

Ultimately, the game is about two concepts which guarantee its future. The first is the determination of the human mind and body to gain control over an inanimate white ball, a challenge of considerable significance in the broad scale of human endeavor. The second concept is image, in which a simple activity represents something else entirely. This was demonstrated by the Mizuno's upscale creation of golf equipment.

Golf, therefore, is a major factor in the global economy by virtue of its intervention in a wide range of human activity. This activity ranges from manufacturing to real estate. Its true complexity and meaning is fully understood only through the comprehension of its growth. Comparative analysis of the social traditions of golf demonstrates the inherent relationship between the form and practice of the game and the context in which it is found. Perhaps most important, it is the sheer human passion for golf that drives this great economic machine. This human desire factor serves as a timely reminder not only for those in the golf industry, but also for those in the sports industry in general.

Notes

[1]Harvey, David. *The condition of postmodernity.* Oxford: Blackwell, 1989.
[2]Geertz, Clifford. *The interpretation of cultures.* New York: Basic, 1972.
[3]*Golf Consumer Profile.* Jupitar, Florida: National Golf Foundation, 1989.
[4]*Australian golf industry reference directory.* Sydney: Federal Press, 1992.
[5]*Golf course news.* (March 1992), pp. 1-20.
[6]*Golf market today.* (September-October 1991), pp. 1-3.
[7]*Golf market today.* pp. 1-3.
[8]Ferrier, Bob. *The world atlas of golf courses.* London: Colour Library. 1991.
[9]Elliott, Allan and John Allan May. *The golf monthly illustrated history of golf.* Sydney: Golden Press, 1990.
[10]Tatz, Colin and Brian Stoddart. *The centenary history of the Royal Sydney Golf Club.* Sydney: Allen & Unwin, 1993.
[11]*Fore.* (May 1987), p. 31.

[12]Williams, Michael. *The official history of the Ryder Cup*. London: Stanley Paul, 1989.

[13]Hagen, Walter. *The Walter Hagen Story*. London: Heinemann, 1957.

[14]Seitz, Nick. "The boys from down under are taking over," *Golf Digest*. 43:2 (February 1992), p. 58.

[15]Braid, James. *Advanced Golf*. London: Methuen, 1908.

[16]Hogan, Ben. *Five lessons: The modern fundamentals of golf*. New York: Barnes, 1957.

[17]Soutar, D.G. *The Australian golfer*. Sydney: Angus & Robertson, 1908.

[18]Mitchell, Abe. *Essentials of golf*. London: Hodder & Stoughton, n.d.

[19]East, J. Victor. *Better golf in five minutes*. New York: Prentice-Hall, 1956.

[20]Leadbetter, David. *The golf swing*. London: Hutchison, 1991.

[21]*PGA teaching manual: the art and science of golf instruction*. Palm Beach Gardens: PGA, 1990.

[22]Maltby, Ralph. *Golf club design, fitting, alteration and repair: The principles and procedures*. Newark, Ohio: Maltby, 1982 (2nd edition).

[23]Fishman, Lew. "A last hurrah for Toney Penna." *Golf digest*. 30:12 (December 1988), p. 90.

[24]*Australian golf industry reference directory*. Sydney: Federal Press, 1992.

[25]*The world of sports*. Tokyo: Mizuno, 1990.

[26]Sommers, Robert. *The U.S. Open: golf's ultimate challenge*. London: Stanley Roberts, 1987.

[27]Cochran, A.J. (Ed.). *Science and golf*. London: Spon, 1990.

[28]Cornish, Geoffrey S. and Whitten, Ronald E. *The golf course*. New York: Routledge, 1981.

[29]Godwin, Stephen. "The godfather." *Golf*. (April 1992).

[30]Johnson, Joseph. *The Royal Melbourne golf club: A centenary history*. Melbourne: RMGC, 1991.

[31]Tatz & Stoddart

[32]*The golf courses of Robert Trent Jones, Jr*. London: Bison, 1988.

[33]Strawn, John. *Drawing the green: The making of a golf course*. New York: Harper Perennial, 1991.

[34]Bourdieu, Pierre. *Distinction: A social critique of the judgement of taste*. Cambridge, Mass.: Harvard University Press, 1984.

[35]*Golf vacations*. Singapore: GV Press, 1992.

[36]*Golf participation in the United States*. National Golf Foundation, FL, 1991.

[37]*Directory of Golf*. National Golf Foundation, FL, 1992.

Part 2: American Sport and the Global Arena

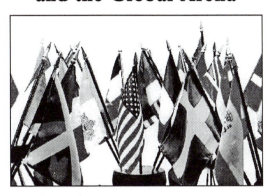

Part 2: American Sport and the Global Arena

The chapters in Part 2 focus on the nature and role of contemporary American sport. From the impact of the American sporting goods industry on the political economy of developing nations; to the recognition, by American universities, of the need to prepare skilled professionals for a rapidly expanding global sports marketplace; a cultural critique of American sport; and a literary analysis of the centrality of sport to American culture — the authors of these chapters provide a clear account of the complexion and significance of sport in modern America and it's position in the New World Order.

George Sage's deeply human analysis of investment by the American sporting goods industry in developing countries of the Caribbean, Central America, and Asia is testimony to the far-reaching impact of American sport in the world today. Though conjuring up emotional images of American unemployment, foreign exploitation, poverty and helplessness, Sage develops a powerful yet rational argument. He contends that export-processing industrialization is motivated by corporate profiteering born of "cheaper land and labor, a non-union workforce, relief from safety and environmental standards, and favorable tax abatements." Providing case studies of the Rawlings Sporting Goods Co., and Nike Inc., assembly plants in the Caribbean and Asia, Sage calls for a greater global awareness for the social outcomes of deindustrialization. Driven by the promise of increased profits, domestic unemployment, foreign labor exploitation, unsafe and unhealthy work conditions, environmental pollution and tax "evasion" are seemingly ignored as necessary casualties of economic growth. The author concludes that the only hope for regulating the operations of large, transnational companies lies with the formation of powerful coalitions, built to represent the concerns of all parties that are targeted by the new global economy.

Once among the most culturally insular of nations, the United States is beginning to recognize the capitalistic potential of an emerging global marketplace. With American Business Schools' international curriculum initiatives dating from the end of the Second World War, Lisa Pike and Ted Fay examine the critical need for a similar shift in emphasis in the preparation of sport business executives. Underscoring the relative youth of sport management programs in American academe, and based upon the findings of a survey, the authors call for the immediate introduction of an international sport management component to contemporary curricular, in order to meet the needs of an ever-expanding global sports market.

The shift toward globalism is only one of the elements considered by Ralph Wilcox in his cultural critique of American sport. Claiming that American scholars have, in the past, been far too deeply immersed in their own culture to draw out the unique characteristics of their sporting world, Wilcox hones in on the inherent contradictions of American sport and culture. Cautioning against an oversimplified, external analysis of American sport, a tendency fueled by its characteristic display of emotion, the author seeks a deeper culturally-based explanation. In structuring his treatise, Wilcox considers the relationship between such fundamental, and frequently oppositional, values as: Nationalism—Globalism; Democracy—Capitalism; Egalitarianism—Elitism; Individualism—Bureaucratization; Tradition—Innovation; and, Rationalism— Emotion. Providing colorful illustrations and abundant data, Wilcox concludes that to understand American sport is to fully appreciate the complexities of American culture.

The intricacies of American sport are matched only by its significance in life. Applying C.L.R. James' centrality of sport model to four contemporary books on American football, Scott Crawford seeks to better explain the role of sport in American society. As with James and Cricket, George G. Mills' *Go Big Red*; H.G. Bissinger's *Friday Night Lights*; Theodore M. Hesburgh's *God, Country, and Notre Dame*; and *Bootlegger's Boy* by Barry Switzer, Crawford shows that more than being merely tales of the grid-iron, they furnished sound evidence to support the centrality of sport in the life of small town America; its common people, high schools and universities.

Chapter 3

Deindustrialization and the American Sporting Goods Industry

George H. Sage

Sociologist C. Wright Mills[1] described the sociological imagination as an attempt to grasp the interplay of history and personal biography, of self and the world. Unfortunately, most of our public discourse does not connect sport with the larger political, economic, and social milieu and its impact on our personal lives. However, following Mills, I take sport to be rooted within the broader stream of political, economic, and social forces of which it is a part. Therefore, I have located this study of the sporting goods industry within the national and international system of unequal economic and political relationships among the developed and less developed countries. My focus is on how this system impacts upon the lives of workers in every factory and office across the world instead of upon athletes, coaches, or sports organizations, which is typically the focus of research in sport studies. My concern is with workers' wages and salaries, working conditions, and benefits, but also the broader social relations of the workplace where sporting goods are manufactured. I evaluate sporting goods manufacturing by the standards of this slogan of organized labor throughout the world, "An injury to one, is an injury to all."

The American sporting goods business is an enormous enterprise. According to the most recent figures, it generates $20 billion in revenue annually.[2] Over 1,500 sporting goods and equipment manufacturers and suppliers are listed in the February 1992 issue of *Athletic Business*. Much of the sporting goods once manufactured in the United States are now manufactured in foreign plants located mostly in Third World countries of the Caribbean, Central America, and Asia. In spite of the patriotic rhetoric and all-American image that the sports world likes to portray, all of the baseballs used in Major League Baseball are made by a Rawlings Sporting Goods Company plant in Costa Rica. Furthermore, 90 percent of shoes worn by major leaguers and 60 percent of the gloves and mitts they use are made outside the U.S. Browse through any sporting goods store and you will find bat bags made in Taiwan, softballs from Haiti, various styles of athletic shoes made in South Korea, the Philippines, and China. Many items, you will discover, are made outside the U.S. Even two-thirds of the uniform U. S. athletes wore in the opening ceremony of the 1992 Winter Olympics were made in foreign countries.[3]

Major structural economic change is sweeping the world and it is represented in the examples described. Several terms are used for this global economic restructuring: deindustrialization, off-shore relocation, export processing, and capital flight. Regardless of the terminology adopted, they all refer to a widespread, systematic disinvestment by multinational corporations of the industrially developed nations and the establishment of manufacturing subsidiaries abroad in Third World countries. Transnational corporations are increasingly tilting the national economies of their home country away from basic industries and transferring the labor-intensive phases of production to Third World nations[4] (see Figure 1). Between 1963 and 1988, the proportion of the world's manufacturing exports accounted for by Third World nations increased from 4.3 to 12.5 percent.[5] In 1950, the annual American direct investment abroad was only $11.8 billion; by 1988 it had mushroomed to $309 billion. Today, over one-third of the earnings of the 200 largest U.S. multinational corporations are from revenues of their off-shore subsidiaries.[6] Figure 1 illustrates this situation for one country—Mexico. Foreign investment by U.S. transnational corporations has eliminated nearly 3 million American manufacturing jobs between 1977 and 1990 — a decline of over 10%.[7]

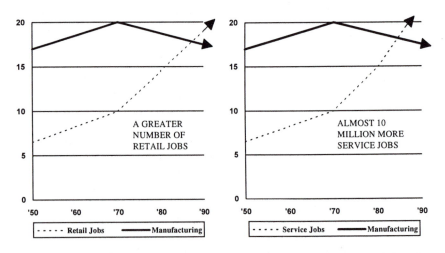

Figure 1—Manufacturing Eclipsed by Lower-Paying Retail and Service Jobs. Adapted from *America: What Went Wrong* (p. 18) by D.L. Barlett and J.B. Steele, 1992, Kansas City: Andrews and McMeel.

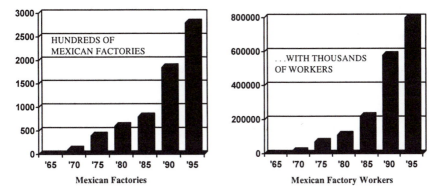

Figure 2—American Corporations are Closing Plants and Shifting Jobs to Mexico. Adapted from *America: What Went Wrong* (p. 34) by D.L. Barlett and J.B. Steele, 1992, Kansas City: Andrews and McMeel.

Export-processing industrialization is a strategy used by multinational corporations to find cheaper land and labor, a non-union workforce, relief from safety and environmental standards, and favorable tax abatements from both the host and foreign countries.[8] For corporations, moving plants and operations off-shore is a way to boost profits. But for American workers and their communities the consequences are usually grim. Closed plants, unemployed workers, community disintegration, and a variety of related afflictions that undermine the nation's social fabric are the results of globalizing manufacturing.[9] Workers faced with plant shutdowns lose much more than wages and benefits. Many lose their homes, their cars, and their savings. Many lose their sense of themselves as productive workers and providers for their families. Increased rates of suicide, homicide, heart disease, alcoholism, mental illness, domestic violence, and family breakup have been linked to the stress of unemployment when plants are closed and productive operations moved off-shore.[10] According to the Office of Technology Assessment:

> Displacement can be devastating for communities and regions as well as individuals. . . . Large losses of employment have ripple effects in the community. A large layoff in one industry also affects workers in supplier industries and workers in local service establishments when laid off workers reduce spending.[11]

Another consequence of globalizing production is that the wages of U.S. working people have been declining steadily for more than 15 years. Among the 14
leading industrial countries, only the U.S. showed a decline in labor costs per
unit of output from 1980 to 1990. By 1990 the average hourly compensation for
U.S. production workers had fallen from first to fifth. Germany, Sweden, Italy,
and France all paid their production workers more (see Table 1).[12]

Table 1
Hourly Wages and Benefits in Manufacturing, 1990[13]

Germany	21.30
Sweden	20.93
Italy	16.29
France	15.25
United States	14.84
Japan	12.84
Britain	12.42

For workers in the Third World, there is overwhelming evidence that multinational investment in assembly production carries with it some heavy burdens
including unjust and inhuman working conditions, sexual exploitation, social
disruption, and distorted economic development. Moreover, attempts to organize labor unions are often violently suppressed by government soldiers. Health
and safety in the workplace are often unregulated, as are pollution and other
environmental protections. Workplace democracy and worker rights are nonexistent. For the Third World, then, the global factory is only the most recent
development in a long history of foreign exploitation and domination.[14] Since
the primary reason multinational corporations relocate overseas is to reduce
labor costs, women are the natural choice for assembly jobs because women
everywhere are paid lower wages than men. The majority of the manufacturing
workforce is young, between 16 and 25 years old. In South Korea, for example,
women between 16 and 25 years of age comprise one third of the industrial
labor force. Actually, many are unable to continue beyond age twenty-five
because of work-related health problems.[15]

Although a handful of Third World countries have benefited from the globalization process, and have made significant progress in industrialization and trade,
the overall gap between First World and Third World nations keeps widening.[16]
Meanwhile, most Americans have no idea about the ill-effects that the multinational corporations of our nation inflict upon the workers of our own country or
upon the workers of Third World countries.[17]

Now it is not just the automobile, steel, and electronics industries where foreign manufacturing has grown dramatically. U.S. sporting goods corporations have also turned to the Third World because an endless supply of cheap labor makes it profitable and because U.S. foreign and trade policies (such as the Caribbean Basin Initiative) provide the corporations with financial incentives. This chapter will demonstrate how corporate flight and plant closings work in the sporting goods industry. Space does not permit any comprehensive treatment of the sporting goods industry, so I'm going to take just two examples: the manufacture of baseballs and athletic shoes.

Rawlings Baseballs

Rawlings Sporting Goods Co., headquartered in St. Louis, has manufactured the baseballs used in Major League Baseball for over forty years.[18] But America's national pastime is no game for women stitching baseball covers. Here is how it is done: Workers squeeze the baseball between their feet, they then bend over and run the needles through the cover, they stand up and, at the same time, jerk the threads high above their head so they tighten at the first draw. They do that 214 times, the number of stitches there are in a baseball, to complete the job for one ball. When they've finished stitching one baseball, they stitch 35 to 40 more the same way during a day's work.[19] As recently as two years ago women who made baseballs the way I've just described got paid 9 to 13 cents per ball— about $2.70 per day. Meanwhile, high profile Major League stars make millions of dollars hitting baseballs made by this process. Nolan Ryan gets $20 for one baseball autographed by him; he earned over $1 million during the 1992 off-season for autographing baseballs.[20]

Prior to 1953 all Rawlings baseballs were manufactured in a plant in St. Louis with unionized labor. In that year, to reduce labor costs, Rawlings shifted manufacturing to Licking, Missouri. At first the Licking plant was non-union, but in 1956 it was organized by the Amalgamated Clothing and Textile Workers Union. The union immediately began efforts to improve wages and working conditions, and Rawlings began looking around for an alternative manufacturing site. In 1964,[21] it moved its baseball manufacturing to an offshore location in Puerto Rico. Advertisements placed in U.S. newspapers by the Puerto Rican Economic Development Administration may explain the benefits Rawlings saw in moving its baseball operations offshore. The advertisements promised, "You're in good company in Puerto Rico, U.S.A." where there are "higher productivity, lower wages and tax-free profits."[22]

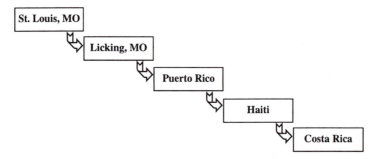

Figure 3—Plant Movements of Rawlings Baseball Manufacturing, 1955-1990

Advertisements like this attracted offshore corporate investment by a number of U.S. firms. But when the initial tax "holidays" for foreign investors ran out and minimum wage laws were implemented in Puerto Rico, many companies left to exploit even cheaper labor in Haiti. Rawlings was one of the first to move to Haiti. In 1969 it closed its Puerto Rican baseball manufacturing plant and relocated in Haiti, the poorest country in the Western hemisphere and one of the 25 poorest in the world. It is also the country in this hemisphere with the lowest wage levels.[23] Put simply, by a Haitian business publication, "Cheap labor is the bottom line in doing business in Haiti: it is Haiti's primary incentive to investment."[24] Rawlings was one of the first export assembly plants in Haiti. Until 1990, in terms of sales and employees, Rawlings was the third largest company on the island, employing close to 1,000 workers. In the 1980s its baseball manufacturing was the second largest assembly industry in Haiti, behind only textiles.[25] Haiti was the ideal setting for Rawlings' offshore baseball assembly operation, even though no one plays baseball in Haiti. There were generous tax holidays, a franchise granting tariff exemption, and the only legal trade unions were those run by the government. Strikes were illegal, and the minimum wage was so low that a majority of Haitians could not derive anything that might reasonably be called a "living" from the assembly plants. Haitians who made baseballs for Rawlings earned less than $3 per day; the weekly average wage was $18. Josh DeWind and David Kinley noted: "Far from creating a way out of poverty, the industry's wages provide the basis for only an impoverished standard of living."[26]

In the late 1980s several human rights group—Pax Christi USA, the Haitian Corporate Campaign, and the Washington Office on Haiti—investigated reports of labor exploitation, denial of workers' rights, and appalling working conditions coming from past and present workers at the Rawlings baseball plant. According to a report prepared by them, the following abuses were documented at the Rawlings plant:

- labor rights violations: discharges for union activity; threats and actual violence against union leaders; army intervention in labor disputes.

- violations of minimum-wage laws: requiring an unreasonably high piece work in order to receive minimum wage; paying a sub-minimum wage during employees' probation period, then firing them when the probation period is over.

- unhealthy working conditions: insufficient access to drinking water and toilets; only two 15-minute breaks per day; no lunch breaks.

- wages of between $.09 to $.13 per ball, when materials are available, and no wages on days when materials are not available.[27]

In November 1990 the Rawlings plant in Haiti was suddenly closed. All baseball manufacturing was moved to a Rawlings plant in Costa Rica. This move represented the fourth time the company's baseball production had been relocated in the past 30 years. In a press release announcing its departure from Haiti, Rawlings' parent company, Figgie International, said the closing of the plant was due to Haiti's "unstable political climate." The three human rights groups identified above saw the move to Costa Rica as a reluctance to adequately address concerns about wages and working conditions at the Haiti plant. They also saw the closing of the plant, just two weeks before Haiti's first democratic elections, as deliberate in that the leading presidential candidate, Fr. Jean-Bertrand Aristide, the candidate who eventually won the election, had spoken out strongly against abuses by multinational corporations in his country.

Actually, Rawlings had been exploring alternatives to its Haitian operations before the actual relocation. According to Leslie Wirpsa,[28] a journalist for the *National Catholic Reporter,* in 1987, Figgie brought three Haitian women to Turrialba, a town about two hours from the Costa Rican capital of San Jose, to teach the art of baseball stitchery. The company began production in a rented warehouse. It opened a newly constructed plant in January 1990. About 600 people, most of them women, are formally employed in the Turrialba facilities.

They classify leather, wrap fibers, sew, stamp and qualify baseballs. The majority of the workers are "sewers." They must stitch 30 to 35 baseballs to earn $5 to $6 a day. The work week is 48 hours long. Approximately 300 Costa Rican women also sew baseballs in their homes, earning 15 cents per ball. Figgie refused Wirpsa access to the Turrialba plant. Everyone Wirpsa spoke to said working conditions were horrible. Workers who have attempted to organize a union have been fired, indirectly violating Costa Rican labor regulations.

Nike Athletics Shoes

Americans are lacing up 388 million pairs of brand-name athletic shoes a year. All told, the market for athletic shoes will reach $10 billion in retail sales this year, and advertising slogans like "Just do it," "Bo knows," and shoe styles like "Air Jordans" fuel the American consumers' appetite for these shoes. Nike, with revenues of $43 billion for the fiscal year that ended in May 1991, is the nation's largest athletic shoe firm, but Reebok, with revenue of $2.7 billion, is in hot pursuit.[29]

Ownership of Nike Inc. is as all-American as you can get. The company was started by current chairman Philip Knight, a University of Oregon graduate, and Bill Bowerman, former track coach at Oregon. Blue Ribbon Sports (BRS) was the original corporate name and the name was changed to Nike in 1978. BRS opened its first American manufacturing facility at Exeter, New Hampshire, in 1974, and it continued to make shoes there until 1984. In 1978 it opened a second American manufacturing plant at Saco, Maine. But within two years, Nike ownership began the familiar corporate pattern of relocating its manufacturing to Third World countries. In 1980, negotiations started with the People's Republic of China for production of Nike shoes there, and a couple of years later it began manufacturing operations in factories in Taiwan and Korea. As manufacturing was shifted offshore, during the 1980s, Nike closed all of its shoe manufacturing plants in the U.S. Presently, all Nike finished footwear is manufactured by foreign suppliers, with South Korea and Taiwan doing the majority of shoe manufacturing, but more and more is being done in China.[30]

The emergence of Nike as a major shoe manufacturer coincided with the emergence of several Asian countries as export processing nations—especially South Korea and Taiwan—whose fundamental industrialization strategy has been the promotion of manufactured goods, concentrating particularly on labor-intensive industries.[31] South Korea's export processing success lay in three areas of comparative advantage over other countries: the combination of low labor costs, long working hours, and the organization of the labor force into a highly efficient system of production.[32] From the 1960s until the late 1980s, the wages of Korean workers were consistently lower than those of workers in other Asian countries. Before unions won big wage gains in the past few years, the hourly pay of Korean manufacturing workers was 11 percent of United States' workers and 14 percent of Japan's,

> But low wages were only one element in the Korean formula for success. Another was the long working day. A 1986 international survey of the International Labor Office found that Korean workers worked the longest hours — an average of 54 hours per week.[33]

While these were the main ingredients of the Korean export processing system for profitability, the contribution of another cost-saving measure cannot be underestimated: minimal investment in safe working conditions. Laws requiring industrial safety, says one authority,

> ...are almost useless in practice... because employers do not follow the rules and regulations set out in the laws... [there is a] lack of proper knowledge of work-induced health hazards, and [there is a] lack of trained professionals and proper equipment to prevent and to treat work-related illnesses.[34]

Not surprisingly, the results of cutting costs on safety have been appalling as "Korea has the world's highest rate of industrial accidents, with an average of 5 workers killed daily and another 390 seriously injured."[35] It is also the leading nation in the world in the rate of occupation-related illnesses.

Korea's economic transformation has been so remarkable that few have bothered to look at the underside of the "miracle." While the so-called Korean "economic miracle" was able to generate impressive growth, it was grounded in the exploitation of Korean workers. Korea's industrial and government elites used a variety of exploitative and repressive measures to depress working conditions in order to accumulate the capital used for economic growth.[36] George Ogle,[37] a noted analyst of Korea's political economy, wrote that South Korea's "great successes were built upon a labor policy that violated the human rights of workers, a labor policy that required pervasive, and often cruel suppression of the nation's working people."[38]

In Taiwan and China, just as in South Korea, young women from rural areas
form the backbone of the labor intensive export industry. It is their low wages
and long hours which make their manufacturers internationally competitive.
Asia's export processing nations have indeed achieved rapid export success. But
they have done so by following a model which places exports over domestic
needs, profits over worker rights, growth over the environment and thus, of
necessity, the interests of the few above the democratic rights of the many.

Summary and Conclusions

Deindustrialization involves serious social costs: broken lives for working people who lose jobs and livelihoods as well as homes and their personal posses-
sions. Entire communities become economically depressed when corporations
relocate in foreign countries[39]. By relocating their manufacturing offshore, First
World corporations are able to exploit the labor and resources of Third World
countries. They are able to pay workers a fraction of what they would have to
pay them at home, and they are able to work them longer hours under unsafe
and unhealthy conditions; they are able to pollute the water, air, and soil; they
are free to dump toxic chemicals, banned pesticides, and drugs that they are prevented from unloading at home; and they are provided tax abatements by both
home and foreign countries.[40] Thus the neocolonial system of unequal economic
and political relationships among the First and Third World countries envisioned by Wallerstein's[41] world-system model of global development becomes
abundantly evident to even a casual observer.

What are some long-term strategies to address the loss of jobs in First World
countries and the exploitation of Third World workers?[42] Presently, we are all
too content to pay discount prices for our baseballs, bats, gloves, and sneakers,
and idolize athletes who make millions of dollars, while the Caribbean, Central
American, and Asian workers who make this possible use up their lives to support our indulgences. Certainly, the challenge for working people throughout
the world is the challenge to confront the transnational corporations, and governments that protect them, forcing them to respect the human needs of workers, communities, and entire nations. As Rachael Kamel has argued,
"Campaigns for enlightened legislation and regulation are key tools in that task,
but they must be complemented by workplace and community organizing
around a host of issues."[43] Both by labor actions and pressure on government,
citizens will have to take direct initiatives to respond to the increasing freedom
now enjoyed by multinational firms. What's important is that people take this
beyond their own place of work or their own community, that they become
committed to struggling for the betterment of other people. "Human solidarity is

not only morally superior to the law of the jungle; it is a matter of practical necessity for working people." Solidarity is how improved incomes and working conditions are won. Solidarity is how people defend their health, their very lives on the job. "Solidarity, not competition, must be the basis of any... strategy in the integrated economy of [the world]."[44] In country after country organizing has begun, creating a courageous challenge to the dominance of U.S.-based corporations and their allies among foreign economic elites. Of course, none of these movements, in the United States or internationally, can succeed alone. Powerful coalitions must be built that can represent the concerns of all who are negatively affected by the new global economy.

<u>Notes</u>

[1]Mills, C. W. *The sociological imagination.* New York: Oxford University Press, 1961.

[2]Comte, E. & C. Stogel, "Sports: A $63.1 billion industry," *The Sporting News,* (January 1, 1990), pp. 60-61.

[3]Dodd, M. "U.S. Olympic wear isn't all-American," *USA Today,* (January 16, 1992), p. 1C.

[4]Bluestone, B., & B. Harrison, *The deindustrialization of America: Plant closings, community abandonment, and the dismantling of basic industry.* New York: Basic Books, 1992; Grunwald, J., & K. Flamm, *The global factory: Foreign assembly in international trade.* Washington, D.C.: Brookings Institution, 1985; Staudohar, P. D. & H. E. Brown, *Deindustrialization and plant closure.* Lexington, MA: D. C. Heath, 1987.

[5]Sklair, L. *The reformation of capitalism: The maquila industry in Mexico and the U.S.A.* Boston: Allen and Unwin, 1989.

[6]"The 100 largest U.S. multinationals," *Forbes,* (July 25, 1988), pp. 248-250.

[7]Glickman, N. J., and D.P. Woodward, *The new competitors: How foreign investors are changing the U. S. economy.* New York: Basic Books, 1989, pp. 176, 186.

[8]Tiano, S. "Maquiladora women: A new category of workers?" In, K. Ward. *Women workers and global restructuring.* Ithaca, NY: Cornell University Press, 1990, pp. 194-223.

[9]Staudohar & Brown.

[10]Kamel, R. *The global factory: Analysis and action for a new economic era.* Philadelphia: American Friends Service, 1990; Perrucci, C. C., R. Perrucci, D.B. Targ, & H.R. Targ, *Plant closings: International context and social costs.* New York: Aldine De Gruyter, 1988.

[11]Office of Technology Assessment. *Technology and structural unemployment: Reemploying displaced adults.* Washington, D. C.: Congress of the United States, 1986, p. 10.

[12]Miller, J. "Silent depression," *Dollars & Sense*, 175 (April 1992), pp. 6-9; "Spiraling down," *Dollars & Sense*, (April 1992), p. 23.

[13]These data are taken from Miller, pp. 6-9.

[14]Kamel; Wallerstein, I. *The modern world-system.* New York: Academic Press, 1974; Wallerstein, I. *The capitalist world-economy.* New York: Cambridge University Press, 1979;and, Wallerstein, I. *The politics of the world-economy.* New York: Cambridge University Press, 1984.

[15]Kamel; Ward.

[16]"Globalization — To what end? Part 1," *Monthly Review*, 43 (February, 1992), pp. 1-18.

[17]LaBotz, Dan. *Mask of democracy: Labor suppression in Mexico today.* Boston: South End Press, 1992.

[18]"Americans in low-wage jobs double in a decade," *The Greeley Tribune*, (May 12, 1992), p. 1.

[19]"Keep your eye on the ball," *Denver Catholic Register*, (July 11, 1990), p. 14.

[20]Jones, D. "Signing the dotted seam," *USA Today*, (April 6, 1992), p. 1B.

[21]Since the 1960s, Rawlings has been owned by conglomerate Figgie International, which is a diversified Fortune 500 company serving consumer, technical, industrial, and service markets worldwide. Sales in 1989 were $1.3 billion.

[22]Fuentes, A., & B. Ehrenreich, *Women in the global factory.* Boston: South End Press, 1983, p. 11.

[23]Robinson, D. "In Haiti, manufacturers take it or leave it," *Journal of Commerce and Commercial,* 386 (December 10, 1990),p. 4A.

[24]Haitian American Chamber of Commerce (HAMCHAM). "Initiative," *Business Haiti*, 2: 2 (1982), p. 31.

[25]Ebert-Miner, A. "How Rawlings use Haitian women to spin profits off U.S. baseball sales," *Multinational Monitor,* 3: 8 (1982), pp. 11-12; Ebert-Miner, A. "Haitians slave to hatch our baseballs." *Business and Society Review*, (Spring 1983), pp. 12-13; DeWind, J., & D.H. Kinley III, *Aiding migration: The impact of international development assistance on Haiti.* Boulder, CO: Westview Press, 1988.

[26]DeWind & Kinley, p. 118.

[27]Marshall, P. *Report on Haitian corporate campaign and interested persons.* (September 15, 1988), pp. 1-9; "Press release," *Pax Christi, USA*, (December 3, 1990), pp. 1-2.

[28]Wirpsa, L. "Where every Rawlings baseball is a foul ball," *National Catholic Reporter,* (December 28, 1990), p. 1.

[29]Strauss, Gary, "Makers say '90s growth is overseas." *USA Today*, (February 18, 1992), pp. 1B-2B; Rudolph, B. "Foot's paradise." *Time*, (August 28, 1989), pp. 54-55.

[30]Johnson, B. "Nike: Don't put too many shoes in one basket," *American Skipper*, 29 (January 1987), pp. 49-52.; Lee, B. "Nike's run for the money," *Savvy*, 7 (May 1986), p. 24.

[31]Bae, K. "Labor strategy for industrialization in South Korea," *Pacific Affairs*, 62 (1989), pp. 353-363.

[32]Bello, W., & S. Rosenfeld. *Dragons in distress: Asia's miracle economies in crisis.* San Francisco: The Institute for Food and Development Policy, 1990.

[33]Bello & Rosenfeld, p. 24

[34]Lee, K. H. "Ours is not to question why," *Business Korea Electronics,* (September 1988), p. 51.

[35]Bello & Rosenfeld, p. 25.

[36]Ogle, G. E. *South Korea: Dissent within the economic miracle.* Atlantic Highlands, NJ: Zed Books, 1990, p. vii.

[37]Ogle.

[38]Ogle, p. 47.

[39]Feagin, J. R. "Corporate location decisions," In, D. S. Eitzen & M. B. Zinn, *The Reshaping of America.* Englewood Cliffs, NJ: Prentice-Hall, 1989, pp. 334-348.

[40]Slater, P. *A Dream Deferred.* Boston: Beacon, 1991.

[41]Wallerstein, *The modern world-system.*; Wallerstein, *The capitalist world-economy.*; and Wallerstein, *The politics of the world-economy.*

[42]Moody, K., & M. McGinn, *Unions and free trade: Solidarity vs. competition.* Detroit: Labor Notes, 1992. See Chapter 8.

[43]Kamel, p. 2.

[44]Moody & McGinn, p. 43.

Chapter 4

Cross-Cultural Studies: Implications on Professional Preparation and Management Training in Global Sport

Lisa L. Pike and Ted Fay

The world is becoming smaller. Moving toward the year 2000, barriers to international cultural exchange will continue to crumble. Already, in the midst of changing global politics, communications are more open and barriers to trade are being lifted. During 1992, much of Europe was expected to become a single market of over 320 million consumers and will rival the trade power of Japan and the United States. In addition, the many nations of Eastern Europe and the republics of the former Soviet Union will continue to undergo vast changes on their political and economic fronts, further opening their boundaries to the global market.

These significant shifts in the global economic and business climate have already begun to open vast opportunities for the sports industry. Sport, be it youth, amateur, or professional, serves as a medium for cultural exchange. Sport is a universal product as language is not a barrier to its social and entertainment value. With such unique qualities, the sports industry should become a prime benefactor of globalization.

Parkhouse and Ulrich have stated that sport requires a new breed of specialists, highly trained managers specializing in one of six sport-related fields: commercial recreation; professional sport; amateur sport; educational athletic administration; arena/stadium management; and promotion, marketing, merchandising, and broadcast media.[1] Although seldom recognized, international management training is an essential element in the preparation of these specialists, as each of these fields is operating in a global market. With the continual blurring of national and continental boundaries, the sports business community must seek competent current and future sport managers with international business capabilities.[2] This practitioner must be prepared to react and respond to cultural nuances and overcome language differences which may otherwise hinder success in this globalization process. Thus, sport managers must be attentive to the inherent cultural issues which will arise as they work to develop multinational sport enterprises and to trade sport, its players, coaches, management personnel, and products throughout the world.

A fundamental thesis of this chapter is that these current global business and economic changes are not being adequately addressed by those in the sport management community. Over the past twenty years colleges and universities have developed curricula and concentrations to prepare students to work in a variety of sport settings. An examination of these curricula and concentrations demonstrates that they lack an international business orientation.[3] A lack of preparation for globalization may deny those in the business of sport the opportunity to prosper in a global marketplace.

Purpose of Study

The purpose of this study is to begin to explore the issues surrounding the preparation of students and training of practitioners involved in the sports industry for a shift from a domestic to more global orientation. The authors' goal is not to present a conclusive study in the area, but rather to build a starting point from which to raise awareness, stimulate discussion, and examine the implications and need for further study. This study involved a comparative assessment of graduate programs in sport management with its business school counterpart, the master's degree in business administration (MBA). The rationale for such a choice was based on the fact that business schools have been actively engaged in educating and training competent managers for the global marketplace for some time. The evolution in business school curricula has fostered a concurrent trend of extending this curricula to practitioners by means of executive training through conferences, exchanges, workshops, seminars, and institutes.

It is apparent that a case can be made that a similar pattern will emerge for international sport management education to be adopted by degree programs and executive training options. Currently this trend is not occurring within the field of sport management per se. As recognized by Hardy,[4] while sport management should not be considered a "proprietary right" of business schools due to the unique nature of sport, sport management must nevertheless adopt the basic elements of the business school model of management if it is to succeed.

In doing so, the field of sport management must seriously examine the validity of incorporating the basic elements of this major paradigm shift in the business school model towards a more international focus. It would be irresponsible, then, to ignore international business education's many stages of development which date back to the late 1950s.[5] Such a comparison may offer us knowledge and provide us with effective models which have sustained over thirty years of modification by some of the best business educators in the world.

A secondary objective of this study was to initiate the development of a survey instrument to be pre-tested for full dissemination at a later time. The objective in designing and pre-testing this exploratory pilot survey on a small sample set was aimed at beginning the process of going beyond an examination of "what is" to a more in-depth inquiry of "what needs to be" in graduate and executive sport management training. A summary analysis of responses from respondents to a pre-test of this instrument to a small sample group of practitioners in the field is provided in Appendix I. It is not the intention of this study to draw any specific conclusions from the responses to this pilot survey at this point.

Review of Literature

Throughout the research the authors' initial suspicions were confirmed: that developments and growth of graduate sport management programs and, specifically, curriculums did not reflect the current trends in curricular changes in management training in business education toward a more international concentration and focus. With the exception of a few current studies still in progress, research in the area of international sport management is largely unexplored. Correspondingly, in the late fifties and early sixties, business futurists began to predict a move toward a global market and suggested that business schools respond by adopting more internationally focused courses in the areas of management, marketing, finance, and accounting.[6] It was during this period that business schools became more directed in their research and experimented with modifications of the traditional business curriculum by shifting the focus to a more international perspective. This shift was reflected in the business research and curricula in such areas as managing in other cultures,[7] negotiating with one's business counterparts in foreign cultures,[8] being fluent in other languages,[9] transacting business in foreign legal and economic systems,[10] and having internship and field experiences abroad.[11]

In seven recent articles evaluating and presenting model sport management curricula, the international business sector was conspicuously absent.[12] Since sport management education is still in the evolutionary process, it is no wonder that international issues have not been raised. Sport management is continuing to conquer issues on the domestic front. Academics in the field are still in the midst of seeking professional acceptance of sport management,[13] emphasizing academic theory and research,[14] defining curricula,[15] and debating standards and accreditation.[16]

Many questions raised by this study directly impact these issues and it would be shortsighted not to also consider the move to globalization when refining the sport management profession. For instance, one needs to consider such issues as: Is the sport management curricula too domestically oriented? Is there a demand from the sports industry for a more "internationalized" sport management curriculum to develop graduates to specialize in international sports business? If so, in what form must this internationalization occur? In other words, is one course sufficient? Should a mastery of one or more languages be a prerequisite for graduation from the program? Should an internship abroad be required? Should exchange programs between domestic graduate sport management programs and universities abroad be developed? Should all graduate students have working knowledge of the global sports industry by the infusion of international issues throughout all courses in the program? And, finally, what training exists or needs to exist for those already at work in sport management positions to prosper in a global sports industry?

In an effort to put a broader face upon the sport management field, Thoma assessed the changes and growth of sport management programs in the United States and Canada, as well as at universities and institutes throughout the world and has exposed and confirmed yet another suspicion. In his remarks, Thoma concluded that there is no evidence that a focus and/or concentration in international sport exists within any sport management program at this time. Currently, only two courses specifically related to the management issues in international sport are known to exist.[17] Critically, both of these courses are taught at the undergraduate level, which further reinforces the concern that master's level curriculum in sport management might not be able to respond adequately to international management-related issues. This is not to suggest conclusively that other courses possessing a full or partial focus on international sport may not exist. It is clear, however, that graduate curricula in sport management are presently not engaged in providing their students with an international perspective or concentration. In order to better understand the rationale and need for serious considerations of such a perspective, a descriptive analysis of the internationalization of the MBA curriculum follows.

Business Schools (MBA Programs)

Since World War II graduate business education in the United States has grown immensely.[18] For example, business schools in the United States in 1960 were graduating about 5,000 students annually and currently that number is between 60-70,000 graduates with MBA degrees.[19] During the 1960s and 1970s, the American MBA model was successfully exported to Europe. Most recently, universities and institutes of East Asia have adopted the American model as a basis for its two MBA programs; one in Japan and one in Hong Kong.[20] This adopted model consists of courses in six key subject areas: (1) Business Strategy, (2) Managerial Economics, (3) Marketing, (4) Human Resources, including Organizational Behavior, Personnel Management, and Industrial Relations, (5) Financial Management, and (6) Operations Management. Both the European and Asian MBA programs have hired faculty educated at U.S. business schools to implement this model.[21] This hiring continues and is reinforced by such examples as Dartmouth College's Amos Tuck School of Business, which offers an MBA program taught by its faculty at the International University of Japan.[22] For the purpose of this comparative study, the authors have limited their focus to the American and European programs, as their numbers and degree of organization far exceed those of the Asian MBA programs.

In comparing the development of the European versus the American model of MBA education, one fundamental difference emerges. When Europeans began adopting the MBA, the key players in the educational venture were not European colleges and universities, but rather businesses. The European graduate business programs were created by businesses seeking to provide top-of-the-line management education in order to help European industry compete internationally. For instance, two of the early Swiss MBA programs were founded by the worldwide Nestlé and Alcan corporations. Incidentally, these programs have recently merged under the name, International Institute for Management Development (IMEDE) and now operate independently from their founding corporations.[23] Similarly, the creation of the French business institute, Institute Européen d'Administration des Affaires (INSEAD), was developed by a group of French businessmen, in 1959, with the help of the Paris Chamber of Commerce and Industry.

The key difference in the organization and educational mission of the European MBA institutes may be that they are now considered the leaders in international graduate business education. The European MBA programs have maintained an international focus from the start. While Europeans historically have preferred on-the-job business training to academic business training, they adopted the MBA to address a specific need: to place European industry in a better position in the international market. In contrast, American MBAs were created as an upper-level business program within previously established university programs which possessed a focus on research and teaching. Thus, in American MBA programs, it can be assumed that international business would be just one of many areas of research and teaching.[24] Schmotter acknowledges that the most evident difference is the institutional flexibility of the European MBA programs.[25] Since they are not affiliated with colleges and universities, there is no regulating body to enforce uniformity in practice, policies and standards. Thus, the Europeans have more freedom on course offerings and requirements, research areas, degrees and certificates granted, faculty hiring, and student administrative procedures. As private institutions, the European programs are free to create an international flavor by imposing language requirements and attracting a diverse faculty and student body, rather than by developing new courses and PhD programs. Students and faculty of such diverse backgrounds create an atmosphere where international business is not a separate subject as in American schools but, instead, is integrated throughout the curriculum.[26]

Some American business schools have begun to adopt such approaches. Recently, the Harvard Business School has increased its international case studies and increased its population of foreign students to 25% representing 50 nations. The University of Maryland requires its professors to focus 50% of the core course material on international case studies. Columbia University has revised its curriculum to develop more international case studies and is altering its hiring practices to recruit faculty with international expertise. The University of Pittsburgh has sent a number of its professors to Eastern Europe to teach and learn in the hope of internationalizing enough faculty to abolish its five-year-old course in international business in favor of an integration of global issues throughout the entire curriculum.[27] Finally, a number of schools have made a semester or an internship abroad with an accompanying language requirement an option, or even a requirement, for graduation.[28]

Additionally, there is another essential difference in the institutional missions between European and American MBA programs. The mission of the American educational institutions is to grant degrees to full-time students. The European institutes, without universities and lacking the large endowments and the taxpayer base of their American counterparts, must focus on executive education so often to produce revenue. For most American universities, continuing executive education is often an afterthought predicated mainly as a revenue-producer and not the main focus of the institution.[29]

In the United States business community, the post-World War II era marked a period of slow change from a predominantly domestic orientation to one of increasing awareness and need of business opportunities abroad. Rather than making deliberate efforts to compete on a global scale, American companies had long been satisfied by creating goods for a solely American market, and considered it a windfall if people overseas happened to want to purchase such products.[30] Faced with the immediate necessity of rebuilding its industrial infrastructure after World War II, and encumbered by the smaller geographic areas of their native markets, European industries were forced to seek larger non-native markets for their goods. Thus, to compete and prosper, Europeans have found it necessary to be sensitive to native cultures when doing business outside of their homelands.

Since Europe is filled with geographic and cultural diversity, preparing students to compete in the European market would demand focusing on such topics as the special need of managing a multinational enterprise, as well as overcoming cultural and language barriers which might otherwise hinder business progress. Thus, European business institute officials argue that international business education must be a requirement, rather than the elective status given to it by American faculty.[31] This belief is emerging in American MBA programs, as the American business community increasingly seeks graduates who possess a global perspective so necessary in a more competitive, rapidly changing business environment.[32]

Now, through changes in economic and political policies as well as communications technology, all companies are competing globally. Not only are multinational companies developing to actively pursue markets beyond the boundaries of the United States, but even companies which compete solely on a domestic basis also are forced to become more aware of global business if they hope to be able to compete with foreign companies which are moving into American markets. As a result of these developments, many companies are giving new emphasis and priority to hiring employees with an international perspective. Gerber suggests that "a 'global manager' is someone with a strong interest in and tolerance for other cultures and who understands how a particular decision might affect a company's many markets or competitors around the world."[33] As Gerber notes, the difficulty arises not in how to define this highly sought-after global business person, but in how to develop a manager with the international capabilities necessary to compete in the changing business worlds.

Currently, debate and experimentation are occurring as academia attempts to reassess its mission in light of complaints from corporate recruiters that the knowledge of its graduates is too theoretical and lacks 'real-world' perspective and global-mindedness.[34] To address the apparent lack of understanding of critical skills necessary in the changing global workplace, innovative business schools such as Wharton and Babson are placing a greater emphasis on internships and work experience while also teaching in modules which bring real world problems into the classroom.[35] Furthermore, since most activity in the workplace is not restricted to one area of business, but overlaps many areas and markets, team-teaching by faculty from different specializations within the business schools is seen as a more realistic preparation for graduation.[36]

Executive Training Programs

As previously noted, executive training is a staple of the European business programs. In America it has developed into a business school revenue-producer and a means for practitioners to stay abreast of changes in their fields. This is particularly true in the area of international business. Many American practitioners were educated at a time when little or no emphasis was placed on global management. Thus, many practitioners are turning to executive training and development to fill in the gaps. These programs are offered in a variety of formats, such as through specialized training programs offered by employers and institutes operating independently or in conjunction with one or more business school program.

The focus of the executive training programs is a statement of the educational needs existing in the business world. Globalization is the most current topic. The training varies from generalized programs, such as "Managing for International Competitiveness" sponsored by the Western Business School, at the University of Western Ontario, and "Strategic Issues Confronting the Global Firm in the 1990s" at the Graduate School of International Relations and Pacific Studies at the University of California at San Diego, to those with a very specific purpose such as "Communicating with the Japanese Business World" sponsored by the J.L. Kellogg Graduate School of Management at Northwestern University, and the "Human Resource Management in Asia" at INSEAD.[37] To put the dimensions of this internationalization process into perspective, the following chart is presented to demonstrate the nature of the course offerings at these international executive training programs:

**Table 1—Common Course Offerings at International
Executive Training Programs**[38]

• Pacific Rim Negotiation Practices	•Steering Change and Managing People
• Pacific Rim Business Etiquette	•Global Organization and Leadership
• The Effect of Various World Cultures	•Global Corporate and Business-Unit Strategy
•The Changing Global Environment	•Global Demographic Trends
•The Global Economic Environment	•Anatomy of a Cross-Cultural Problem
•The Global Political Environment	•Incorporating Diversity in the Workplace
•Government -Business Relations	•World Views and Managerial Functions
•Hidden Pictures of Prejudice and Discrimination	•Managing Across Boundaries
•International Joint Ventures Risks and Rewards	•The Experience of Being in a Different Culture
•International Marketing Strategy	•Product Development in the Global Firm
•Analytical Framework of International Relations	•International Finance Strategy
•International Organization Strategy	•Evaluation of International Competition
•Cross-Cultural Management: Challenges and Opportunities	•Corporate Structure and Culture
•Cultural Values and Attitude toward Work and Achievement	

It is evident that the direction or intent of many of these offerings is efforts to respond to the more immediate needs of practitioners immersed in a rapidly changing business world. In many cases these courses reflect extensions or modifications of traditional functional areas commonly offered in MBA programs. Using these management models as a comparative standard, it is the intent of this study to examine graduate programs and executive training in sport management to determine the potential for a similar paradigm shift toward a more international perspective.

Sport Management Graduate Programs

In just over a decade, the number of graduate programs in sport management has quadrupled. In 1978, there were 20 programs offering graduate degrees in sport management.[39] Currently there are more than eighty such programs in

North America.[40] Historically, sport management programs have grown out of physical education programs which evolved to meet changes in student interest and demands of the market for graduates with business training to operate sport organizations.[41]

Sport management programs are, however, still in evolutionary stages. Many stumbling blocks exist in the development of sport management as an academic pursuit. For instance, a lack of uniformity in curricula and career development, as well as a need for accreditation, are present. Review, refinement, and consolidation of curricula and programs in sport management with other disciplines on campus are still occurring for under its umbrella varied specializations within sport-related fields sit. Due to inconsistencies and the broad labeling of programs, the title sport management does not accurately indicate a uniform offering within the field.[42] One may assume that much of the disarray exists because sport management has grown out of various disciplines. While the majority of programs have grown out of physical education (and recreation),[43] others have evolved from business, health, and human performance. Thus, curricula and career development may differ by department and may not always maintain a sport business focus. For instance, in a review of sport management curricula one may often find a greater number of foundation and activity courses in physical education and recreation than sport business courses. Likewise, business courses in sport management programs housed in the business schools may be offered without attention or focus on the unique nature of sport. In terms of career specializations beyond the business scope, one may also find specialization in coaching, athletic training, exercise physiology, and cardiovascular rehabilitation.[44] On the other hand, academic majors in "Facility Management," "Corporate Fitness," or "Health Promotion and Recreation" may be housed in other departments while possessing curricula which would appear acceptable as part of a sport management program. Therefore, an initial hurdle in the development of sport management as an accepted, accredited academic program is the full transition from its predecessor programs into a more business-oriented program without the loss of the sport experience.

While the management of sport dates back to ancient times, it is a relatively new and continually evolving academic subject. Over the past two decades there have been significant changes in the sport management curriculum. For example, the 1971 curriculum of the nation's second graduate program, implemented at the University of Massachusetts at Amherst, included a foundation of physical education courses: history, philosophy, psychology, and sociology of sport, as well as an internship. Today, the curriculum has evolved to better represent the business side of sport as all required and elective courses are presented from a management perspective and foundation. Throughout the evolution of this particular program, one constant has remained: the emphasis on the application of classroom learning to the workplace through the requirement of an internship as a capstone experience. Exceptions to the required internship are granted to students who opt to write a master's thesis. Often, this choice is made because a particular student is planning on pursuing doctoral work. Even in such a case, unless a student has extensive work experience, it will be strongly recommended for a student to complete both an internship and a thesis. Due to the competitive nature of the sport industry, an internship offers a critical dimension and perspective which further distinguish graduates from others entering or reentering the job market without such an experience. Table 2 provides a capsule of the UMass master's curriculum as it presently exists:

Table 2—University of Massachusetts Master's Curriculum

REQUIRED COURSES	ELECTIVE COURSES
•Sports Marketing	•Sport Business and Finance
•Sport and the Law	•The Athletic Director
•The Sport Enterprise	•Labor Relations in Sport
•Sport Management Policy	•Television Sports: A Business
•Managerial Accounting in Sport	Analysis
•Computer Applications in Sport	•Event Management
•Internship or Thesis	•Facility Management

The following courses are offered on a tutorial basis only:

•Historical Foundations of Sport	•Social Psychology of Sport
•History of Sport in the United States	•Athletics: A Philosophic Inquiry

This model is being presented only as an example of a program which has gone through a number of stages of evolution experienced by other programs of a similar age and size. It is also important to note that despite the recognition by faculty of the need for a shift to a more international curriculum, the UMass program only offers a single upper level undergraduate course in international sport management at this time. Serious discussion is currently taking place among faculty with respect to adding an international sport management course as a graduate elective in the near future.

Better defining the scope of the academic subject area is also a necessity. As Parkhouse notes, the term "management" can be misleading.[45] Taken in the business school context, it exists as one area of study, limited to subject matter which focuses on the planning, organizing, directing, and controlling functions of business. In the context of sport management, however, the term is more broadly construed to include all areas of business, economics, and law as they apply to the operation of a sports organization. If one adapts these areas of study to the sport industry, then it is logical to also adapt international business perspectives. As most sport entities move toward, or are already operating at, some level of significance in the global arena, a parallel trend must exist with respect to the development of graduate courses or career specialization in international sport management to help serve this shift in the industry. This is reinforced by the sport management curricular evaluation and needs assessment study conducted by DeSensi, Kelley, Blanton and Beitel. It is interesting to note that there was a lack of any direct reference to international sport as a relevant sport management category in their assessment. Further review of their study revealed no mention of an international perspective or course as based on their analysis of the typical courses offered in sport management programs.[46] It is obvious that curricular review and assessment over what the core requirements of this field are/or should be is currently undergoing serious debate. The process of infusing an international perspective and/or focus into these existing and evolving curricula is at best a problematic enterprise at this time within the field of sport management.

II. Executive Training Programs in Sport Management

A couple of factors are contributing to the growing popularity of executive training in sport management. First, due to the relatively recent acceptance and growth of sport management as an academic pursuit, many of the field's practitioners do not hold degrees in the area. Second, due to the competitive nature of the business and scarcity of positions in the field, those who hold positions seem reluctant and perhaps unable to take a year or more off to pursue a graduate degree.

One of the foremost executive training programs is The Sports Management Institute Executive Program sponsored by the athletic departments and business schools of the Universities of Southern California, Notre Dame, and North Carolina. The program is a seven-month course, which includes three weeks in-residence, and was developed to satisfy the needs of mid- and upper-level managers in collegiate and professional sports. The three-week in-residence course curriculum presented in Table 3 is rooted in seven functional areas and predicated on the MBA model. Note, once more, the curriculum is void of international focus:

**Table 3—Curriculum Outline of the Executive Training Program
of the Sports Management Institute**

•Marketing	•Managing Human Resources
•Managing Financial Resources	•Behaving Legally and Ethically
•Managing Physical Resources	•Managing Information Resources
	•Managing Strategically

As sport management is still in its transitionary stage of development, formal executive training programs are few and many of the conferences are billed as continuing education opportunities. In considering one such conference, the International Conference on Sports Business, offered for the third time this year, it is interesting to again note the very limited emphasis on international sport management. Billed as an international conference, it has at most 12 of its 74 presentations and discussions dealing with issues which transcend national boundaries. While conferences focusing on international sport and conferences on international business exist, there is not one which is truly devoted to the international business issues present on global sport. The curricular offerings relative to international sport management presented at the 1992 Conference of the North American Society of Sport Management (NASSM), while being high-lighted as a key area in the conference program, cannot be said to have occurred in any significance among over 40 presentations and poster sessions listed. Likewise, the number of sessions dealing with sport management issues at "Sport in the Global Village," the 8th Biennial Conference of the International Society for Comparative Physical Education and Sport, represented less than 5% of the listed conference offerings.

Recommendations

Conferences in the late 1950s provided the impetus for systemic change for business school education's possession of an international dimension.[47] An international movement within the business field has been influenced by the establishment of international business institutes and executive training programs. Since international sport management issues are now beginning to be discussed at conferences, and among educators and practitioners in the sports management field, a similar route may be pursued by the sport management profession. Assuming the conferences serve as forums for current issues facing the field, the very titles "Sport in the Global Village: Comparative Perspectives" and "The International Sport Business Conference" indicate that international sport is a topic receiving greater attention by those in the profession.

Considering also that the evolutionary process of educating for globalization within business schools has occurred over the past 30 years and is still not complete, it seems that the discussion for those educators in sport management ought to begin by drawing upon research conducted by those in business. In simplistic terms, international business education has followed an evolution which began with the inclusion of a broad and general elective course, moved into more specialized forms of required courses, such as international finance, moved to include language requirements and international internship experiences, and is now moving toward a full integration of international issues into every course in the curriculum.[48] It is likely that integration of international business in sport management education will follow a similar road, and therefore there is no need for sport management, as a business-related discipline, to reinvent the wheel.

Due to its youth, sport management education is facing additional problems of status, accreditation, consistency, and agreement as to curricular and career development. Further, there are few programs in sport management located outside of the United States and Canada. These were not issues facing business when it began developing an international dimension. Thus, without substantial research conducted as to the curricular needs of a systematic movement toward international sport management training, sport management programs may be climbing an even longer ladder than that of business education.

It is expected that this preliminary study will confirm that little research or implementation exists for curricular development in a global sports market. Valuable, yet unsubstantiated work is occurring daily in the field as practitioners move toward globalization. The sport management profession has a duty to act on this area of research if students, practitioners and educators are to successfully move to globalization . Time and energy must be devoted to research and to the implementation of programs to better develop the global sport manager.

Appendix I[49]

Pilot Study: Findings and Implications
The pilot survey instrument consisted of 99 questions divided into three parts: I) training/competencies considered essential for a professional involved in international sport management, II) information about the career, education, and training of the survey respondent who is involved in international sport management, and III) an organization profile of the international sports organization with which the respondent is associated. The following is a brief description of the subsections of Section I:

Sub-section I: General Educational Background Included questions related to level and type of degree earned (Questions #1-6).

Sub-section II: Educational Coursework and/or Special Training
Included questions related to the desired type of coursework and/or special training which might be relevant for a professional involved in international sport (Questions #7-19).

Sub-section III: Cultural/Language Background
Included questions related to the desired cultural and language background which might be relevant for a professional involved in international sport (Questions #20-33).

Sub-section IV: Sports Background
Included general questions related to the desired sports background relevant for a professional involved in international sport (Questions #20-33).

Sub-section V: Management/Work Background
Included general questions related to the desired management and work background relevant for a professional involved in international sport (Questions #41-56).

This pilot survey was tested prior to the "Sport in the Global Village" conference in Houston. The pilot survey was targeted to 35 practitioners (alumni and associates of the Sport Management Program at the University of Massachusetts) who are currently managing or were recently affiliated with international sports organizations. The profile of the 12 respondents included seven from the U.S.A. and one each from Canada, Australia, Belgium, Holland, and Japan. This group consisted of respondents holding positions ranging from assistant director to CEO.

Due to the small sample size (N=12), application of advanced statistical techniques to the data was deemed inappropriate. Therefore, the analysis phase was limited to a preliminary assessment of the means and standard deviations. Using this approach, two general questions (Questions 70 & 71) which addressed the perceived needs of the field appear to provide interpretable results. These questions were constructed with a basic bi-polar response option (yes or no) and revealed fairly consistent positive agreement among respondents. In Question #70, 88% of the respondents agreed that there is a need for colleges/university programs in sport management to offer a focus or concentrations in international sport. The responses to question #71, regarding perceived need for development of executive and middle management training programs in the area of international sport management for current practitioners, also showed a high level of agreement (75%). These results were further supported by 12 additional respondents who returned an abbreviated version of the instrument distributed at the "Sport in the Global Village" conference. These respondents typically represented academic institutions and were attendees at the conference at which this study was presented. Despite the small size, these preliminary findings seem to indicate there is an agreement regarding the need for the field of sport management to provide an increased cross-cultural focus during professional preparation and training of practitioners.

A more in-depth examination of the specifics of such a need was addressed by way of Part I of the survey. Unfortunately, the size of the sample greatly limited the ability to draw meaningful conclusions regarding questions which utilized the Likert scale format. Arbitrary cutoff points of ≥ 5.5 or ≤ 3.5 were used to determine which questions warranted further investigation. Only 10 out of a possible 59 questions qualified using these criteria:

When hiring a new staff member involved in a management position, how essential would it be for him/her to have:

		Mean	St. Dev.
#1	a bachelor's degree?	6.545	0.687
#5	a specific degree in the task are for which they are being hired?	6.000	0.894
#6	relevant work experience for the position for which they are being hired?	6.091	0.831
#20	relatives still living in another culture?	2.100	1.197
#21	a strong personal or family relationship to another culture (i.e., immigrant, marriage, etc.)?	2.400	1.71
#38	competed in and/or coached a sport at a national level?	3.200	1.814
#39	competed in and/or coached a sport at an international level?	2.800	2.044
#40.	competed in and/or coached a sport at the professional level?	3.500	2.506
#41.	demonstrated management experience?	5.900	1.370
#55.	held a financial position in a national or international business?	3.273	1.679

$$M \geq 5.5 \text{ or} \leq 3.5$$

While the responses to these questions were deemed significant using our cut-off points, the high standard deviations (Questions 21, 38, 39, 40, 41, 55) placed any interpretation of these results under suspicion. While these high standard deviations would appear to indicate a strong lack of agreement among respondents, another factor could have skewed these results. Specifically, the use of the term "essential" in the Likert scale might have led to interpretations by respondents not intended by the authors. It is likely that the inclusion of the word "essential" forced respondents to make absolute judgments as to the need for international sport managers to have specific qualifications. In contrast, use of the terms "helpful" or "important" would elicit responses related to the relative degree of appropriateness of certain qualifications. This change would facilitate a better discrimination of preference by the respondent, as well as improving consistency across the different subsections of questions in Part I.

While the small sample size of this pre-test precludes the statistical testing of hypotheses, it should be noted that eight specific hypotheses have been developed for testing during the primary phase of this research. These hypotheses are intended to create a basis from which to discuss the implications for training and professional preparations of sport managers. It is expected that significant differences will occur based upon eight primary independent variables:

V 1: The national origin of the respondent.
V 2: The type and level of the academic background of the respondent.
V 3: The type and level of the sport background of the respondent.
V 4: The type and level of the language background of the respondent.
V 5: The type and level of the management background of the respondent.
V 6: The nature and type of organization which the respondent works for.
V 7: The number of continents in which the respondent's organization conducts business.
V 8: The size of multinational staff of the respondent's organization.

Notes

[1]Parkhouse, B.L., & D.O. Ulrich. "Sport management as a potential cross-discipline: A paradigm for theoretical development, scientific inquiry, and professional application." *Quest*. 31: 2, pp. 264-276.

[2]Parkhouse & Ulrich. Global examples, using the Parkhouse and Ulrich model (1979), include:

• Commercial industry, including sporting goods, leisure and fitness, involve the import and export of goods and services as well as international resorts.

- Professional teams are competing internationally; for example, the World League of American Football operates across two continents, the Australian Baseball League, a minor league operated by America's Major League Baseball, and the National Football League and the National Baseball Association both hold exhibitions abroad.

- Amateur sports organizations, such as national governing bodies for Olympic sports, compete internationally as big business.

- College and high school teams are beginning to hold exhibitions abroad, as well as to sponsor cultural exchange games/sporting events.

- Many arena/stadium management companies are involved in multinational enterprises.

- Marketing, merchandising, promotions, and the broadcast media have moved into an international market with the advances in communications technology, reaching and building larger markets creating a broader fan-base.

[3]Zanger, B.K., & J.B. Parks (Eds), *Sport management curricula: The business and education nexus.* Bowling Green State University, School of Health, Physical Education, Recreation, 1984, pp. 97-109; Mullin, B.J. "A graduate curriculum in sport management: Considerations before taking the plunge," In Zanger & Parks, pp. 110-113; Parks, J.B., & R.J. Quain. "Sport management survey: Curriculum perspective," *Journal of physical education, recreation, and dance.* pp. 22-26; Hardy, S. "Graduate curriculum in sport management: The need for a business orientation," *Quest,* 39, pp. 207-216; DeSensi, J.T., D.R. Kelley, M.D. Blanton, & P.A. Beitel. "Sport management curricular evaluation and needs assessment: A multifaceted approach," *Journal of sport management,* 4, pp. 31-58; Fielding, L.W., B.G. Pitts & L.K. Miller. "Defining quality: Should educators in sport management programs be concerned about accreditation," *Journal of sport management,* 5, pp. 1-17.; Lipsey, R.A. (Ed.) "College and university programs in sport management," *Sports marketplace 1992.* Princeton, NJ: Sportsguide, 1992, pp. 537-46.
[4]Hardy, pp. 207-216.
[5]Otteson, S. F. (Ed.). *Internationalizing the traditional business curricula.* Bloomington: Indiana University, 1968, pp. 89-98.
[6]Otteson.
[7]Hall, E.T. (Ed.) *International business classics.* Lexington, MA: Lexington Books, 1988., pp. 89-102; Lee, J.A. (Ed.) *International business classics.* Lexington, MA: Lexington Books, 1988., pp. 89-102; Wadia, M.S. (Ed.)

International business classics. Lexington, Ma. Lexington Books, 1988., pp. 79-97; Otteson, ; Kolde (Ed.). *Environment of international business.* Boston: Kent Publishing Co., 1985, pp. 416-429; Albaum, G., J. Strandskov, E. Duerr, & L. Dowd. (Eds.) *International marketing and sport management.* New York: Addison-Wesley Publishing Co., 1989, p. 62.

[8]Hall; Lee; Kolde; Ferguson, J., *Tomorrow's global executive.* 1988, pp. 204-225; Moran, R.T. (Ed.). *Global business management in the 90's.* New York: Beachum Press, 1990, pp. 17-23.

[9]Kolde; Gregor, A. "Southern California job market; surviving in the '90s: languages can translate into global mobility: The international business world needs multilingual workers. Universities, specialty school, and companies offer solutions," *Los Angeles Times.* September. 25, 1990, p. 12; Child, C. "Business colleges become more international," *Crain's Detroit business.* 7: 18 (May 6, 1991), p. 10; Updyke, T. "Spirit of the MBA corps: students trained to serve in Eastern Europe, " *Atlanta Journal and Constitution.* 1: (July 30, 1991); P. "Monterey Institute makes language fluency a key part of its international curriculum: Many required courses given in foreign tongues," *Chronicle of Higher Education.* (July 1, 1992), pp. A33-34.

[10]Otteson; Albaum, Straudskov, Duerr, & Dowd.

[11]Gregor; Child; and Updyke.

[12]Mullin; Parkhouse; Zanger; Parks & Quain; Hardy; DeSensi, Kelly, Blanton, & Beitel; Fielding, Pitts, & Miller.

[13]Parkhouse & Ulrich.

[14]Parkhouse & Ulrich; Parkhouse, B.L., Ulrich, D.O., & D. Soucie. "Research in sport management: A vital rung of this new corporate ladder," *Quest,* 34: 2 (1982) pp. 176-186.

[15]Mullin; Parkhouse & Ulrich; Zanger; Parks & Quain; Hardy; DeSensi, Kelly, Blanton, & Beitel; Fielding, Pitts, & Miller.

[16]Fielding, Pitts, & Miller.

[17]Thoma, J. "Sport management education: Who is doing what and what are they doing? Paper presented at "Sport in the Global Village: Comparative Perspectives," The Eighth Biennial Conference of the International Society for Comparative Physical Education and Sport, Houston, June 1992.

[18]Bradsher, K. "The Pacific: Looking west for an MBA: Japan, whose management techniques have long been touted, enlists Dartmouth professors to teach business program," *Los Angeles Times*, 3 (May 16, 1988); Otteson.

[19]Bradsher.

[20]Bradsher.

[21]Bradsher; Schmotter, J.W. "Business education's cross-Atlantic currents," *Wall Street Journal.* (October 9, 1989), p. A12; Greenhouse, S. "Americans discover international business schools in Europe," *Chicago Tribune,* (July 7, 1991), p. 7A.

[22]Bradsher.

[23]Schmotter.

[24]Schmotter.

[25]Schmotter.

[26]Greenhouse.

[27]Deutsch, C.H. "Global issues in every classroom.," *The New York Times.* (August 25, 1991), p. F25.

[28]Patillo, D. M. "A cooperative approach to international business training," *Business America.* (March 31, 1986), p. 1; Gregory; Byrne, J.A. "Wharton rewrites the book on b-schools," *Business Week* . 43 (May 13, 1991); Child; Opdyke; Hemp, P. "Remaking the MBA: Babson College curriculum may become business school prototype," *Boston Globe.* 33 (August 23, 1992), p. 39.

[29]Schmotter.

[30]Gerber.

[31]Greenhouse.

[32]Hemp.

[33]Gerber, p. 32.

[34]Byrne; Deutsch; and Hemp.

[35]Byrne; and Hemp.

[36]Hemp.

[37]*Peterson's Guides. Bricker's international directory 1992*; Volume 1. Princeton, NJ: *Peterson's guides*, 1991. (4th Ed.) pp. 48, 167, 179, 187-88, 201, 422.

[38]*Bricker's international dictionary* 1992, Volumes 1 & 2, 23rd Edition, *Peterson's Guides,* 1991.

[39]Parkhouse & Ulrich.

[40]Lipsey.

[41]Kjeldsen, E.K.M. "Sport management: An emerging profession," *Arena review.* 4 (1980) p. i; Mullin; Parkhouse & Ulrich; Parks & Quain.

[42]Parkhouse.

[43]Kjedson; Mullin; Parkhouse & Ulrich; Parks & Quain.

[44]Lipsey.

[45]Parkhouse & Ulrich.

[46]DeSensi, Kelly, Blanton & Beitel.

[47]Otteson.

[48]Bradsher; Schmotter; Gregor; Byrne; Child; Deutsch; Greenhouse; Hemp.

[49]Special thanks to Mark McDonald, Lecturer, Sport Management Program, Department of Sport Studies, University of Massachusetts at Amherst, for editorial assistance with Appendix I.

Chapter 5

Of Fungos and Fumbles: Explaining the Cultural Uniqueness of American Sport, or A Paradoxical Peek at Sport: American Style

Ralph C. Wilcox

This chapter seeks to uncover the unique elements of sport in the United States of America and to explain its appearance in terms of the nation's dominant system of cultural values. Unlike so many before, it is *not* the intent of this author to build a case around the frequently oversimplified "sport as a mirror of society" or "agent of social change" frameworks, neither is an attempt made at pursuing solely politico-economic explanations for the nature and function of American sport, nor to test a variety of historical theses concerned with the process of modernization. Rather, this chapter will place sport against the broader, sometimes contradictory, backdrop of American culture.

With regard to the importance of this study, it is quite clear that America has redefined the meaning of sport in the post-industrial world. Moreover, the identification and explanation of the unique elements of American sport has been inadequately addressed by American scholars who, for the most part, have taken them for granted. One exception is George Sage's brilliantly perceptive *Power and Ideology in American Sport. A Critical Perspective,*[1] which is the first book to begin to penetrate the undulating shell of American culture as it provides a deeper understanding of the creation and metamorphosis of American sport.[2] As the world moves ever closer to the reality of a global village and the terms "new world order," "cultural homogenization," and "westernization" find increasing usage in the vocabularies of more and more nations, the potential export of Americanization (that being the nation's dominant value system) through sport needs to be better understood.[3] With the potential for a growing stream of zealous converts to American sport, caution must remain the watchword. Further, this chapter will respond to the culturally naive and often vacuous criticism targeted at American sport around the world today.

No one in contemporary American society is untouched by sport. From the metaphorical "doublespeak" of sport so apparent in both American politics and the colloquial tongue,[4] to the print and broadcast media blitz of the ballfield, the immortalization of sporting legends in Hollywood's celluloid "halls of fame," regular sporting celebrations hosted in the rose garden of the White House by the nation's president, the "little league" rites of passage for young American boys, and the flood of sports consumer products (ranging from "Baby Ruth" confectionery to "Major League Fantasy" vacations), the centrality and significance of sport to American culture is abundantly clear. Necessarily, however, the focus of this chapter will rest primarily with elite sport for there exists no organized equivalent of egalitarian "Sport for All" programs as may be found elsewhere in the world. Because American culture is no easy phenomenon to comprehend it follows that any attempt to appreciate the meaning of sport should neither be taken too lightly nor too superficially. The complex politico-economic paradox inherent in American sport has, perhaps, been no better demonstrated in recent months than by the actions of the United States government which, after granting "favored nation" status to the People's Republic of China for trade purposes, was instrumental in defeating Beijing's bid to host the Olympic games in the year 2000 as the Congress publicly voiced its abhorrence of China's record of ongoing human rights abuses. Throughout the remaining pages of this chapter, sport will be examined in the context of the following predominant cultural contradictions, value relations that, while appearing in opposition to one another are, in reality, central to American culture:

Nationalism	—	Globalism
Democracy	—	Capitalism
Egalitarianism	—	Elitism
Individualism	—	Bureaucratization
Tradition	—	Innovation
Rationalism	—	Emotion

In effect, American sport is examined here in the context of cultural symbolism. Finally, while comparisons with other national and cultural systems of sport are not drawn explicitly, clearly for one who has lived, studied, competed, and generally imbibed a wholesome dose of sport in several countries, implicit comparison is inevitable. Indeed, were it not for the author's growing appreciation of sport in a variety of national settings, the identification and explanation of the cultural uniqueness of American sport would not be possible.

The World League and the World Series: Cultural Imperialism and National Insularity in American Sport

The United States is a nation barely emerging from infancy wherein its identity is weak and veiled in a shroud of uncertainty. A nation wherein five-year-olds find themselves unknowingly coerced into the daily ritual of pledging their allegiance to the flag, where participants and spectators alike, across all levels of sport, raise their eyes to the "stars and the stripes" and their voices to the national anthem, in what has become a familiar, albeit monotonous, nationalistic celebration. Ever searching for a national game to call its own, and all too willing to proclaim "World Champions" in domestically contested sports, patriotism remains an all powerful element throughout American sport. Sporting spectacles have become favorite scenarios for paramilitary displays, and have attracted armed services sponsorship of television sports coverage.

It is the National Football League's (NFL) Super Bowl which leads all contenders for America's leading single sport event. In considering its unifying purpose Mike Weisman, Executive Producer of NBC sports, described the Super Bowl as an undeclared "national holiday" and went on to say:

> ... more people come together to watch a Super Bowl than for any other event. The World Series is not just one game, New Year's Eve takes place at different times in different time zones and Presidential elections just don't compare. I wouldn't get into what that says about this country but it's a fact that we are really a united nation on this day.

Yet the world is changing and so is American sport. While baseball, basketball and volleyball have long been used as tools of American imperialism, football's more recent venture onto the world scene has been culturally revealing. Starting in Tokyo in 1975, and traveling to Mexico City (1978), and later London (1983), the

NFL eventually debuted its World League of American Football (WLAF) three years ago with franchise teams in Canada, England, Germany, Spain and the United States. Despite global expansion plans for the future, its relatively slow success (coupled with the NFL's own domestic crises), has resulted in the temporary suspension of League operations for the 1993 season. With the American Broadcasting Corporation (ABC) reportedly losing half of its $10 million contract to televise games during the 1992 season, serious questions regarding the future of this international sport initiative remain. Cross-cultural intolerance (not unlike that leveled at the opening of EuroDisney on the outskirts of Paris in 1992), combined with the desperate need for "marquee" players with whom the world might identify, has left the once novel sport of American football a global orphan. Sharing a similar experience has been the story of professional soccer in America. Although the United States will be the site of the 1994 World Cup, the fully fledged sport of Association Football has had a mottled history in America. Yet, emerging out of this nation's reluctance to embrace alien values characterized by the demise of the professional North American Soccer League (NASL in 1985), the Major Indoor Soccer League (later the MSL) appeared to satisfy the unique cultural needs of the nation's sports consumer through a bastardized version of the sport described by one British observer as "A zippy, splashy organized riot of sport... An extravaganza that would make P.T. Barnum envious."[5] With plans to expand into Europe in 1993 the old adage of "exporting coal to Newcastle" or "sand to Saudi Arabia" rang true as Graham Walker, MISL consultant for international expansion, confidently stated, "This is the McDonald's of Soccer... The English will take to it like American fast food."[6]

Out of the Cotton Fields and into the Football Fields: Opportunity and Exploitation in American Sport

This section could equally have been titled "The parable of the cheerleader, the dumb jock, and the shuffleboard player," for while democracy remains the most proudly proclaimed ideal it is also the most deeply entrenched myth in American culture. Indeed, the observation that contemporary American culture is emblematic of "Liberty's gift—Liberty's legacy" remains one for the ideologues, at least in sport. One need not excavate too deeply beneath the crust of American sport to uncover widespread inequities born of age, race, gender, and socioeconomic means. Whether as participant or consumer, most would concede that access to sport has widened over the years although such opportunity is not balanced nor are status and power proportionately shared among groups.

Indeed, this most patriarchal of cultures continues to restrict access and opportunity to women despite legislative change, the efforts of health promoters and the media, as well as the frequently unheralded accomplishments of America's sportswomen. While many socially constructed, physiological myths pertaining to women's athletic performance have been broken down there remains in America, a generally pervasive, condescending attitude toward women. Reinforced by *Sports Illustrated*, the nation's highest circulating multi-sport magazine, and other media outlets which frequently portray women as passive, sex symbols scantily clad in skintight Spandex, any serious coverage of the sportswoman is left to those activities determined by men to be gender appropriate for women most notably gymnastics, figure skating, diving and swimming, tennis, and volleyball, sports which share a distinct collective character.[7] This reality was reinforced in a recent national survey in which former gymnast Mary Lou Retton (a medalist in the 1984 Olympic games), and figure skater Dorothy Hamill (a medalist in the 1976 Olympic games), beat out the likes of Michael Jordan (basketball), Joe Montana (American football), Nolan Ryan (baseball), Wayne Gretzky (ice hockey), Arnold Palmer (golf), and Martina Navratilova (tennis) as the most popular sports figures in America today.[8] Even Linda Kohl seemingly succumbed to the dictates of male America when, excited at the new found acceptance of the American sportswoman she wrote, "Thanks to 'Flo Jo,' it has become socially acceptable for women to perspire in public. She has made us realize that women can be strong and sultry at the same time."[9]

American sport has long been held a sacred bastion of masculinity wherein western machismo has been readily promoted along with the seeming requisite denigration of women and homosexuality. Once considered to be safely preserved in a heterosexual environment where sportsmen dress, fraternize, shower, travel, and sleep in the same room, such fundamental values have recently been threatened by the increasing athletic success of gay men and lesbians in American sport. It is interesting to note that while stereotypical images of lesbians competing in sports traditionally identified as non-gender appropriate have been readily perpetuated throughout America, male athletes who find success in certain sports have been faced with similar labels. This is particularly evident in male figure skating where the recently publicized incidence of Human Immunodeficiency Virus (known to be high among gay male populations) leading to AIDS was treated very differently from more celebrated cases in the sports of baseball, basketball and American football.[10] In a nation that continues to struggle with a deeply entrenched sense of homophobia, made evident by the ongoing domestic debate on gays in the military, it appears that gay male and lesbian athletes have generally chosen to conceal their sexual orientation in favor of retaining social approval and commercial sponsorship. While it seems reasonable to assume that the proportional representation of gay men and lesbians in sport is little or no different from that of the larger society, this group remains one of the least talked about yet most discriminated against in American sport.[11]

Potentially one of America's greatest strengths, yet also the cause of repeated social dislocation is the diverse heterogeneity of the population based upon the variables of race, ethnicity, national origin, and religious affiliation. Conflict with indigenous peoples continues to grow in the sporting arena as, showing little sensitivity to the promulgation of native American stereotypes, professional and collegiate sports teams readily adopt such nicknames as Braves, Chiefs, Redmen, Savages, and Warriors replete with mascots, logos, and symbolic gestures. Indeed where else in the global sports arena could one partake of elite athletic competition between Redskins and Cowboys, or the Spartans and the Trojans? This is, in many respects, sport made for Hollywood and only that institution has done more to perpetuate the negative perception of native Americans.[12]

Since the settling of the New World by Europeans in the seventeenth century, the power base, status and influence in America has unmistakably remained with the white, Anglo-Saxon Protestant male. Today, with black Americans accounting for approximately 15% of the American population, their apparent overrepresentation in Major League Baseball (MLB—32% of the playing personnel), the National Football League (68%), and the National Basketball Association (NBA—77%) is tempered by their frequently low status in sport. "Stacking" remains a familiar problem in American sport. Position ascription on the basis of race, while undergoing some reform on the playing field remains deeply entrenched at the executive level of sports administration. The Rainbow Commission for Fairness in Athletics led by former Presidential candidate Jesse Jackson, together with the Center for the Study of Sport in Society at Northeastern University, have recently drawn attention to the fact that ethnic minorities account for only 17% of "front office" employees in MLB, 10% in the NFL, and 16% in the NBA. The story is little different among coaches, managers, referees and owners.[13] Furthermore, this pattern is replicated in the infrequent appearance of black Americans within the arenas of sport consumerism. Commonly referred to as "turnstile apartheid," black Americans account for 6.8% of MLB, 7.5% of NFL, and 17.0% of NBA fans.[14] In Major League Baseball, such 'hidden' racism reared its ugly head recently as Marge Schott, owner of baseball's first professional team the Cincinnati Reds, was sanctioned for referring to a former player as her "million dollar nigger." Suspended for one year, fined $25,000.00, and ordered to attend a multicultural training program Schott's behavior was characterized as including "...language that is racially and ethnically offensive [which] brought substantial disrepute and embarrassment to the game—and [was] not in the best interest of baseball."[15]

Nor is discrimination against athletes limited to gender, sexual orientation and race. Ownership of the athletes in both the collegiate and professional ranks remains a jaded reality in a nation that continues to struggle with its plantation heritage. Many universities readily exploit young men and women athletes under the pretense of providing them an education (for they are most surely not graduating at an acceptable rate), with the promise of collecting the recognition and riches that national sporting success brings. It appears that student-athletes from high school to college are increasingly being viewed as dispensable commodities. Nationwide reforms have been slow in coming. It is quite common to hear stories of children held back in school and "red shirted"[16] in order that they may mature physically and thus compete with chronologically younger athletes. In 1984, led by businessman and recent Presidential candidate H. Ross Perot, House Bill 72, the so-called Educational Reform Act, was passed by the Texas State Legislature. Affectionately known as the "No Pass No Play" rule, it has become the blueprint for many other states, has survived numerous legal challenges and is generally considered to have been moderately effective in ensuring that high school sports team members (as well as other extracurricular participants) receive an education through offering some protection against the abuses of Texas high school athletics.

Similarly, at the college level, an overemphasis on athletic excellence driven by simply outrageous monetary rewards has resulted in scandalous levels of academic performance by student athletes. With excessive hours spent at practice and "on the road," student-athletes are provided little encouragement to study. For example, in the autumn of 1987, the California State University at Fullerton football team logged 18,238 air miles while playing in all five American time zones from Florida to Hawaii.[17] The most recent statistics show that while 43% of male basketball players earned their degree within six years, and seven top-flight men's basketball programs (including the private universities, Duke, Northwestern and Villanova) saw 100% of their players graduate within six years, 15 other Division 1 programs (including such public universities as Alabama, Houston, Long Beach State, and Massachusetts) failed to graduate any of their players within the same period. The story is little different in the case of American football as the University of Notre Dame (86%), Duke University (84%), and Boston College (83%) topped the list, and the University of Houston (11%) and Long Beach State University (13%) fell to the bottom of the class! Complicated by such variables as race, gender, level of competition, degree pursued, and the uniqueness of the university culture the story, nevertheless, remains a sad one.[18] Today the call to share, in more equitable fashion, the multimillion-dollar fruits of victory with student athletes (the majority of whom are leaving universities with neither a degree nor a professional sports career) is being heard more loudly around American college campuses.[19] Fears that such action would compromise the amateur traditions of American collegiate sport appear unfounded in a capitalistic world in which thousands of young men and women are already receiving "Pay to Play" through the awarding of athletic scholarships. Central to this debate is a deep belief in the need for structure, discipline and retention of power *over* the athlete which necessarily mitigates against displays of individual freedom and improvisation both on and off the field.

The history of effective player associations, organizations and unions in American sport has been a poor one. Over the past decade, American professional sports have been wracked by ongoing labor disputes between owners and athletes resulting in nationwide strikes. Only recently has the NFL and its players' union agreed to the terms of a labor contract (after being without one for six years!) that provides players with improved benefits and will modify the terms of free agency.[20] Though limited by space, it is important to recognize that cultural stereotypes associated with age impact upon sport as athletic participation by the aged in America is frequently seen as a manifestation of eccentricity. Furthermore sports such as golf, sailing, skiing and equestrianism have maintained a particular exclusivity through the demand for discretionary income and time. Such sports remain the privilege of the upper socioeconomic strata of American society. Summarily therefore, in a nation that proudly claims to be the leader of the free and democratic world, tension born of demographic differences, and status inequities continue to leave a significant scar on American sport.

"Winning Isn't Everything, It's the Only Thing": Competition, Capitalism, Commercialism and Sport in the Consumer Culture

Capitalism is the most pervasive, fiercely contested and frequently understated element of American culture. The "ME generation" is, perhaps, a contemporary reflection of the traditional American belief in rugged individualism. This central phenomenon is manifested in sport through increased role specialization in team sports,[21] the MVP (Most Valuable Player), All American and All-Star, the high profile of the coach, the awarding of "varsity letters," the "retiring" of players' numbers, and a growing emphasis on the measurement of individual performance in team sports (e.g., ERA, RBI, assists, errors, plus/minus ratios, and % of goals scored), creating profiles of individual ability which become all-important at the time of contract negotiation.

America's relentless pursuit of victory has found cultural support from a deeply entrenched work ethic, characteristic bold tenacity and a sincere belief in industry. Religious adherence to hard work and the "No pain, no gain" idiom has resulted in hyperconditioning and overtraining in American sport and, consequently, physiological and psychological harm to athletes. Meanwhile, winning has become the be-all and end-all of life in America, including sport wherein elitism has emerged as a dominant force. Roy Blount has pointed out that "In this country today, 220 books are in print whose titles begin with the word 'Winning.' ... How can anybody in America relax and have a good time anymore, [he adds] if every morning presents anew the question, 'Am I going to win today?'"[22] Coming in second place is just not good enough in American sport. In their relentless pursuit of victory American athletes and sports leaders have gone to seemingly ridiculous lengths. In 1988, Westfield High School of Houston sought a Texas State District Court decision on the outcome of a high school football game. Sharing an identical win-loss record with another team, a 20-20 tie in their game with one another, and the same number of penetrations past the 20-yard line (the parameters used to judge which team should advance to the State playoffs), the judge was left to make a decision.[23] "Tie breaking" and "sudden death" strategies have been creatively introduced to ensure a guaranteed outcome within time limits, and with the ready acceptance of tryouts, cuts and benching there appear to be little genuine interest in and support for the egalitarian provision of "Sport for All," the idea of deferred gratification, or a belief in the instrumental benefit of sports participation. Yet, in this most highly competitive arena, there remains a mysterious adherence to respecting the opponent in not "running up the score."

In America, success is measured in a material sense. Sport is both entertainment and big business. The free entrepreneurial spirit has created a vast sports industry, one which includes franchised teams, individuals, sporting goods, television, and wagering. This author believes that Leigh Steinberg, one of America's most prominent sports agents, said it best when he wrote, "There is an interplay between the worlds of sports, business, and entertainment, a synergy that is the playing field of the truly powerful."[24] Anyone who doubts this key relationship need only look to the case of Rhyne Sandberg of the Chicago Cubs baseball team who, in 1992, signed a four-year contract extension worth $28.4 million; the prize money of $6.5 million going to each of the two college football teams that appear in the annual Rose Bowl game; the estimated $12 million that Patrick Ewing brought to Georgetown University in the years that he played there[25]; the $1.7 billion in revenue paid to Nike shoe company shareholders in 1992; or the $500 million spent by the Philip Morris company on advertising and promotions in sport during 1991.

Once more a cultural paradox comes into play as it would be easy for the naive outsider to be blinded to the deeply serious fiscal nucleus of sport by its somewhat trivialized and superficial displays of emotion. Many American professional sports teams are unable to keep pace with demand and retain extensive waiting lists for season tickets. The Washington Redskins, of the NFL, have sold out every home game since 1966 and estimate upward of 40,000 potential season ticket holders are waiting "in the wings." Today, the average ticket price in MLB is $9.57, $25.16 in the NBA, $25.96 in the National Hockey League (NHL), and $27.19 in the NFL. *Team Marketing Report* has formulated a "Fan Cost Index" to track the growing cost of live spectator sport consumption in America. Using a family of four, which would have to park, purchase tickets, two beers, four hot-dogs, four soft drinks, two baseball caps, and two programs, their calculations show that the average total cost to attend a MLB game is now $90.87 (ranging from $116.00 for the Toronto Blue Jays at SkyDome to $77.31 for the Cincinnati Reds at Riverfront Stadium) compared to the NFL (1993) at $173.33 (ranging from $207.00 for the San Francisco 49ers to $143.87 for the Cincinnati Bengals), and the NBA (1992-93) at $158.17. The generally high demand for tickets remains, so much so that Chicago officials have recently offered Bulls and White Sox tickets in exchange for the voluntary surrender of handguns and assault weapons, the cause of so much violent crime in that city.[26] The law of supply and demand, however, represents a delicate balance which requires careful adherence to such elements as the "salary cap" and the "draft," each carefully designed to maintain a degree of homeostasis and parity within sport. Nevertheless, a variety of creative and ingenious financial arrangements (including signing bonuses, incentive clauses, and credit lines), seemingly the hallmark of American business, have begun to capitalize on loopholes by circumventing the fundamental principles involved thus threatening the future of the leagues.[27]

One need not look far from the American sports venue to begin to appreciate its broader economic impact. In his recent book, *Playing the Field: Why Sports Teams Move and Cities Fight to Keep Them,* Charles Euchner provides a compelling argument for sport as the economic mainstay of many communities. From high school, to college, and professional sports the calculation of financial influence demands a complex equation. The many small towns, particularly in climatically favorable Florida and Arizona, which have invested millions of dollars in the construction of facilities for baseball's annual ritual of spring training, bear testimony to the economic payoff. Likewise, each year more and more cities in America go to great expense in their attempt to attract sports teams. Offering new stadiums, expanded television markets, sizable franchise fees, tax incentives, and other attractions it would appear that professional sports leagues throughout America are never short of new "expansion" suitors.[28]

The most publicized dollar amounts in contemporary American sport are, without question, the players' skyrocketing salaries. Presently the average annual salary of players in MLB is $1,012,424.00, $1,208,000.00 in the NBA, $643,000.00 in the NFL, and $379,000.00 in the NHL (1992-93). Among the leagues' highest paid players are Barry Bonds, who earns $7,291,667.00 annually playing for MLB's San Francisco Giants (as part of a six-year $43.75 million contract), Hakeem Olajuwon, who signed a six-year $38 million contract with the Houston Rockets of the NBA; John Elway, quarterback of the NFL's Denver Broncos, who has a four-year contract worth $20 million, and Wayne Gretzky of the NHL's Los Angeles Kings, who recently signed a three-year contract worth $25.5 million.[29] When compared with the average salary of a male, American worker ($29,421.00) the figures appear outrageous yet set in the company of other entertainers such as Bill Cosby (who earned $40 million in 1992), Michael Jackson ($26 million), and Madonna ($24 million), they are less remarkable.[30] Yet salaries do not tell the full story. When combined with product endorsement contracts the annual earnings of many sportsmen and women can multiply. Presently, Michael Jordan, who has recently announced his retirement from the NBA's Chicago Bulls, leads the way with $32 million worth of annual endorsements, followed by golfer Arnold Palmer ($11 million), Shaquille O'Neal of the NBA's Orlando Magic ($10 million), tennis player Andre Agassi ($9 million), golfer Jack Nicklaus ($9 million), and Joe Montana, quarterback of the NFL's Kansas City Chiefs ($8 million). O'Neal, the 21-year-old basketball sensation, furnishes endorsements for Pepsi-Cola ($10-13 million), Reebok ($20 million over five years), Spalding ($6 million for five years), and at least ten other national sponsorships for a total earnings of $32 million. The downside of such arrangements frequently emerges with the athlete's contractual ownership by the producer. In the case of O'Neal, Pepsi-Cola has recently refused to allow USA Basketball to market his likeness, effectively preventing him from representing the national team in international tournaments.[31] Today, even those players hoping to represent the United States in FIFA's 1994 World Cup are signing long-term contracts with the United States Soccer Federation, as American Olympians compete with the promise of $15,000 prize money for a gold medal victory and reduced increments to $5,000 for a fourth place finish.[32]

Neither should the owners' profiteering be ignored as so often has been the case in the past. The financial accounting of the NFL, finally made public in the free-agency trial of 1992, revealed something of the hidden wealth in American professional sports ownership. Among *Forbes'* most current list of the nation's 400 richest figures appeared 21 who owned at least 30% of one or more professional sports teams. This elite group includes Miami Heat partner Ted Arison (with a wealth estimated at $3.3 billion), Portland Trailblazers owner Paul G. Allen ($3.1 billion), Atlanta Braves and Hawks owner Ted Turner ($2 billion), Orlando Magic Chairman Rich DeVos ($1.5 billion), New York Giants co-owner Robert Preston Tisch ($1.5 billion), and Washington Redskins owner Jack Kent Cooke ($1 billion).[33]

While not all these businessmen garnered their wealth on the playing field, American professional sports have clearly represented a sound investment in the twentieth century. In their book, *Pay Dirt: The Business of Professional Team Sports,* economists James Quirk and Rodney Fort calculate the investment growth of MLB (1901-90) at 7.5%, the NBA at 16.5% (1950-90), and the NFL at 20.4% (1920-90), compared with a growth in common stocks of 10.3% (1920-90).[34] The current worth of the 10 most wealthy professional sports franchises[35] in America today is shown below:

Rank	Team	League	Estimated Worth (in $ millions)
1	Dallas Cowboys	NFL	165
2	New York Yankees	MLB	160
3	Toronto Blue Jays	MLB	155
4	Los Angeles Lakers	NBA	155
5	Philadelphia Eagles	NFL	149
6	New York Giants	NFL	146
7	New York Mets	MLB	145
8	Miami Dolphins	NFL	145
9	San Francisco 49ers	NFL	139
10	Buffalo Bills	NFL	138
103	Winnipeg Jets	NHL	35

It has long been said that American universities field "the best teams money can buy." Rife with fiscal mismanagement, scandal, and corruption despite attempts at strict regulation by the National Collegiate Athletic Association (NCAA), there is no denying that sport is the biggest business on American campuses today.[36] With championship money amounting to multimillions of dollars in American football and men's basketball, athletes are treated as prima donnas and it is common to find head coaches earning twice the salary of college presidents and Nobel prize winning professors. When Don James, the head coach of the University of Washington football team, stepped down in August of 1993 he gave up $161,000.00 in base salary, $163,000.00 in television and radio show earnings, a share of a $35,000.00 Nike shoe contract, $1,000.00 each time he wore a particular hat during a televised game, and an estimated $100,000 in speech and appearance fees.[37] Yet even this pales in comparison with the four-year, $4.7 million shoe contract that Dean Smith, head men's basketball coach at the University of North Carolina, recently signed with Nike or the $375,000 annually for the next 15 years that Mike Krzyzewski, head men's basketball coach at Duke University, will earn for ensuring that his players wear Nike rather than Adidas shoes on court.[38] Given the limited job security associated with coaching professional and college sport teams, such negotiated rewards are to be expected as one is reminded constantly of the shallow words of support, "Remember, Coach, we're right behind you — win or tie!"

Given these economic realities, it is easier to comprehend why American commercial sport has focused on its creation of a viable consumer product. Promoters see sport first as a commodity which they carefully design, package, and sell to a consumer society where demand regularly exceeds supply. From innovatory changes in traditional sports, which include the implementation of shot/play clocks, one/two/three point scoring options, and illegal defense rules, to the establishment of new commercial products such as the MISL or Arena Football, the latter "an off the wall hybrid" of the gridiron game first unveiled in 1987 in which "There are real fireworks after touchdowns to heighten the incendiary atmosphere, [and] loudness is the word from the striped uniforms by Zubaz to the sound effects,"[39] and the birth of such "garbage sports" as the Superstars, the professional World Wrestling Federation (WWF), or the more recent American Gladiators wherein seemingly chemically induced beings wage battles of strength with one another to the delight of a growing cult of TV consumers, it becomes abundantly apparent that profit margin is the primary consideration in American sport today.

Television necessarily enjoys a critical, commercial reciprocity with American sport. From the introduction of Rod Dixon's "helmet cam" and Bill Rodgers' pulse monitor during the 1985 New York City Marathon, to the use of indoor and outdoor blimps, helicopters, electronic chalkboards, "scuba cams" (in the most recent America's Cup), on-screen graphics, and the audio-visual wiring of participants in the WLAF, American television executives find themselves constantly challenged to provide novel ways in which to enhance their consumer product. Depending as they do on recouping contractual and production expenditures from advertisers (and thus the consumer!), a competitive and appealing product is critical, one which will claim and retain the sports consumer's attention. Perhaps the cultural naiveté and innocence which was highlighted earlier is all too well demonstrated by the British Broadcasting Corporation's Dan Maskell, who covered Wimbledon for more than 30 years. A model of British restraint and understatement, speaking of cross-cultural styles in sports commentary, he wrote:

>We have a very different attitude than you
>Americans. Your approach would not go
>here I'm afraid. Talking through rallies
>breaks our golden rule. Once the service
>ball is delivered, unless something extraor-
>dinary happens, we keep our mouths shut.
>We have a television audience that is fairly
>knowledgeable about tennis. Our job is to
>enlighten, inform and involve them in a
>subtle sort of way that provides a deeper
>enjoyment of the pure spectacle of the
>match. It seems to me that commentators in
>America are there much more to entertain.[40]

The American television sports consumer need never go hungry. Recently, the nation's first 24-hour all sports channel, ESPN, chose to debut a second channel. The broadcast medium remains a key element in the continued success of the American sports business enterprise. Currently, major league television revenues amount to approximately $912 million (from five networks) for the NFL experience currently billed as "America's Passion," $365 million (from ABC, NBC, and ESPN) for MLB, and $219 million (from NBC, TNT, and TBS) for the NBA, representing the leading source of income for all teams.[41] Since the 1976 Olympics in Montreal, American network television companies have essentially underwritten the centerpiece of the International Olympic Committee. In 1992, the National Broadcasting Corporation (NBC) paid $401 million for the rights to broadcast, exclusively, the world's largest multisport festival in America.[42] With an additional $210-225 million spent on production and marketing, NBC's innovative "Triplecast" pay-per-view package which provided consumers with 1,080 hours (24 hours a day) of commercial-free Olympic coverage for $29.95 a day (or $125 for the complete package) fell far short of expectations. Recouping a portion of the expenditures through advertising revenues ($425 million), affiliate subscriptions ($30 million), "Triplecast" subscriptions ($7 million), and Cablevision loss share ($50 million), the network registered an overall $99-114 million loss on its coverage of the Barcelona games.[43] Despite this poor debut for pay-per-view its future seems assured as a 1992 poll revealed that 56% of viewers would subscribe to such service to watch the NFL's Super Bowl, 49% the World Series of MLB, 39% the NCAA Final Four (men's collegiate basketball), 36% the Summer Olympics, and 34% the NBA Finals.[44]

To the American television executive who receives little, if any, financial subsidy from the government commercial advertising rates represent the primary source of revenue. Seemingly unperturbed by, and even accepting of, the incessant barrage and delays wrought of commercial "breaks" in television sports coverage,[45] the consumers appear content to sit back and let someone else pay for their entertainment seldom realizing that indeed, they are paying the indirect cost of the broadcast. This reality is no better represented than in the annual broadcast of the NFL's Super Bowl. Compared to the $260,000.00 charged per 30-second commercial slot on ABC's live *Monday Night Football* program, the $850,000.00 rate for the 1993 NFL Championship game might, at first, appear to be in error. Yet, with Pepsi-Cola and Anheuser Busch leading the way and spending $6.8 million apiece on television advertising, Reebok ($3.4 million), Lee jeans ($3.4 million), 7 Up ($2.6 million), Nike ($2.6 million), Subaru ($2.6 million) and others followed until every available second of commercial time was sold, expenditures which must inevitably be turned over to the product consumer. In 1994, NBC will be charging $900,000.00 for each 30 second slot during the Super Bowl and has already sold time to Anheuser Busch, Miller Brewing, Pepsi-Cola, and Converse.[46]

Michael Hiestand's statement that "Sponsors make sports bigger, richer and more telegenic as they wage the priciest competition in sports: the scramble for fans' brand loyalties,"[47] underscores the solid recognition by the nation's corporate powerbrokers that sport is, perhaps, the most seductive cultural instrument available in American marketing today. Corporate expenditures on sport have been estimated at $22 billion annually shared among sports related corporate overheads, sales promotion, public relations and event signs ($6.7 billion), corporate entertainment at sports events ($6.2 billion), advertising on television ($3.4 billion), advertising in the print media ($3.3 billion), and sponsorship fees ($2.4 billion). Among the leading American corporate sponsors in 1987 were Philip Morris Co., which spent $351 million on sport, Anheuser Busch ($350 million), General Motors Corp. ($310 million), RJR Nabisco ($174 million), Ford Motor Co. ($145 million), Chrysler ($131 million), the U.S. Armed Forces ($115 million), IBM Corp. ($102 million), AT&T ($82 million), and Gillette ($70 million).[48] Today, a number of large companies including Federal Express, Mobil, Jeep Eagle, Weiser Lock, Thrifty Car Rental. Poulan Weed Eater, John Hancock, Outback Steakhouse and Blockbuster sponsor, and even give their name to, postseason college football games (or "bowls"). Similarly, that longtime bastion of amateurism, the Olympic movement, has openly succumbed to the attraction of widespread sponsorship. During the summer of 1992, American consumers were presented with a variety of products blessed by the Olympic family including the official Olympic pain reliever (Nuprin), water (Evian), timer (Seiko), hair-care product (Clairol), cosmetics (Max Factor), medal award suit (Reebok), snack food (Snickers), coffee (Maxwell House), sunglasses (Ray-Ban), hotel (Hilton), bike helmet (Bell), clothier (J.C. Penney), and swimming ear plug (Santa Barbara Medco's Ear Putty). Humorous though it may sound, there is no mistaking the world of big business wherein alcohol and tobacco companies are generally provided the fullest consideration.[49]

Neither are the communications industry and corporate promotion executives the only ones that have capitalized on the American population's embracing of sport. The sporting goods industry and sports merchandising are engulfing an increasingly significant portion of the nation economy. Case in point is the highly competitive American athletic footwear market. In 1992 Philip Knight, Nike's Chairman, was selected as the most powerful person in sport by *The Sporting News* claiming that his company "is unquestionably the most powerful and influential organization in the sports world."[50] During the previous year, having weathered broad-based criticism surrounding the use of cheap labor in developing countries and its role in the creation of "a fantasy-fueled market for luxury items... [that] led to a frightening outbreak of crimes,"[51] Nike recorded a 30% share of the American market with revenues in excess of $1.7 billion. Reebok (23% with $1.3 billion), LA Gear (8% with $465 million), and Keds (6% with $345 million) followed. Today as Gary Strauss has noted, "The athletic-shoe war is escalating. And the battleground is more global than ever"[52] as Nike claimed 27%, and Reebok 32%, of their revenue from overseas. From Hula-Hoops to in-line skates, the modern history of the American sporting goods industry has been characterized by mass production, mass consumption and unparalleled growth. Today, the licensing and merchandising of sportswear and products appears to be one of America's most rapidly expanding enterprises and is projected to become a $10 billion industry in 1994. All major and minor sports leagues together with universities have recognized the potential rewards in both licensing fees and product sales. With black and teal blue representing the contemporary American consumers' colors of choice it is not surprising that the Los Angeles Raiders (with 16.8% of the NFL market), Dallas Cowboys (15.9%), the Chicago White Sox, Colorado Rockies, and Florida Marlins of MLB, together with the Charlotte Hornets of the NBA and the NHL's San Jose Sharks are among the leading sports franchises based upon merchandise revenue.[53] No one was surprised then, when the Mighty Ducks of Anaheim, the Walt Disney-owned newcomer to the NHL, decided to include teal in their team colors.

The hoarding of sports memorabilia and the childhood hobby of collecting baseball cards have turned into major sources of investment for many, bearing witness to the diverse reach of American sport. Today, the National Sports Collectors' Convention draws upward of 100,000 participants annually. While relics used and signed by athletic legends are in greatest demand, in 1992, the ball that went through Bill Buckner's legs (during game six of MLB's 1986 World Series) sold for $93,500.00. One year earlier, a 1909-11 Honus Wagner baseball card sold for $451,000.00 at a Sotheby's auction.[54] While it would be beyond the bounds of this chapter to further explore the extent of the American sports enterprise, the picture painted has been an accurate one sketched upon a complex, cultural fabric of business, mass media, and the consumer's delight in athletic display.

Liberty and Justice for All: Tradition and Innovation in American Sport

Despite recent events in California there remains, in America, a sincere belief in a judicial system that allows all individuals the right to be heard and to be fairly judged. It is interesting that each day the newspaper *USA Today* includes a "Jurisprudence" section among its sports pages. Ranging from the case of a young girl who challenged the right to play on a boys' team, to the question of free agency, and the right of professional team owners to move their franchises from one market to another, the courts seem to cover the broad spectrum of sport law on a daily basis. Penalties range from the overturning of sports results, to dollar fines, suspensions, television broadcast restrictions, and a variety of other sanctions including the "death penalty" in college athletics which effectively destroys a university sports program's ability to raise revenue. In 1986, a professor of English at the University of Georgia was fired for openly claiming that some of the institution's football players had received preferential treatment in remedial classes. Subsequently awarding the professor $2.5 million in back pay and punitive damages, the university president was forced to admit that some of the athletes involved were functionally illiterate.

The much heralded cases of Katrina Krabbe (in Germany) and Butch Reynolds (in America) present an interesting set of scenarios for cross-cultural study inasmuch as they both challenged the decisions of the International Amateur Athletic Federation (IAAF) and other governing bodies but through contrasting judicial systems. While it may be difficult for those outside of America to understand Reynold's prolonged battle with the international governing body of track and field, waged in the American courtroom which would appear to have no jurisdiction over the global sports arena, the outcome says it all as the plaintiff has already recouped some of his award from American corporate sponsors of the IAAF.

Increasingly, legal notices are finding their way into American newspapers. In June 1993, notice of a class action law suit filed against Auburn University on behalf of the University Women's Soccer Club sought a program upgrade and adequate funding for the sport, financial damages, and enforcement.[55] Earlier, the following notice[56] (in advance of the much publicized free agency court case) appeared:

LEGAL NOTICE

IN THE UNITED STATES DISTRICT COURT
FOR THE DISTRICT OF MINNESOTA

——————————————————————————X

REGGIE WHITE, et al.,	:	
	:	Civil Action No.
Plaintiffs,	:	4-92-906
	:	
v.	:	Judge David S. Doty
	:	
NATIONAL FOOTBALL LEAGUE, et al.,	:	
	:	
Defendants.	:	

_ _X

SUMMARY NOTICE OF HEARINGS ON PROPOSED
SETTLEMENT OF CLASS ACTION

TO ALL PERSONS: (1)WHO HAVE BEEN, ARE NOW, OR WILL BE UNDER CONTRACT TO PLAY PROFESSIONAL FOOTBALL FOR A MEMBER CLUB IN THE NATIONAL FOOTBALL LEAGUE AT ANY TIME FROM AUGUST 31, 1987 TO THE DATE OF THE FINAL JUDGMENT IN THIS ACTION AND (2) ALL COLLEGE AND OTHER FOOTBALL PLAYERS WHO, AS OF AUGUST 31, 1987 TO THE DATE OF FINAL JUDGMENT IN THIS ACTION, HAVE BEEN, ARE NOW, OR WILL BE ELIGIBLE TO PLAY FOOTBALL AS A ROOKIE FOR A MEMBER CLUB IN THE NATIONAL FOOTBALL LEAGUE (THE "CLASS").

You are hereby notified, pursuant to an Order of the Honorable David S. Doty of the United States District Court for the District of Minnesota, dated February 26, 1993, that a hearing will be held on April 16, 1993 at 9:00 A.M. in Courtroom 4 of the United States District Courthouse, 110 South Fourth Street, Minneapolis, MN. 55401 for the purpose of determining whether a proposed settlement of the above-captioned action should be approved by the Court as fair, reasonable and adequate.

If you are a member of the Class described above, your rights will be affected by this settlement, in which antitrust and other claims on behalf of the Class are being dismissed. In exchange, settlement payments are being awarded to the Class to be allocated among certain categories of Class members, and modifications are being made to the National Football League free agency rules, college draft, NFL Player Contract minimum salary amounts and other rules concerning the compensation and rights of professional football players employed by the NFL clubs.

If you do not receive a detailed notice, which is to be sent to all known members of the Class at the direction of the Court, you may obtain a copy by writing to James W. Quinn or Jeffrey L. Kessler, Class Counsel, at Weil, Gotshal & Manges, 767 Fifth Avenue, New York, New York 10153. If you wish to object to the terms of the settlement, you must expressly state your objections in writing to be received by the Court by no later that April 2, 1993. Further information on making such objections may be obtained from Class Counsel.

TO PROTECT YOUR LEGAL RIGHTS, PLEASE ACT PROMPTLY.

Dated: March 8, 1993   Clerk of the Court
         Minneapolis, Minnesota   United States District Court
                                      District of Minnesota

Furthermore, the rapid growth of the American sporting goods retailing industry has made legal action inevitable. In 1992, the active footwear company LA Gear paid $1 million to rival Reebok International in settlement of a patent infringement suit over Reebok's inflatable shoe technology called "The Pump."[57] Given the current trend of expansion across all elements of the American sports enterprise any cessation, or even reduction, of litigation in the foreseeable future is altogether unlikely.

Technological innovation has had at least as great an impact upon changing the complexion of American sport as has legislation. Seemingly less rooted in tradition (perhaps with the exception of baseball) than in other cultures, science and technology have ushered in a new athletic era. The impact on equipment, training techniques, and officiating are particularly apparent as the computer, space age materials, and medical advances have each made their mark on American sport.[58] The use of "Cyclops," a high-tech electronic eye "line judge," in tennis has been superseded by the Tennis Electronic Lines (TEL) system which uses magnetic coils buried beneath each line to detect the contact made by specially manufactured balls. The result of declining confidence in human judgment, and greater fruits of victory, the NFL has also experimented with technological intervention in officiating. However, the current disenchantment with "instant replay" (in which television footage is replayed frame by frame to determine the "correct call") seems to be primarily based on economic reasons. In 1992 owners voted 17-11 to retain "instant replay" but it was not enough to convince the League Commissioner's office which had become concerned that the resulting breaks in action (although providing additional time for commercials and thus increased advertising revenue), would extend the length of the game therefore negatively affecting the viewer ratings.[59] Finally, in the spirit of fair play and in order to counteract the impact of home crowd noise on visiting teams (particularly in covered stadiums), the NFL is experimenting with a voice amplifying-device called the "Audiblizer." Providing a wonderful example of the impact of technology on sport, an electronic transmitter worn in a quarterback's padding carries his voice from a shock-proof microphone in the chinstrap of his helmet, and broadcasts his "call" over the roar of the crowd thus neutralizing the impact of the fans.[60] While American sport remains a contradiction, exemplified by comparing the physical, communicative contortions of coaches in baseball with the high-tech headsets and aerial photographs of opposing defenses faxed to the sideline in football, attempts at regaining "control" over sport are becoming increasingly commonplace in America.

Gaining and Losing Control: Rationality and Emotion in American Sport

The well-developed structure and order apparent in the mechanical organization of American sport and culture stands in stark contrast to the colorful displays of emotion present in the nation's sporting spectacle. While set plays, game clocks (now timing in 100ths of a second), time-outs, and incremental team penalties for crowd misbehavior and other "field" infractions seem to suggest rational control as well as elements of preciseness and rigidity, Mike Franklin, a British journalist, paints a picture of the other side of American sport in describing the gridiron version of football as "... one of the most exciting games in the world [he adds] ...no one need be an aficionado to enjoy the thrills and spills. American football is an emotional experience... and even as a spectator it can be a draining experience."[61] Rock and roll music, "tailgate" parties, half-time shows, cheerleaders, fireworks, marching bands, laser shows, smoke screens, mascots, big screen televisions, and giant sound systems, comprise the razzmatazz so commonly associated with American sport. While the observation of such spectacles is common it is sometimes difficult to explain when set against the seemingly rational order of the sport itself.

It has been said that "capitalism begets quantification." Clearly in American sport, where statistics of every imaginable kind are liberally communicated with actor and audience alike, such a belief is borne out. "Box scores" first appeared in *The Sporting News* in 1886. Since then a vast array of figures cover the sports pages daily adding to the American sports lexicon such terms as "assists," "saves," "shutouts," "turnovers," and "winningest." How amusing it sounds, to the uninitiated, when during a Monday night MLB television broadcast the commentator kindly informs the audience that a batter "has an average of 2.74 against left-handed pitchers, in the Astrodome, on Monday nights in June," and the passive armchair spectator is expected to believe it! Even Woody Hayes, a late football coach at Ohio State University, voiced some skepticism by stating, "Statistics always remind me of the fellow who drowned in a river whose average depth was only three feet." Today *The Sporting News* is marketing a "Sportrax" handheld monitor to consumers for $495.00 each plus a monthly service subscription rate of $79.50. This device provides fans with up-to-the-minute electronic information on schedules, betting odds, injury reports, weather forecasts, scores, highlights, statistics, headlines, signings and transactions from nearly every corner of the sports world. Moreover, American sports' apparent intent to rid themselves of all elements of chance through such strategies as the construction of indoor, climate-controlled arenas, refereeing by "committee" and the utilization of "instant replay" and other high-tech devices in officiating, supports an increasing shift toward rationalization in the games itself. Finally, the ranking of teams in the vast morass of American sport today is no longer as easy as calculating wins-losses, and point differentials as it is not possible for one team to play all others of similar rank across the nation. Placing the utmost confidence in mathematical explanation Jeff Sagarin, of *USA Today*, has generated a rating scale intended to be:

> ... a numerical measure of the team's strength. To determine a hypothetical margin of victory in a game [one should] compare the ratings of the two teams after adding four points to the home team's ratings.

> Each team's schedule strength is the numerical average of the ratings of the opponents it has played (taking into account whether each game was played at home, away or on a neutral court). A team rating is determined by the schedule strength in combination with the scores in [Division I] games played.

> There is a diminishing returns principle
> built into the system that prevents a team
> from building up its rating by running up
> large margins of victory against weak
> teams. Instead, it rewards teams that do well
> against good opponents.

Of course, the emerging statistics find increased utility among the wagering fraternity. Although there is no federal government control over sports betting in America only five states offer legalized gambling on human athletic endeavors while 36 states do sanction pari-mutuel betting on horse racing or jai alai. Gambling on sport in America is not as simple as picking a winner and loser based upon predetermined odds. Rather, the challenge of "covering the point spread" by selecting the margin of victory has created a tarnished history of "point shaving" scandals.[62] Given the national media's common disregard for the limited legality of sports gambling, as "betting lines" are daily published and broadcast for the consumer, estimates that $3 billion were wagered illegally on the outcome of the last Super Bowl are quite believable.[63]

The deep cultural significance afforded sport in America has ushered in other patterns of social deviance. The recent slayings of international visitors to Florida has painted a national profile steeped in violence. In the past, America's seemingly insatiable appetite for violence has been fed by brutal outbursts *on* the court, rink and field for, as Scott Crawford has suggested, the athletic arena has come to represent "... a privileged sanctuary allowing ritualized crimes to go on in a sanctioned, approved, and legitimate fashion."[64] Sometimes induced by drugs, frustration, taunting and retaliation, as well as the sheer physical size of the American sportsman, of greater concern today is the increasing incidence of fan violence *outside* the field of play. For American sports leaders who could once state with a certain smugness that the malady of European and South American soccer would never reach their shores, today there remains very real cause for concern. On October 14, 1984, one person died and eighty were injured as fans of the Detroit Tigers celebrated their victory in the World Series. Six years later, the same city witnessed eight deaths and 127 injuries in riots after the Detroit Pistons won their second consecutive NBA Championship. Fans of the Chicago Bulls celebrated in like fashion, in 1992, resulting in 1,000 arrests. Finally, a parade in honor of the 1993 NFL Super Bowl Champion Dallas Cowboys ended with two dozen people hospitalized with shooting and stab wounds.[65] How then could James Michener write, in 1990, "I take great pride that up to now our public behavior at games is infinitely superior to that shown by English ruffians, Italian partisans and Peruvian rioters."?[66] Today the message is clear: Sport holds a deeply significant yet complex meaning to the American psyche. Although the conditions may be different to those faced elsewhere in the world the potential for an escalation in fan violence is high. Civic and sports leaders of the future should beware.

The Seventh Inning Stretch: Contemplating the Future of American Values and Sport

It is entirely likely that American sport will move into the new millennium with a growing emphasis on capitalistic elitism. Despite the efforts of Democrats in Congress, pay-per-view sports consumption across an expanded global market will necessarily develop and attract interest from multinational corporate owners. The day of "Rollerball" waged in vast "theaters of sport" may not be far off. This scenario suggests a pessimistic view of sport with an increased emphasis on the ultimate goal of winning wherein technological advance, pharmacological and scientific intervention, and violence will become endemic. The alternative is to resist change and risk the perceived demise of American sport, a condition all too familiar to those in Major League Baseball today.

In conclusion, it must be recognized that America's headlong individualism and emphasis upon capitalistic gain are *not* conducive to nurturing the simplistic gospel of "esprit de corps" and amateurism, values rightly perceived as archaic in American sport. Citizens of the global village must understand that to embrace American sport, as part and parcel of an ongoing universal homogenization of culture, is to accept American values. International scholars must take more care to contextualize their criticism of American sport by first making a greater effort to understand the subtleties and complexities of American culture. Finally, to return to the title of this chapter. A fumble may be observed when the pigskin is snapped and handed off to the tailback who works a reverse with the split-end who, in turn, fails to maintain possession, while a fungo may be spotted amidst pepper, pop flies and line drives radiating from the diamond. If the reader is none the wiser, do not fret for of greater consequence than knowing what is understanding why—why this sometimes crazy, brash and always colorful spectacle called American sport is the way it is.

Notes

---

[1]Sage, George S. *Power and Ideology in American Sport. A Critical Perspective*. Champaign, IL: Human Kinetics Books, 1990.

[2]That is not to say that there are any number of very fine books written by American scholars which systematically examine and document the nature and significance of sport in American society. While a cursory review of the American sport sociology literature will reveal the extent of such volumes most assume an insider's view of American culture and hence fail to provide a unique cultural explanation, to their readers, for the condition of American sport.

[3]See Ralph C. Wilcox, "Imperialism or globalism? A conceptual framework for the study of American sport and culture in contemporary Europe," *Journal of Comparative Physical Education and Sport.* XV: 1 (1993), pp. 30-40.

[4]From "ballpark figure" to "striking out," an extensive vocabulary of sporting metaphors has entered the daily speech patterns of Americans.

[5]Chadwick, Bruce. "Soccer - loved and ignored," *Inside Sports.* (July 1984), p. 67.

[6]Quoted in Roscoe Nance, "MISL expects to expand into Europe in 1992-93," *USA Today.* (February 21, 1992), p. 10C.

[7]Dvorchak, Robert. "Newsstand sales sizzle," *Houston Chronicle.* (February 19, 1989), p. 13K.

[8]"Survey: Retton, Hamill best-loved," *USA Today.* (May 17, 1993), p. 2C; See also, Cardiss Collins, "Women in sports: No more 'wait till next year,'" *USA Today.* (February 10, 1993), p. 11A; Wieberg, Steve. "Universities discover good intentions not enough," *USA Today.* (June 8, 1992), p. 10C.

[9]Kohl, Linda, "Flo Jo. She's fast becoming a role model." *Houston Chronicle.* (Sunday October 9, 1988), p. 10L. A winner of three gold medals and one silver medal at the 1988 Olympic Games in Seoul, Florence Griffith-Joyner has recently been appointed Co-Chair of the President's Council on Physical Fitness and Sport, the American federal government's quasi-political agency which has traditionally sponsored youth fitness and sports programs throughout the nation's schools.

[10]The generally held assumption here is that while Magic Johnson, the former National Basketball Association star, must certainly have contracted the disease through promiscuous heterosexual behavior, thus barely slipping in status in the minds of the American public, the ice skaters' malady was a direct outcome of their culturally implied homosexual deviance.

[11]Brady, Erik. "The credo; Don't ask, don't tell," *USA Today.* (June 24, 1993), pp. 1-2C. It is interesting to note that Gay Games IV, an Olympic style festival offering more than 31 events is scheduled to be held in New York during June 1994. See also, Michael A. Messner and Donald F. Sabo, *Sport, Men, and the Gender Order. Critical Feminist Perspectives.* Champaign, IL: Human Kinetics Books, 1990; and Brian Pronger, *The Arena of Masculinity: Sports, Homosexuality and the Meaning of Sex.*

[12]Sandefur, Gary. "Promoting stereotype debases achievement," *USA Today.* (April 29, 1993), p. 12C; and Dorsey, Valerie Lynn, "State legislators look at issue," *USA Today.* (April 29, 1993), p. 12C.

[13]Dodd, Mike. "Baseball gets 'C' on 'Racial Report Card'," *USA Today.* (July 9, 1993), pp. 1-2C; and, Dorsey, Valerie Lynn, "Training viewed as useful tool," *USA Today.* (July 9, 1993), p. 2C; "Race in sports: A black and white issue," *USA Today.* (December 18, 1992), p. 3C; and Dodd, Mike, "Survey finds minorities rare in 'Power Positions'," *USA Today.* (January 11, 1993), p. 6C.

[14]Staples, Brent. "Where are the black fans?" *The New York Times Magazine.* (May 17, 1987), pp. 26-34, 56; Beitiks, Edvins, "Turnstile apartheid in the city," *Newsday.* (May 17, 1987), p. 13; Interestingly, black viewership of Monday Night Football (ranked 16th) has proven to be lower than viewership of the television program across all households (ranked 8th). See, "Black viewership," *USA Today.* (April 5, 1993), p. 3D.

[15]Dodd, Mike, "Schott accusations expand," *USA Today.* (December 2, 1993), pp. 1C, 3C; and "Selig's statement on suspension," *USA Today.* (February 4, 1993), p. 3C.

[16]The term "red shirt" refers to a student-athlete who is held out of competition for a year to allow for greater maturation and an additional year of eligibility to compete. See, B.J. Phillips, "Fattening them up for football," *Time.* (March 9, 1981), p. 44.

[17]*The NCAA News*, (September 28, 1987).

[18]Lederman, Douglas. "43% of male basketball players earned degree within 6 years," *The Chronicle of Higher Education.* (May 26, 1993), pp. A32-33; Wieberg, Steve, "Data can guide students, spur schools to improve," *USA Today.* (May 20, 1993), p. 10C; Blauvelt, Harry. "Adapting socially proves to be tough hurdle to overcome," *USA Today.* (May 20, 1993), p. 10C; Blume, Debra E. "Graduation rates of scholarship athletes rose after Proposition 48 was adopted, NCAA reports," *The Chronicle of Higher Education.* (July 7, 1993), pp. A42-44.

[19]King, Billie Jean, "A radical proposal: Let's pay college athletes," *Women's Sports and Fitness.* (January 1986), p. 60.

[20]"NFL, players' union settle on 7-year deal," *USA Today.* (May 7, 1993), pp. 1C, 9C.

[21]The complex division of labor in American sport continues to become more specialized as NFL teams, for example, are moving away from the signing of utility players in preference to "situational" athletes who meet the specific demands of "short yardage" plays, indoor/outdoor venues, and field goal/punting requirements.

[22]Blount, Roy. "Winning: Why we keep score," *The New York Times Magazine.* (September 29, 1985), Part II, pp. 24-27, 46.

[23]*Houston Chronicle.* (November 5, 1988), p. 1.

[24]Steinberg, Leigh, "Power brokers," *Inside Sports.* (March 1993), p. 64.

[25]*Chronicle of Higher Education.* (January 8, 1986), p. 29.

[26]Castle, George. "You could fill a stadium with some season-ticket waiting lists," *Sport.* (April 1989), p. 13; Brown, Ben. "Supply and demand set ticket prices," *USA Today* (May 11, 1993), p. 8C; "NFL on a budget," *USA Today.* (September 7, 1993). p. 2C; Hiestand, Michael. "Cost for day at ballpark not increasing as rapidly," *USA Today.* (April 2, 1993), p. 12C; Ward, Sam. "On the tab," *USA Today.* (May 13, 1993), p. 6D; *USA Today.* (October 6, 1993), p. 4A.

[27]Seemingly running counter to the fundamental principles of free enterprise, the emergence of dynastic monopolies has been shown, historically, to be counter-productive to the fiscal health of American sport. Recent decisions on "free agency" (guaranteeing greater freedom for athletes to seek their market worth), it has been argued, threaten the very balance of American professional sports. Yet, with confidence placed on the "salary cap" (in the NBA, this ensures that the players can receive up to 53% of the team's gross revenue), and the "draft" (in which the rights to eligible 'newcomers' are shared equitably among a league's teams), some degree of parity is presently assured. See, DuPree, David. "Teams learn to survive within salary cap limits," *USA Today.* (October 7, 1992), p. 12C; Shuster, Rachel. "Sports world adjusts to life under the cap," *USA Today.* (August 19, 1993), p. 8C.

[28]Cohen, Eliot. "Spring training is big business," *Sport.* (April 1989), p. 14; Brown, Ben. "Luring pro franchises costly venture," *USA Today.* (September 21, 1993), pp. 1-2C; Hiestand, Michael. "Economic impact studies viewed with skepticism," *USA Today.* (September 21, 1993), p. 9C; Euchner, Charles. *Playing the Field: Why Sports Teams Move and Cities Fight to Keep Them.* Baltimore: John Hopkins University Press, 1993; and Quirk, James, and Rodney Fort. *Pay Dirt: The Business of Professional Team Sports.* Princeton, N.J.: Princeton University Press, 1992.

[29]With contract negotiations ongoing, it is difficult to identify the highest paid player in a league at any particular point in time. Bobby Bonilla earned $6.2 million playing for MLB's New York Mets this season as 262 other MLB players earned more than $1 million and 99 exceeded $3 million. A more striking example may be the case of 45-year-old Nolan Ryan who earned $4.5 million pitching for the Texas Rangers in 1993 and, during the off-season, signed 90,000 baseballs at a cost of $20 each netting him an additional $1.2 million. Jones, Del. "Signing the dotted seam," *USA Today.* (April 6, 1992), p. 1B. Similarly, Shaquille O'Neal's $40 million over seven years, playing for the NBA's Orlando Magic, and Reggie White's $17 million over four years playing for the NFL's Green Bay Packers are among the highest salaries in professional sport. See Brown, Ben. "Are athletes overpaid?" *USA Today.* (May 11,

1993), pp. 1-2A, 8C; "Sports fans feel the pinch," *USA Today.* (July 14, 1992), p. 12C; Allen, Kevin. "Kings make Gretzky NHL's highest-paid," *USA Today.* (September 22, 1993), p. 1C; Mihoces, Gary. "Reggie White unpacks bags in Green Bay," *USA Today.* (April 7, 1993), p. 1A; "O'Neal's $40 million pact largest in sports history," *Houston Chronicle.* (August 8, 1992), p. 7B.

[30]Myers, Jim. "Wage gap expanding dramatically," *USA Today.* (May 11, 1993), p. 8C.

[31]"Top athlete endorsers," *USA Today.* (March 22, 1993), p. 1B; Potter, Jerry. "Nicklaus has golden touch off links, too," *USA Today.* (July 8, 1992), pp. 1-2C; Moore, Martha T. "Shaq attack on Madison Avenue," *USA Today.* (February 22, 1993), pp. 1-2B; Strauss, Gary. "Rookie scores big on Madison Avenue," *USA Today.* (November 18, 1992), p. 10B; and, Strauss, Gary. "Going for the green," *USA Today.* (August 7, 1992), pp. 1-2B.

[32]Nance, Roscoe. "Thirteen players agree to national team deals," *USA Today.* (January 8, 1993), p. 12C; Woodward, Steve. "Money-for-medals faces scrutiny," *USA Today.* (June 4, 1993). p. 10C; and Strauss, Gary. "Olympian prospers," *USA Today.* (September 14, 1992), p. 6B.

[33]"Undaunted by recession, rich get richer," *USA Today.* (October 5, 1992), p. 3B.

[34]Quirk & Fort.

[35]Extracted from *Financial World.* (May 25, 1993); Also see, "Profits and losses," *USA Today.* (July 9, 1992), p. 10C.

[36]Schuster, Rachel. "Compliance officers become more common as scrutiny grows," *USA Today.* (April 1, 1993), p. 5C; Schuster, Rachel. "Going by the book not simple task for schools," *USA Today.* (April 1, 1993), p. 5C.

[37]"James' loss," *USA Today.* (August 25, 1993), p. 1C.

[38]*USA Today.* (October 4, 1993), p. 1C. In addition, Kryzyzewski earned a $1 million signing bonus, while Smith donated his $500,000.00 bonus to charity.

[39]Mihoces, Gary, "Arena league puts ball in fans' hands," *USA Today.* (May 28, 1992), pp. 1-2C.

[40]Quoted in Bob Rubin, "This Bud's not for tennis purists," *Inside Sports.* (July 1984). pp. 8-10.

[41]Brown, Ben. "Business as usual is over for pro game," *USA Today.* (May 11, 1993), pp. 1-2A, 8C; Hiestand, Michael. "Sports rock," *USA Today.* (September 19, 1993), pp. 1-2C; Bodley, Hal. "New ABC-NBC partnership will change TV game forever," *USA Today.* (May 10, 1993), p. 5C; Kimmelman, Gene. "TV sports: Fans lose, cartel wins," *USA Today.* (May 13, 1993), p. 15A; and "How the leagues compare," *USA Today.* (September 22, 1993), p. 3C. These dollar amounts break down to $6.5 million per team in MLB (a decline from $14 million per team in the previous contract), $30-33 million per team in the NFL, and $10.2 million per team in the NBA.

[42]This compares with $90 million paid by European networks, $62.5 million from Japan, $33.8 million from Australia, and $16.5 million from Canada.

[43]Cox, James. "Future for pay-per-view getting tryout," *USA Today*. (July 21, 1992), pp. 1-2A; Martzke, Rudy. "Triplecast might drag NBC to all-time loss," *USA Today*. (July 27, 1992). p. 4E; and Woodward, Steve. "Networks bid on '96 with eye on wallet," *USA Today*. (July 23, 1993). pp. 1-2C.

[44]"Sports fans feel the pinch," *USA Today*. (July 14, 1992), p. 12C.

[45]For where else in the world of sport can 15 seconds of action take 15 minutes to complete and broadcast?

[46]Moore, Martha T. "Super Bowl, super price," *USA Today*. (July 12, 1993), p. 3B; Moore, Martha T. "Advertisers try different game plans," *USA Today*. (January 29, 1993), pp. 1-2B; "Super Bowl ad meter," *USA Today*. (January 27, 1992), p. 3B; Moore, Martha T. "Panel flips for Nike's 'Hare Jordan' ad," *USA Today*. (January 27, 1992), p. 3B; Moore, Martha T. "Basketball battle beats jeans," *USA Today*. (February 1, 1993), p. 3B; Moore, Martha T. "Pepsi's Super Bowl ad money well spent," *USA Today*. (February 2, 1993), p. 1B.

[47]Hiestand, Michael. "Sponsorship: The name of the games," *USA Today*. (June 16, 1993), pp. 1-2C.

[48]*Sport Marketing News*. 3: 4 (February 15, 1988), p. 1.

[49]Strauss, Gary. "The Olympics brought to you by...," *USA Today*. (July 21, 1992), pp. 1-2B. See also, Mihoces, Gary. "Tents are centers for corporate hobnobbing," *USA Today*. (June 16, 1993), p. 9C; Dodd, Mike. "New baseball TV deal changes playing field," *USA Today*. (June 16, 1993), p. 9C; Potter, Jerry. "Automakers target buyers with golf," *USA Today*. (June 16, 1993), p. 9C; Guy, Pat. "Nike puts full-court press on NBA Finals," *USA Today*. (June 7, 1993), p. 1B; Kelley, Michael, "Corporate sponsors going for the gold at sporting events," *Houston Chronicle*. (April 5, 1992), p. 7F; Moore, Martha T. "Bo still knows a good pitch. Hip surgery doesn't derail ad career," *USA Today*. (May 28, 1993), pp. 1-2B; and Woodward, Steve. "Corporations woo clients with Games," *USA Today*. (August 6, 1992), pp. 1-2B. Presently, World Cup USA 94™ has secured Canon, Coca-Cola, Energizer, Fujifilm, Gillette, GMCtruck, JVC, MasterCard, McDonald's, Philips, and Snickers as official sponsors, and Adidas, American Airlines, Budweiser, EDS, ITT Sheraton, Sprint, Sun Microsystems, and Upper Deck Trading Cards as marketing partners. "World Cup tickets. History will be made. Don't miss it for the world," *USA Today*. (October 8, 1993), p. 9C. Anheuser Busch, Miller Brewing, Coors, Virginia Slims, Winston, and Copenhagen/Skoal (smokeless tobaccos) are among the nation's leading sponsors of sport.

[50]Quoted in, *USA Today*. (December 19, 1992), p. 11C. Also see, Michael Hiestand. "Is Nike too powerful?" *USA Today*. (December 2, 1992), pp. 1-2C;

Hersh, Phil. "Flights of fancy. Do high-tech sneakers live up to hype?" *Houston Chronicle.* (February 14, 1993), pp. 1B, 11B; Walker, Blair S. "New Balance owner sets own pace," *USA Today.* (October 14, 1992), p. 10B; and Strauss, Gary. "Pump up your wallets for $200 sneakers," *USA Today.* (February 8, 1993), p. 1A.

[51]Telander, Rick. "Senseless," *Sports Illustrated.* 72: 20 (May 14, 1990), pp. 36-38, 43-44, 46, and 49. During the early 1990s, Nike, Reebok, and other "leading players" in the American sports shoe market found their basic morality and business ethics challenged by civic leaders who argued that corporate insensitivity and greed represented the root cause of an unrealistic elevation of "sneaker status" prompting young males to mug and shoot one another for the "shoes on their victim's feet."

[52]Strauss, Gary. "Global race for athletic shoes," *USA Today.* (February 18, 1992), pp. 1-2B.

[53]Mihoces, Gary, "Trying to get a handle," *USA Today.* (September 17, 1993), p. 6C.

[54]Warnes, Danielle. "Baseball greats' items in big demand." *USA Today.* (September 7, 1993), p. 7B; Williams, Pete. "Uncertain future weighs in industry," *USA Today.* (July 9, 1992), p. 8C; and, Williams, Pete. "Collectors gathering for fun, nostalgia," *USA Today.* (July 22, 1993), pp. 1-2C.

[55]"Legal Notice. To: All Auburn University female undergraduates and graduates in the classes of 1991, 1992, and 1993," *USA Today.* (June 24, 1993), p. 4D.

[56]"Legal Notice. To: All persons (1) who have been, are now, or will be under contract to play professional football for a member club in the National Football League..., and (2) All college and other football players...," *USA Today.* (March 8, 1993), p. 5C.

[57]"Pump suit settled," *USA Today.* (November 13, 1992), p. 1B.

[58]Waggoner, Glen. "It's a whole new ballgame! PCs and baseball," *PC Computing.* 2: 6 (June 1989), pp. 61-73.

[59]Goldstein, Jody. "Computerized line calls will debut at US Open," *Houston Chronicle.* (August 23, 1993), p. 11B; and, Schuster, Rachel. "No great clamor for the return of instant replay," *USA Today.* (September 23, 1992), p. 9C.

[60]Weisman, Larry. "Tests set for system to battle crowd noise," *USA Today.* (August 19, 1993), p. 8C.

[61]Franklin, Mike, "Grid Iron: The hard men of '86," *Hot Air.* 10 (1986), pp. 10-11,13.

[62]Carroll, Bob, Pete Palmer and John Thorn. "The thinking man's guide to football betting," *Sport.* (December 1988), pp. 79-83; McGarvey, Robert. "Sports gambling '90s style," *Sport.* (April 1989), pp. 57-59. "Point shaving" is the practice of players (corrupted by the promise of payoffs) who deliberately

ensure that the outcome of a sporting contest results in a team's inability to cover the projected margin of victory/defeat.

[63]In contrast, it is estimated that in the state of Nevada approximately $50 million was wagered on the 1993 Super Bowl between the Dallas Cowboys and Buffalo Bills, *USA Today.* (January 24, 1993), p. 1E.

[64]Crawford, Scott A.G.M. "Values in disarray. The crisis of sport's integrity," *Journal of Physical Education, Recreation, and Dance.* 57: 9 (November/December 1986), pp. 41-44; See also, B.G. Gregg. "Ballgames become embattled," *USA Today.* (June 16, 1992), p. 10C; and B.G. Gregg. "Society's turbulence is the major culprit," *USA Today.* (June 16, 1993), p. 10C.

[65]Weir, Tom. "Rioting celebrants defy reasonable logic," *USA Today.* (June 22, 1993), p. 3C; Edmonds, Patricia. "No-win mix for sport. Thrill of victory, agony of violence," *USA Today.* (June 22, 1993), p. 3A.

[66]Michener, James. "A walk into the 21st century," *Newsday.* (January 7, 1990), p. 23.

Chapter 6

C.L.R. James and His Centrality of Sport Model: Possible Applications in an American Setting

Scott A.G.M. Crawford

On June 2, 1989, C. Gerald Fraser writing an obituary in the *New York Times* reviewed the life and career of an 88-year-old Trinidadian C.L.R. James. Fraser described James as a "prodigious and eclectic intellectual."[1] James, however, was much more than a brilliant, if eccentric, scholar. He was an international figure who saw cultural interweaves as more critical than social origins, political ideologies and ethnic roots. He debated with the Soviet exile Trotsky in Mexico and, in 1952 during the McCarthy era, he was interned on Ellis Island and eventually deported. From 1970 to 1980, he was on the faculty of Federal City College of Washington, D.C. Earlier in his career, in the 1930s and after World War II, he came under the wing of the doyen of all cerebral cricket writers, the art critic, Neville Cardus. James flourished as a cricket writer for the *Manchester Guardian*[2] and eventually came to write what many people feel is the finest cricket book of all times. Intriguingly, the *New York Times* committed a frequent error in naming James' book, *Beyond a Boundary* and the change from the definite to the indefinite article is of no little philosophical importance. James' world was not one of compartments with boundaries and divisions, but rather a heaving, ever-changing stage with shifting borders. His wife, Selma Weinstein James, said that "he saw the world, literature, sports, politics, and music as one totality."[3]

The *Times* of London described this leader of the Pan-African movement as "the black Plato."[4] James, as a militant Marxist and confidant of Paul Robeson, might have been somewhat amused at the juxtaposition of his obituary in the *Times*, a centuries-old newspaper with a powerful history of conservative affili-

103

ations. Above James was a tribute to the exploits of Squadron Leader "Ginger" Lacey, a World War II flying ace. Beneath him, an elegant essay of the life of the great Yugoslavian dramatic soprano, Zinda Milanov. There in the center is the profile of James who, at one and the same time, was philosopher, social historian, political scientist, cultural anthropologist, and cricket aficionado.

Beyond a Boundary

The book was originally published in Great Britain by Stanley Paul in 1963, and Pantheon Books of New York brought out an American edition in 1983. Robert Lipsyte, an American journalist, in an introduction to the 1983 volume, commented on the way in which James articulated a sporting "universality of... experience."[5] In many respects, Beyond a Boundary is an amalgam of biography and social commentary. In the opening chapter James described his early years in Tunapuna, a village of 3,000 people only eight miles from Trinidad's capital, Port of Spain. An elder aunt, Judith, is recalled with a certain quizzical affection. She dropped dead at a very advanced age during the feeding of the local cricket team, "Yet she had never taken any particular interest [in cricket]."[6]

James was given a cricket bat and ball on his fourth birthday[7] and before his teens was a voracious reader of Charles Dickens, as well as the various local sporting newspapers. Characters from Vanity Fair were accorded the same youthful awe as cricketers W.G. Grace and C. B. Fry.[8] For James, his world was energized by the two forces of books and cricket. As a six-year-old, he could stand on a chair, look out the window and watch the cricket matches. He could also, by standing on tiptoe reach his library on the top of the wardrobe:

> Recreation meant cricket, for in those early
> days [circa 1918], except for infrequent ath-
> letic sports meetings, cricket was the only
> game.[9]

James won a prestigious scholarship to Queen's Royal College and in school cricket found a game of similar serious intent to the Latin, Greek and French of the classroom. Cricket was education and life:

> On the playing field we did what ought to
> be done. Every individual did not observe
> every rule. But the majority of the boys did.
> The best and most respected boys were pre-
> cisely the ones who always kept them.

> When a boy broke them he knew what he
> had done and, with the cruelty and intoler-
> ance of youth, from all sides our denuncia-
> tions poured in on him—Eton and Harrow
> had nothing on us.[10]

In 1918, James attempted to join an English regiment to see service in World War I. The recruiter "took one look at me, saw my dark skin and, shaking his head vigorously, he motioned me violently away."[11]

James had a passion for all things to do with cricket. He immersed himself in the history, statistical flotsam and personalities of cricket as a global institution, at least within the remnants of the old British Empire. And it was cricket that shaped his ethical core and created his "sense of conduct and morals."[12] In a chapter entitled "The Light and the Dark," James analyzed the racial composition of the West Indies and the color/ethical social class base of the various cricket clubs ranging from the Queen's Park Club (part white, well established, wealthy) to the working class, blue-collar Stingo Club, "Totally black and no social status whatever." James joined the Maple Club, an organization devoted to a middle class, neither white nor black, but brown-skinned.[13] James relished re-telling the heroic feats of those he felt were the all-time best West Indian cricketers. There was George John, the great fast bowler of the post-1914 period and an athlete seen as an invincible folk idol. "When John was routed, every-body talked of it, as people must have talked of Napoleon's defeats."[14] During the same period Wilton St. Hill was a superb batsman. James wrote of him as "beautifully erect"; he "flicked the ball away like a conjurer" and "his spirit was untamable."[15] The third figure in James' cricketing litany of excellence is Learie Constantine, whose career spanned the years 1921 to 1939. Constantine played for the West Indies and commuted backwards and forwards to England where he played professional cricket. He was much in demand as a public speaker:

> The people in Lancashire had an inordinate
> appetite for asking Constantine to come to
> speak to them, most often in church and
> similar organizations.[16]

Eventually Constantine came to be a spokesman against racial discrimination.

Although James speaks of the Australian Don Bradman as being the best bats-man of all time, he makes the case that West Indian George Headley was nearly as good. James explores the thesis that it was not so much what cricketers like

George, John, Wilton St. Hill and George Headley did but rather what qualities made their achievements possible:

> If life were not so urgent I would be willing to spend a year talking to a great batsman asking him questions and probing into all sorts of aspects of his life on and off the cricket field. If he and I hit it off the result would be a book such as had never yet been written, which physiologists, anthropologists and psychologists would read more eagerly than cricketers.[17]

In chapter twelve of *Beyond a Boundary,* entitled "What do Men Live by?," James pens a poignant plea for the acceptance of "British sport" history as a key academic discipline:

> ...not a single English scholar, historian or social analyst of repute had deemed it worth his while to pay even the most cursory attention to these remarkable events (the cultural diffusion of British sports) in which his own country played so central, in fact, the central role.[18]

James sets the scene for his lively mini-biography of the Victorian cricketer, W.G. Grace, in a prolegomena[19] that encompasses William Hazlitt, Charles Dickens, Thomas Arnold, and Thomas Hughes. The chapter on W.G. Grace has been frequently excerpted over the years. Suffice to say that in it, James outlines the social origins and athletic feats as well as the cultural importance of Grace as he strode towards mid-1885 when, in his forty-eighth year, he scored his one hundredth century. James is fascinated not so much by the stellar athletic achievements of Grace but, rather, by the manner in which these accomplishments excited and electrified a nation. James claims that this "spontaneous, unqualified, disinterested enthusiasm and goodwill of the community" is the "most potent of all forces in our universe."[20]

Another "favorite" chapter of James found in anthologies on sport and literature is his philosophical commentary, "What is Art?" In this, he argues that while games in general are dramatic, cricket creates a more specific type of drama. His drama epitomizes the best of the theatrical tradition inasmuch as two star characters — the batsman and the bowler — "are pitted against each other in a conflict that is strictly personal but no less strictly representative of a social group."[21] On a second level, James advances his thesis of the artistic uniqueness of cricket as a result of its structural unity. The game of cricket he sees as a series of perfectly contained segments. And, for the spectator, these sub-plots or plays within the game have meaning and significance. "What matters in cricket, as in all the arts," he wrote, "is not finer points but what every one with some knowledge of the elements can see and feel."[22]

James repeatedly harkens back to what he felt was the civilized and cultured age of Greece where an educated "leisure" class was schooled in the muses as well as skilled physical activity. Society sustained itself by being informed observers and participants:

> The popular democracy of Greece, sitting for days in the sun watching "the Orestei," the popular democracy of our day, sitting similarly, watching Miller and Lindwall [famous Australian pace bowlers] bowl to Hutton and Compton [celebrated English batsmen]— each in its own way grasps at a more complete human existence.[23]

In much of his writing James produces word pictures based on a series of light, anecdotal, cerebral brush strokes. In "Proof of the Pudding" it is a James of a different mettle. His fire and brimstone campaign, carried out in 1960 in the columns of *Nation* to combat discrimination was, in his own words, unfair and full of "untutored vulgarity." It seemed as if the authorities would select a white West Indian (Alexander) as captain while James advocated a black West Indian, Frank Worrell. James said he was fueled by anger and a "fifty year knowledge of discrimination behind it."[24]

On the final page of *Beyond a Boundary*, James, in a final tribute to the charisma and athleticism of Frank Worrell, who had captained the West Indian team on their tour of Australia, underscores the impact of cricket as theater on a global stage:

> ...a quarter of a million inhabitants of Melbourne [came] into the streets to tell the West Indian cricketers good-bye, a gesture spontaneous and in cricket without precedent, one people speaking to another.[25]

Centrality of Sport

In a 1990 North American Society for Sport History tribute to James, Alan Metcalfe stressed the debt owed to James. Metcalfe made the point that James, in his treatment of cricket, presented a convincing argument for the centrality of sport. This chapter then takes the Metcalfe thesis—the James centrality of sport model—and applies it in a speculative fashion to examine the role of football in American society as reflected by four contemporary football narratives:

A Centrality of Sport Model[26]

Cricket	Cultural Resonance
Cricket as a "many splendored thing"	"What do they know of cricket that only cricket know?" (James)
Cricket as a game of wider significance	Sport interwoven with the major forces of society, economy and politics
The role of the individual in cricket	The worth of the athletic folk-hero and the informed spectator
Cricket as life	"The cricket field was a stage..." (James)
Cricket as a bridge	"History was not an artificial, academic experience divorced from the realities of life but an ongoing experience rooted in life's experiences" (Metcalfe).
Cricket as paradox	The necessity to conform and behave (the team player) yet only survive by innovation (the agent provocateur)
Cricket as an expressive avenue for the alienated common man	From W.G. Grace to Garfield Sobers the successes of cricketing greats buoyed up the working classes
The unity of cricket	The game was not a staccato collection of compartments but an integrated whole

Cricket as art   "It [cricket] belongs with the theater, ballet,
                                        opera, and the dance" (James)

The Story of a University of Nebraska Football Player

George G. Mills, in *Go Big Red* describes the Cornhusker legacy of athletic
excellence on a campus where football success has been inextricably tied to the
name, status and reputation of the University of Nebraska. What is unusual, perhaps unique about the narrative, is that Mills recounts the story of an average
player who, while he may have had dreams of future glory on the gridiron,
quickly came to realize that, because of a variety of happenings, stardom was
not to be his.

Mills describes being recruited by Nebraska and arriving on the campus in 1971
to see the football team go undefeated and win a second consecutive national
championship. At 6 feet 5 inches and 228 pounds the defensive tackle had every
reason to be confident of doing well. However, in 1976 when he graduated,
greatness had eluded him, injuries had plagued his career and all he had to show
was memories of a cultural milieu dominated by sports. Happily, Mills is neither the reverential voice eulogizing the heroic properties of college football nor
the "angry young man" bitter at the illusory chimera surrounding football. As
Randy Roberts notes in the foreword, Mills takes a middle ground. What
emerges is, à la James, another study on sport's centrality.

Although "big" games are recalled, the evocation is of a sense of place and time
for as Roberts noted, "the small joys of life—the first sight of an ocean, the
camaraderie on the team bus, the feeling of belonging."[27] Towards the end of his
biography Mills, without meaning to, underscores the larger than life aura of big
time college football. In 1976, Mills decided to try out with, and was signed by,
Calgary of the Canadian Football League:

> I didn't like it compared to playing at the
> University of Nebraska, Calgary wasn't as
> nice. The stadium wasn't as big, the locker
> room wasn't as modern, nor was the equip-
> ment as nice... Besides that, the Canadians
> had accents. Why that bothered me, I didn't
> know. All I knew was that I didn't like what
> I was seeing and I was already homesick
> and ready to leave.[28]

This vignette, perhaps more than any other, encapsulates the Jamesian notion of the pieces of a tapestry that tie in with other cultural and societal elements. C.L.R. James of Tunapuna, Trinidad, and George Mills in Lincoln, Nebraska, shared one unusual characteristic. They allowed themselves to look back and shape something more than a collage of reminiscences and autobiography. James, in his preface, emphasizes that he posed the question "What do they know of cricket who only cricket know?"[29] On a much less profound "level" Mills attempted, and to a degree succeeded, in posing his question "What do they know of football who only football know?"

Friday Night Lights—A Town, a Team and a Dream

H. G. Bissinger, the author of *Friday Night Lights,* has impressive credentials as a writer. After seven years on the desk of the *Philadelphia Inquirer* he was a Nieman Fellow at Harvard University from 1985 to 1986. As a recipient of the Pulitzer Prize, one would expect to find the author's writing insightful and analytical. Bissinger's remarkable book is about small town American high school football as a microcosm of race, politics, economics, and education. In a dust jacket promotional, author David Halberstam sums up the book's magic:

> By choosing to write about something
> small—the culture of high school football in
> a Texas small town—Bissinger has ended
> up writing about something large, the core
> values in our society.

Just as film maker Peter Bogdanovich did so masterfully with Larry McMurtry's *The Last Picture Show*, Bissinger lets his eye wander over the workings of a piece of Texas. Odessa, like so many small towns across America, has seen better days. Real estate values are not what they once were, the young mostly migrate and relocate to find work, and the town has an air of neglect. Odessa after all was "in the severely depressed belly of the Texas oil patch"[30] in West Texas. But on Friday nights in the fall, the town becomes energized and the economic gloom evaporates. The Panthers of Permian High School play football in front of 20,000 partisan spectators, and these faithful fans (as well as the coaches and the players!) find, in the games, something transcendent and invigorating. In 1989, one of the Panther stars, Brian Chavez, was admitted to Harvard and in the fall of that year, he tried out for the freshman football team. He quit after one day:

> When he [Chavez] went out for the team at
> Harvard, it no longer felt right. It wasn't the
> purpose of his being there, and for the first
> time in his life he was in an environment
> where football had no special cachet. When
> he was at Permian... he had once received a
> standing ovation at an elementary school
> assembly, with all those gaping nine and ten
> year olds wanting to desperately to be just
> like him someday. But when he stepped out
> onto the playing fields of Harvard in the
> Fall of 1989, he knew such moments were
> over.[31]

Bissinger quotes a young man's description of an Odessa football game forty
years earlier. George Bush, on graduating from Yale where he played baseball,
lived in Odessa for a year with his wife. Bush spoke of a "feverish" night, wild
fans "rattling the stands from the opening kickoff" and an experience that eventually was described as a "quasi-religious experience."[32] In an acceptance
speech for the Republican nomination for president, George Bush propagan-
dized verbal images of American wholesome living:

> ...in time we had six children; moved from
> the shotgun to a duplex apartment to a
> house and lived the dream—high school
> football on Friday nights...[33]

Bissinger points out just how special Odessa was. In 1987, *Money* magazine
placed Odessa as the fifth worst city (out of 300) to live in. A year later,
Psychology Today ranked Odessa seventh out of 286 metropolitan areas as the
most stressful place to live in terms of alcoholism, crime, suicide and divorce.[34]
Despite its myriad houses of worship (sixty-two Baptist churches, nineteen
Church of Christ churches, twelve Assembly of God churches, eleven
Methodist churches, seven Catholic churches, and five Pentecostal churches),
Bissinger wonders if this aura of religion and correctness did not veil "social
beliefs in racial and gender bigotry," and foster a communal temperament more
insulated than isolated.[35] Nevertheless, true faith had its central arena in the cul-
tural calendar:

> In the absence of a shimmering skyline, the
> Odessas of the country had all found some-

thing similar in which to place their faith. In
Indiana, it was the plink-plink-plink of a
ball on a parquet floor. In Minnesota, it was
the swoosh of skates on the ice. In Texas
and dozens of other states, it was the weekly
event simply known as Friday Night.[36]

James and Bissinger testify to the celebration of community and the transfigura-
tion of sport into popular theater. The Tunapuna Cricket Club and the Panthers
of Permian High School symbolize a game where the onlookers live out their
own hopes and dreams.

God, Country, and Notre Dame

The Reverend Theodore M. Hesburgh was handed a key to a university office in
1952 and found himself at work as the new President of Notre Dame. At a university known for its academic traditions, Hesburgh found himself somewhat
surprised that there he was appointed as its spiritual and academic leader without convocation, installation or speeches. Under Hesburgh's rule Notre Dame
survived the student unrest of the 1990s, gave up its religious governmental
autonomy, and went co-educational. However, during his tenure as President,
Notre Dame stood as a beacon for excellence in academia and athletics.

Chapter five of *God, Country, Notre Dame* is entitled "On the Playing Field."
The opening half paragraph is a synthesis of the ideal-romantic underpinning
that justifies the educational embrace of interscholastic and intercollegiate athletics:

Sports are an important microcosm of life,
for on the playing field all of the important
values of life come into play in a tightened,
heightened framework called the rules of
the game. You win or lose on the playing
field in front of thousands of spectators and
they see, too, how you play the game. It is a
fine training ground for developing character and responsibility in youngsters, which
often derives from the character and integrity of the coach and the college or university
behind them.[37]

In this chapter, Hesburgh describes "bringing the athletics department to heel"[38] and his "athletic" role as President to vouchsafe that honesty and integrity were neither clichés nor recruiting ploys. Players were seen to be student-athletes (in that order), all players were expected to graduate, and cheating by players or coaches would result in immediate dismissal. Hesburgh makes the point that Notre Dame "is an athletic institution and it will continue to grow and prosper as long it continues to do an outstanding job academically."[39] Nevertheless, Notre Dame rid itself of football coach Gerry Faust in the late 1980s because he simply did not win enough games. His reputation in every other respect was impeccable.

Father Hesburgh and C.L.R. James could hardly have been more dissimilar in terms of background and professional calling. Yet both shared a passion for maintaining sport as something good, wholesome and pure. In the 1950s James was profoundly shocked by a national basketball scandal in the USA which revealed collusion between players and bookmakers to "arrange" final scores. Hesburgh in 1989 joined the Knight Foundation for the express reason of revamping university sport with a mission statement to achieve academic integrity, and fiscal integrity:

> We [the Knight Commission] have high
> hopes of eliminating once and for all the
> various kinds of duplicity and fraud that
> seem to pervade college sports from time to
> time... .[40]

Bootlegger's Boy

In 1989, Barry Switzer's world began to implode. Three Oklahoma University football players were charged with rape. Another player faced accusations of shooting a friend, and a fifth player found himself denying charges of dealing in cocaine. Then stories surfaced that Switzer had falsified the Oklahoma University football drug testing program. Switzer was forced to resign.

At the end of *Bootlegger's Boy*, Switzer is full of bittersweet reminiscences. "If life were like a football game, as a coach I would be able to figure out why I had lost."[41] At a United States Olympic Festival in August 1989, two months after his resignation, Switzer was introduced to 76,000 people at Oklahoma's Memorial Stadium. Switzer wondered how the crowd would react:

> As I stepped into the spotlight, I heard the
> steady rumble from the crowd begin, turning
> into a tremendous, ear-shattering standing
> ovation. It moved me with a terrific, warm
> excitement that made me want to laugh and
> cry at the same time.[42]

In many respects, the most moving part is Switzer's recollections of his youth. As with James, the memories of childhood are vivid and propelled with larger than life characters. Switzer's father was a bootlegger and home was a shotgun house built on log supports. There was no electricity, no telephone, no running water, and chickens, dogs, and hogs shared various spaces with the Switzer family. The toilet was a "three-holer outhouse"[43]; entertainment was listening to "the Grand Ole Opry" on a battery radio on Saturday nights. In 1959, Switzer suffered the heartbreak of being at home when his mother committed suicide. In 1972, his father was shot by an angry girlfriend and, in a car wreck on the way to the hospital, they were both burned to death.

Switzer received a scholarship to play football at the University of Arkansas:

> ...the University of Arkansas offered me a lot
> more than just football. I started hitting the
> books and eventually made the dean's list in
> the business department. I learned to be a
> leader and get along with people at the same
> time.[44]

In a foreword to *Bootlegger's Boy*, Penn State's coach, Joe Paterno, underscores the lack of hypocrisy, the deep concern for African American athletes and the candor which were Switzer's hallmarks. Nevertheless, the sheer importance of football at Oklahoma State—in every sense the dominating centrality of its position in the cultural life of the campus and the Norman community—clouded moral judgments:

> It [*Bootlegger's Boy*] is the story of a tough
> man determined to overcome all odds and
> who at times gives way to self-serving ratio-
> nalization to support the rightness of many of
> his actions. It is the story of excesses of
> strong-willed individuals caught up in the
> exhilaration that surrounds great athletes,
> great teams, and being number 1...[45]

Switzer and James eventually found themselves to be controversial spokesmen for the rights of minority athletes. It should be reiterated that it was James, more than any other individual or institution, who paved the way for Frank Worrell to be the first black captain in the history of West Indies representative cricket.

Conclusion

Of the many reviews and retrospectives on the life of C.L.R. James, the vast majority are by white middle class intellectuals. An exception is an essay by fellow West Indian Jervis Anderson. Writing in the *American Scholar,* Anderson gives a marvelous synthesis of what makes *Beyond a Boundary* so special. James gives us an athletic example that deserves application in other cultural milieu and, as this chapter has argued, with other sports. Replace if you will the sport "cricket" with the sport "football" and employ the Jamesian paradigm in the context of the football biographies discussed in this chapter:

> It [*Beyond a Boundary*] is about cricket and more. It is as much about the techniques of cricket as it is about the sociology and psychology of the game. It is about the role that cricket played in the formation of James' character and outlook; about cricket as a medium of entertainment and aesthetic expression; about cricket as a reflection of English manners and temperament and as a model for personal and public ethics.[46]

Notes

[1]Fraser, C.G., "C.L.R. James," *New York Times.* (June 2, 1989), p. D15.

[2]In many of the portraits of James, much is made of his cricket writing duties with the *Manchester Guardian* (1933-1938). However, in *Beyond a Boundary* James notes that he also had a stint with the *Glasgow Herald* (p. 149). The cultural interweave here is fascinating—a West Indian writing about cricket for a newspaper founded in a community where cricket, at best, was a minor sport and with the newspaper's editorial office within walking distance of the homes of soccer giants Glasgow Rangers and Glasgow Celtic. Further studies are called for (if, indeed, they are not already completed), cataloguing, classifying, and analyzing James' total body of written work in the *Manchester Guardian* and the *Glasgow Herald.*

[3]Fraser.

[4]Tennant, I. "C.L.R. James dies," *Times*. (June 1, 1989), p. 44. The obituary to James is in the same issue, p. 16.

[5]Lipsyte, R. "Introduction," to *Beyond a Boundary*. by C.L.R. James. New York: Pantheon Books, 1983, pp. xi-xiv.

[6]James, p. 22.

[7]James, p. 19.

[8]James, p. 26.

[9]James, p. 16.

[10]James, p. 35.

[11]James, p. 40.

[12]James, p. 43.

[13]James, p. 56.

[14]James, p. 82.

[15]James, p. 103.

[16]James, p. 126.

[17]James, p. 148

[18]James, pp. 152-153.

[19]James, p. 168.

[20]James, p. 182.

[21]James, p. 192.

[22]James, p. 194.

[23]James, p. 206.

[24]James, p. 232.

[25]James, p. 252.

[26]This model is based solely on the author's interpretation of Alan Metcalfe's essay on C.L.R. James that appeared in the *Canadian Journal of Sport History*. Any errors or misrepresentations are the responsibility of the author. See, Metcalfe, A., "C.L.R. James' contribution to the history of sport," *Canadian Journal of Sport History* (1989).

[27]Mills, G.R. *Go Big Red!* Urbana: University of Illinois Press, 1991.

[28]Mills, p. 225.

[29]James.

[30]Bissinger, H. G. *Friday night lights - A town, a team, and a dream*. Reading: Addison-Wesley, 1990.

[31]Bissinger, p. 344.

[32]Bissinger, p. 182.

[33]Bissinger, p. 193.

[34]Bissinger, p. 31.

[35]Bissinger, pp. 33-35.

[36]Bissinger, p. 35.

[37]Hesburgh, T.M. & J. Reedy. *God, Country, Notre Dame*. New York: Doubleday, 1990.

[38]Hesburgh & Reedy, p. 81.

[39]Hesburgh & Reedy, p. 89.

[40]Hesburgh & Reedy, p. 91.

[41]Switzer, B., & B. Shrake. *Bootlegger's boy*. New York: Jove Books, 1990.

[42]Switzer & Shrake, p. 383.

[43]Switzer & Shrake, p. 25.

[44]Switzer & Shrake, p. 38.

[45]Switzer & Shrake, p. viii.

[46]Anderson, J. "Cricket and beyond: The career of C.L.R. James," *American Scholar*. (Summer 1985), pp. 345-359.

Part 3: Professional Sport in Global Perspective

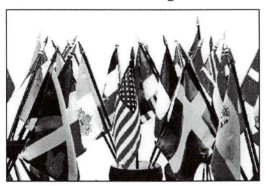

Part 3: Professional Sport in Global Perspective

In the later part of the twentieth century professional sport has undergone rapid and profound changes. Sport owners and producers have attempted to establish footholds in previously untapped markets, elevate the exposure of their product and increase existing market share. The sporadic attempts to establish the World League of American Football in Europe, the Canadian Football League's foray into NFL strongholds and the rise in basketball's global spectator appeal readily exemplifies this position. While the debate over the impact of such cultural imperialism rages on, there can be little dissent over the international fascination with, or heightened cross-cultural awareness of such activities. The exploits of Michael Jordan, Monica Seles, Greg Norman and Jackie Joyner-Kersey are no longer confined merely to the sporting environment. Aided by rapid advancement in technology they are now celebrities on a global stage.

However the relationship between producers and consumers and the resultant delivery of the product is not the only dimension of professional sport that has altered. Increased entrepreneurial activity and changes to the nature of the relationship between labor and management have further internationalized the character of sport. While the former has directly led to a meteoric rise in the commercialization of professional sport and a significant increase in the revenue it produces, the later, in many instances, has resulted in an ongoing struggle between owners and players. Furthermore any gains made by the athletes have been modest and painstakingly achieved.

The two papers in this section illustrate this point well. Braham Dabscheck's study of player associations and unions in Australian sport, and Siegfried Gehrman's work on the rise of professional soccer in Germany, both illustrate numerous historical and organizational impediments to the athletes' desire to be equitably recompensed for their labor. Furthermore these studies illustrate the lack of an active voice on the part of the players in the decision-making process.

Dabscheck draws attention to the irony that although Australia is heavily unionized this has not carried over into the field of sport. He divides the numerous attempts at the establishment of player associations into three groups and classifies them as follows: Organizations with such limited support they did not get off the ground, groups that have had a brief shelf life but eventually faded into oblivion, and those associations that have stood the test of time. This later group is rather small numbering only four. Two are Australian Rules Football groups with the third being the Rugby League Players union of the NSW Rugby League. All three groups are regionally situated which results in a geographical concentration of potential membership. The fourth group is the fledgling player's association of the National Basketball League.

Dabscheck argues that there are two fundamental problems facing Australian player associations. One, the lack of a development of internal effectiveness within the associations and, two, the inability of the groups to establish an external relationship with the relevant governing bodies. Obviously the second is predicated upon the first and this has mitigated against any real development. However the author believes that gains are being slowly made in Australian Rules Football and Rugby that bodes well for the athletes in the respective codes.

Siegfried Gehrman casts his work against the backdrop of a developing homogenous European society and ponders significant questions. He explores the existence of a tendency toward similarities in social profiles and importance of sport consumption in a European culture. Further, he contemplates at what time during the development of sport forms in various countries does sport shed its indigenous characteristic and develop a degree of sameness.

To interpret his framework Gehrman uses the decision of the DFB to introduce professional soccer into Germany highlighting the major components of the decision making process. The author argues that the move was a watershed in the history of German soccer and such a pronouncement would be difficult to refute considering the evidence. There is no doubt that the consolidation of 74 teams in five regional leagues to 16 teams in one superleague is indeed a radical step. However, the argument is well made that the significance of the action lies not in its occurrence but that it took so long to happen. Given reasons for the development of the league are well constructed. Devotees of cricket will see a number of parallels between the development of professional soccer in Germany and changes in professional cricket over the past three decades. The debate in both instances was ideological, revolving around the amateur—professional dichotomy.

Gehrman discusses at length the impact of the decision on the athletes. The enhanced skill level, increased payments and the potential for greater spatial and social mobility are all noted. He also draws attention to the increased interest on the part of the general public in the league. The author concludes that Germany has now caught up with the rest of Europe on the soccer pitch and suggests the same may have occurred in both the social and economic sphere.

If the major characteristics of professional sports are fully explored it is easily determined that there are numerous similarities irrespective of geographical location. Initial resistance to change, lack of empowerment to workers by owners and management, unionization, public acceptance and the development of sport celebrities are features of sport that have little regard for national boundaries. Braham Dabscheck and Siegfried Gehrman have collectively illustrated the above noted conditions very well. They have also demonstrated that there are still significant questions to be analyzed and discussed by sport scholars.

Shayne P. Quick

Chapter 7

Player Associations and Sports Unions in Australia

Braham Dabscheck

Australia is usually regarded as a nation which has a relatively high degree of unionization.[1] While there is evidence that the level of unionization has fallen in recent years, it is estimated that between 40 and 55 per cent of the Australian workforce is unionized.[2] This relatively high level of unionization is generally attributed to the existence of industrial tribunals which, throughout the twentieth century, have regulated relationships between the buyers and sellers of labor. Industrial tribunals have provided unions with legal recognition (virtually eliminating recognition disputes) and a forum for resolving disputes with employers.[3]

While Australia may be regarded as having provided an environment which is conducive to the formation and operation of unions, player associations have not assumed a role of any major significance in the running or governance of their respective sports. From the early decades of this century there have been sporadic, and largely unsuccessful, attempts by the players of a variety of team sports to form associations to protect and advance their collective rights and interests. There are examples of player associations limping on for several years in frustrating, if not vain, attempts to improve the lot of members. There are only two player associations with any longevity in Australia—the Australian Football League Players' Association formed in 1973[4] and the Rugby League Players Union formed in 1979[5]—formed among the players of Australian Rules Football and Rugby League, the two most popular spectator team sports in Australia.

Player associations in Australia are still in their infancy, seeking to carve out a role for themselves in the governance of their respective sports. They have not experienced the success, nor assumed the stature of player associations in other countries such as English soccer's Professional Footballers' Association, or the various associations in the major North American team sports. At worst

125

Australian player associations constitute a minor irritant to club and league officials; at best they are at a stage in their development similar to that of the Professional Footballers' Association in the 1950s and North American player associations in the 1960s, where the respective player bodies developed the skill and verve to obtain a variety of benefits for members.[6] The successful challenge, of the Rugby League Players Union in 1991, in blocking the introduction of an internal draft, the Adamson case (see below), by the New South Wales Rugby League may suggest that some Australian player associations are on the verge of emulating the achievements of their counterparts in English soccer and North American sport.

This chapter will be organized into four sections. Section one will examine various labor market rules which have been introduced by different leagues to control and restrict the employment rights of players. Section two will survey different attempts by players in a variety of competitions to establish player associations. Section three will identify various issues and problems which have dogged player associations in developing the wherewithal to represent and improve the lot of members. Information concerning recent activities of player associations will be presented in section four.

<u>Labor Market Controls in Australian Sport</u>

Australian player associations have sought to pursue the collective interests of players in the context of an unusual or peculiar labor market — a labor market unique to the operation of professional team sports. The leagues and clubs of a variety of sports have instituted a series of labor market controls which have restrained, or restricted, the economic freedom and income earning capacity of players. Distinctions can be drawn between three broad types of labor market controls. They are the recruitment of players, movement of players between clubs, and the use of wage maxima. The major method used in Australian sport to recruit players has been a system of zoning. Under zoning, clubs are granted an exclusive right to recruit players in a designated geographic area. In the 1980s, the Australian Football League[7] introduced various systems of drafting to recruit players, a procedure which it borrowed from professional sports in North America. Under drafting, new players are notionally placed into a common pool where clubs choose players in order, with the club which finished last having first choice, the second last club second choice, and so on with the top club having last choice. This process is repeated a stipulated number of times.[8] This procedure, for drafting new players, has been described as the external draft. The New South Wales Rugby League introduced a similar external draft before the commencement of the 1991 season.

The employment rules of Australian sport traditionally stipulated that once a player signed with a club he was bound to that club for the rest of his playing life under the transfer, or reserve and transfer system. Even following the expiration of his contract a player could not take up employment with another club without first obtaining the permission of his original or 'owning' club. For quality or star players, and even players of lesser ability, such a release usually necessitated the payment of a transfer fee.[9] Prior to the abolition of transfer fees by the Australian Football League in 1988, star players were traded for amounts in the vicinity of $250,000. The New South Wales Rugby League was forced to develop a new system of employment rules in the early 1970s following a High Court decision in the Tutty case, which found its retain and transfer system to be an unreasonable restraint of trade.[10] It subsequently introduced the thirteen import rule which allowed clubs to employ up to thirteen players from outside their zone. In 1983, following negotiations with the Rugby League Players' Union,[11] transfer fees were reintroduced with the size of the fee determined according to an agreed scale, and added measures to safeguard the rights of players.

The Australian Football League revised its employment rules after Mr. Justice Crockett of the Victorian Supreme Court, in the 1983 Foschini case[12], declared its transfer system to be an unreasonable restraint of trade. After a series of experiments, the Australian Football League in 1988, introduced an internal draft to reallocate players between clubs. Unwanted or non-contract existing players[13] could be drafted by clubs according to the same principles which govern the external draft as described above.[14] The New South Wales Rugby League adopted an internal draft before the beginning of the 1991 season. This resulted in a souring of relations with the Rugby League Players Union when it challenged the legality[15] of the internal draft before the Federal Court of Australia (see below).

The officials of various leagues have introduced different systems of maximum wages to control or limit the income of players. Traditionally, limits were placed on the level of income that an individual could earn. In 1985, the Australian Football League introduced a salary cap to limit the total income that clubs could spend on players. The introduction of the salary cap was based on an agreement between the (North American) National Basketball Association and National Basketball Players' Association in 1984.[16] The salary cap enables clubs to negotiate different levels of remuneration with different players, subject to an overall spending limit. At the end of the 1980s both the New South Wales Rugby League and the National Basketball League introduced salary caps. For the 1992 season the Australian Football League had a club salary cap of $1.5

million (with a 52-man roster[17]); the New South Wales Rugby League $1.6 million (57-man roster); and the National Basketball League $375,000 (12-man roster).[18]

Player Associations Down Under

Research so far indicates that there have been eighteen attempts by the players of a variety of different Australian team sports to form player associations. These eighteen attempts can be divided into three distinct categories. First, there is the situation where an attempt is made to form an association; however the person or persons proposing the development of such an association are unable to attract enough interest and support from players to bring the association into being. Or, to borrow a term from baseball, the attempt fails to reach 'first base'. Second an association is formed, operates for a period of time, experiences problems which it is unable to overcome, becomes moribund and/or subsequently disbands. The third situation is those associations which have survived the test of time.

Ten examples of the first type of player association can be identified. Sandercock and Turner, in their pioneering work on the development of Australian rules football in Victoria, mention three unsuccessful attempts by players to form a union or association in 1913, 1931, and 1944.[19] Rugby League's 1952/53 Kangaroos[20] discussed the possibility of forming a union to advance the interests of Rugby league players.[21] Following the formation of the Australian Football League Players' Association in 1973 there was an attempt by former Hawthorn player Bob Keddie to establish a similar body for players of the South Australian National Football League.[22] In 1974 there was also talk amongst players of the New South Wales Rugby League on forming an association on similar lines to those of the Australian Football League Players' Association.[23] John McQuaid, of the Australia Theatrical and Amusement Employees' Association, maintained that players would benefit from being covered by an award of an industrial tribunal.[24] At the end of 1978 Redcliffe player Bob Jones mooted the possible formation of a union in the Brisbane Rugby league competition.[25]

In February 1960 the (English soccer's) Professional Footballers' Association received a letter from a Mr. R. Haddington, a former Manchester City player, of his intention to form a players' association for Australian soccer players.[26] In 1989 goalkeeper Tony Pezanno, and former international player John Kosmina, spoke of the need for players of the National Soccer League to form a players' association.[27] Peter Allen, the executive director of the Australian Football League Players' Association, has informed the author that he has received a number of requests from players of the National Soccer League concerning problems they have experienced with their employment and contracts. East Perth player Glen Bartlett, who at the time was in the employ of the Federated Clerks Union, attempted in 1988 to establish an association of players, umpires and trainers in the Western Australian Football League. Umpires were experiencing difficulties with football administrators over payments. However, once this issue was resolved the umpires lost interest in the idea of an association, as did the trainers, which put an end to the formation of such a body.[28]

Four examples of players associations which fall into the second category can be identified, two in Australian rules football, the third in cricket, and the fourth in soccer. In 1914 players of the Victorian Football League and the Victorian Football Association[29] formed the Victorian Footballers' Council. The Council wished "to assist, in full loyalty, at all times, the club committees in the protection of both the game and the players, and to raise funds by donations, subscriptions, etc, to provide (1) retiring allowances to members, and (2) to assist members, when the executive may decide, in case of accident or illness."[30] The Council folded with the advent of World War I.

In 1955 former St. Kilda player Tom McNeil sought to organize players of both the Victorian Football League and Victorian Football Association into the Australia Football Players' Union. He decided on this course of action following an overseas trip where he had come into contact with a number of European soccer players' unions. The Australian Football Players' Union found it difficult to attract members, with a total membership of 178, or a unionization rate of approximately 20%. Moreover, it experienced difficulties in obtaining recognition from clubs, the League, and the Association. Following an unsuccessful attempt to obtain recognition as a trade union under the (Commonwealth) *Conciliation and Arbitration Act* of 1904, the union disbanded in 1956.[31]

During the early and mid 1970s, Australia's leading cricketers believed that they were inadequately compensated for the time they devoted to cricket, and that the Australian Cricket Board did not take account of their needs when making decisions. Under the leadership of Ian Chappell, the players felt that their position would be enhanced by forming a players' association. During the mid 1970s they had discussions with Bob Hawke, president of the Australian Council of Trade Unions, to discuss ways and means to enhance the welfare of players. In 1977 business magnate Kerry Packer capitalized on this player discontent in forming World Series Cricket, a rival competition (or breakaway league). Packer's decision to develop his own competition followed the refusal of the Australian Cricket Board to grant his television network rights to televise international or Test Match cricket.[32]

With the advent of World Series Cricket, players formed the Professional Cricketers' Association of Australia, with Packer providing a $10,000 loan to aid in its establishment! In early 1979 the Cricketers' Association was registered under the New South Wales *Companies Act* 1961. In 1979 Packer and the Australian Cricket Board negotiated a truce whereby Packer discontinued his rival competition in exchange for the rights to televise Test Match and One Day cricket.[33] Following this merger the Cricketers' Association sought to expand its membership to Board[34] players. At its height the Association had 67 members, or approximately seventy-five per cent of regular first class players. The Cricketers' Association was mainly constrained by the problem of having a small membership evenly distributed across six states in a continent as large as Australia. In addition, the Australian Cricket Board's use of a player representation system in a Cricket Sub-Committee,[35] and the appointment of a coordinator to act as an intermediary between the Board and players frustrated the Association's attempts to be recognized by the Board. The Cricketers' Association was moribund by 1982, and officially wound up in 1988.[36]

In 1976 a group of Western Australian soccer players held a meeting in the Norwood Hotel, East Perth and formed the Soccer Players' Association. The founder of this body was Reg Davies, who had formerly played in the United Kingdom and had been a member of the Professional Footballers' Association. In forming the Soccer Players' Association Davies sought advice from his former union. The Constitution of the Soccer Players' Association bears a striking similarity to that of the Professional Footballers' Association. The Soccer Players' Association was registered under the Western Australian *Association Incorporation Act* 1895. The major functions performed by the Soccer Players' Association were to represent players in contract and employment disputes with clubs, to organize an end of season mini-'World Cup' between players of different nationalities in the form of a social get-together, and to provide an award for a players' player of the year. At its height the Soccer Players' Association had 308 members, a unionization rate of approximately ninety per cent with the Western Australian Soccer Federation having a ten-team competition with three grades. With the passing years, however, the Soccer Players' Association found it difficult to recruit members, and find replacements for committee members who retired from the game. Eric Marocchi, a former leading official describes the players, body as being 'currently dormant', though he is hopeful that it will be revived in the future.[37]

Australia currently has four player associations. The oldest body is the Australian Football League Players' Association formed by Essendon player Geoff Pryor at the end of 1973.[38] Since its formation the Association has represented approximately between sixty and seventy per cent of players, having, at different times, experienced problems with North Melbourne, Geelong, Richmond, and Brisbane Bears in being able to recruit players. In negotiations completed in 1990, concerning a Standard Playing Contract, the Australian Football League agreed that all clubs should provide access to the Association to enable it to recruit members,[39] which in turn has led to an increase in membership. At various times the Australian Football League Players' Association has flirted with the idea of affiliating with the Australian Council of Trade Unions, or seeking registration as a trade union under industrial relations legislation.[40] This latter objective will be difficult to achieve under 1991 amendments to the (Commonwealth) *Industrial Relations Act* of 1988, which impose a minimum registration level of 10,000 members.[41]

While the Australian Football League Players' Association has been recognized by the Australian Football League it would not be too unfair to state that it has found it difficult to obtain or wrest concessions from the League. At various times it has threatened the use of strike action. In 1974 it indicated its preparedness to strike when the League foreshadowed the abolition of the ten-year rule—a rule which enabled players with ten years' service with a club to seek employment with other clubs free of the encumbrance of the transfer system. The League ignored the threat and duly abolished the rule; the players' association did not act on its threat.[42] In late 1980/early 1981 the League withdrew recognition of the Association. A threat by Essendon and Fitzroy players not to play in the opening round of the night competition, however, resulted in the League backing down and agreeing to again recognize the Association.[43] In 1988, the League and the players' body agreed to the introduction of a Standard Playing Contract. In 1989 and 1990 the Association threatened strike action in negotiating changes to the Standard Playing Contract. Notwithstanding its ability to obtain some concessions this agreement, which the Australian Football League heralded as 'A Moratorium' (on challenges to its employment laws) and the Players' Association as 'A Collective Bargain', enshrined the League's zoning, drafting, and salary cap rules, as well as enabling clubs to cut players and their payments during the life of a contract.[44]

Western Australian Ian Miller played with Fitzroy in the Australian Football League in the 1970s, being a member of the Players' Association. After returning to the west he formed the Western Australian Football League Players' Association in 1979. The organization did not experience problems attracting members; however, it found it difficult to develop a bargaining relationship with, and secure concessions from, the Western Australian Football League. Following the announcement that the West Coast Eagles would enter the

Australian Football League,[45] the players' association went into limbo in 1986[46], and only continued to exist by virtue of some monies held in a bank account. As already mentioned above, East Perth player Glenn Bartlett unsuccessfully sought to form an association of players, umpires and trainers in 1988 (apparently unaware of the association that had operated in Western Australian football). In 1990 it was suggested that the balance of the Western Australian Football League Players' Association funds, held in the bank, could be used to help pay Western Australia's costs of competing in the Teal Cup (a junior interstate competition). Bartlett, as a club captain and senior player, was contacted to see if these funds could be made available for the Teal Cup side. His answer was no and he initiated action to revamp the players' association. A new committee was elected in 1991 and recognition was obtained from the Western Australian Football Commission. With the retirement of several senior players, however, the Association experienced problems in filling committee positions at the beginning of the 1992 season. At this stage it is unclear what the future of the Association will be.[47]

In 1979 a group of players, former players, coaches, accountants and lawyers formed the Rugby League Players' Union in the New South Wales Rugby League. Following the election of coach Jack Gibson as President, in 1980, the Union experienced growth and development. It was registered under the New South Wales *Trade Union Act* of 1881, in 1980, and the *Industrial Arbitration Act* of 1940, in 1984. Notwithstanding its registration, the Rugby League Players' Union has only recently begun to make use of industrial tribunals in New South Wales. In 1990 the New South Wales Industrial Commission was activated in resolving an intra-union dispute when Kevin Ryan replaced John Adam as leader, on a ticket of opposition to the New South Wales Rugby League's proposed introduction of drafting.[48] Following its subsequent victory in challenging the legality of the draft the Union has initiated action before the industrial tribunal to obtain an award specifying minimum terms and conditions of employment for players (see below).

The Union has, generally speaking, had in excess of ninety per cent of players enrolled as members. Despite some initial problems the Union obtained recognition from the New South Wales Rugby League. Between 1982 and 1989 the two bodies experienced cordial relations with Union representatives being appointed to the League's General and Judiciary Committees (the latter is concerned with determining the innocence or guilt, and penalties, of players accused of rough play). Following the New South Wales Rugby League's announcement of its intention to introduce a draft, relationships between the two substantially deteriorated. There were also disputes between the League and the Union, during 1990, concerning the administration and rights of players associated with drug testing.[49] In 1991 the Union affiliated with the Labor Council of New South Wales.

Players in the National Basketball League formed the Basketball Players' Association of Australia, in 1989. Led by international representatives Larry Sengstock and Damian Keogh the Association has achieved between forty-five and seventy per cent of membership coverage, and has been recognized and enjoys a good working relationship with League administrators. The players have representatives on basketball's salary cap and competition management committees. There has been some talk of the basketball players making use of, or sharing, the administrative structure of the Australian Football League Players' Association[50] (both organizations use the same firm of solicitors). Kevin Ryan, of the Rugby League Players' Union, believes that eventually there will be a single union covering persons from all sports in Australia.[51]

Problems Confronting Australian Player Associations

Player associations have experienced a number of problems in seeking to defend and advance the rights and interests of members. These problems can be broadly distinguished into two categories: the development of internal effectiveness, and the ability, or inability, to develop an external, or bargaining, relationship with the clubs and leagues of their respective sporting competitions. The two, of course, are highly interdependent. A player body lacking internal effectiveness will find it difficult to obtain concessions for members from clubs and the league and, at the same time, an inability to obtain concessions from employers will make it difficult for the player body to demonstrate its usefulness and relevance to players. The discussion will begin with an examination of issues associated with the internal organizational effectiveness of player associations.

Other than the peculiar labor market arrangements which govern the employment of players of professional team sports (see above), the most distinctive feature of the employment of players is the shortness of their playing life. With the unremitting pressure on maintaining form and the ever-present risk of injury, only a small number of highly skilled players last in the game for ten years or more, and/or are still playing in their thirties. In the Australian Football League, for example, as of July 1 1992 only 39, or approximately five per cent, of senior listed players were over thirty years of age.[52] When a young player enters the game he may easily be carried along by the game's glamour and kudos, with his thoughts directed to establishing a regular first-team place, rather than worrying about issues associated with employment rights. Moreover, club management will assure our young hopeful that the club will always do the right thing by him, as long as he realizes his unlimited promise. In addition, the payment of relatively 'high' incomes to star players may convince a young player that life can be fairly sweet for those who excel at professional sport. With the passing years the glamour of the game may begin to wear off. Players may start to think more seriously about their profession and the associated conduct and operation of their sport. However, by now they may be near the end of their career, and will become concerned about what life and future employment (and income) prospects await them once they retire from the game.

The implications of this phenomenon for player associations are twofold. First, there is a relatively high degree of apathy among players concerning their employment rights and the role and function of player associations. In the words of John Adam, a former President of the Rugby League Players' Union:

> It must always be remembered that players are extremely apathetic and they will not rally to any cause unless they are directly affected... Players... will not turn up to meetings... and provide little input.[53]

Second, the constant turnover of players/members means that player associations experience difficulties in developing any sense of continuity, and impose costs with having to educate new members as to the needs or rationale of having such an association.

The membership of Australian player associations is, and has been, small. The 1955 Australian Football Players' Union only attracted 178 members. The Professional Cricketers' Association of Australia, in the early 1980s, had a maximum membership of 67, spread across the length and breadth of the Australian continent! The (Western Australian) Soccer Players' Association had a maximum membership of 308. The maximum membership of the Rugby League Players' Union is 912 (16 teams by a 57-player roster), 796 for the Australian Football League Players' Association (13 by 52, and the Sydney Swans and Brisbane Bears by 60), 156 for the Basketball Players' Association of Australia (13 by 12), and up to 500 for the Western Australian Football League Players' Association.

All player associations have, or have had, low membership subscriptions. The membership fee of the Soccer Players' Association was $5. During its first regency between 1979 and 1986 the Western Australian Football League

Players' Association initially set its membership fee at $10 for senior players (less for juniors), which it subsequently increased to $12. Following its revival, under the leadership of Glenn Bartlett, joining fees were set at $2, with an annual fee of $10. The cricketers initially determined their membership fees at $50, and lowered them to $25 following the compromise/merger between Kerry Packer and the Australian Cricket Board. The basketball players have set their fees at $20. Throughout the 1980s Rugby league players had an annual fee of $20, which increased in 1991 to $100 for senior, and $30 for junior, players. In 1992 the Australian Football League Players' Association increased its membership subscription to $90. Player associations have also supplemented their income by sponsorships and product endorsements.[54]

A small or low membership base and low subscription levels translate into low incomes, which reduce the ability of player associations to provide services for members and pursue issues on their behalf. As a result of low income player associations have experienced leadership problems. They have not generated enough revenue to employ persons who could devote all their time, and provide them with the necessary wherewithal, to pursue the needs of players. Individual players have either performed these functions themselves, in addition to their commitments as players, and other obligations or, alternatively, they have relied on former players and other individuals, to work on behalf of the association in an honorary, but nonetheless part-time capacity. For example, both John Adam and Kevin Ryan, the current and previous Presidents of the Rugby League Players' Union, both of whom were former players, have performed their functions in the spare time provided by working in a legal practice. Peter Allen, who has guided the affairs of the Australian Football League Players' Association since 1980, has performed this function in the context of a business which is devoted to sports promotion.

Player associations have also experienced difficulties in obtaining recognition and/or developing a bargaining relationship with the clubs and leagues of their respective sports. The 1955 Australian Football Players' Union failed to gain recognition from the Victorian Football League and the Victorian Football Association. The Australian Cricket Board used a Cricket Sub-Committee and a cricket coordinator to deflect the establishment of a bargaining relationship with the Professional Cricketers' Association of Australia. Both the Basketball Players' Association and the revamped Western Australian Football League Players' Association have received recognition from their respective leagues. However, developments in both sports are embryonic at this stage, and more time will need to pass to determine the tone of the bargaining relationships that may develop.

Except for a period in the early 1980s, the Australian Football League Players' Association has been recognized by the Australian Football League. While the Association can point to some gains it has achieved,[55] and in 1990 secured some modifications in negotiations concerning Standard Playing Contracts (see above), it has nonetheless found it difficult to obtain concessions from the League. The League has been able to introduce major changes to labor market arrangements governing the employment of players, with little or limited involvement from the players' association. Such examples would be the abolition of the ten-year rule in 1974, introduction of the salary cap, determination of the size of salary caps, and the introduction of various drafting systems.

Following its desire to re-introduce transfer fees in 1983, the New South Wales Rugby League was prepared to enter into negotiations and discuss various issues with the Rugby League Players' Union. This preparedness to negotiate with the union, however, could be interpreted as an attempt by the League to use collective bargaining to shield themselves from any legal attacks which may have been mounted against the new transfer system in light of the High Court's decision in the Tutty case. Relationships between the two bodies substantially deteriorated when the League announced its intention to introduce drafting.

Recent Developments

Undoubtedly the most significant development which has occurred in Australian sports industrial relations has been the Rugby League Players' Union's legal challenge to the introduction of the internal draft. Under the internal draft, current players who had not negotiated a new contract with their club were placed into a pool, to be drafted or selected by clubs, with the worst performing club having first choice, and the first place club last choice, with the procedure repeated a number of times. The Rugby League Players' Union was initially unsuccessful in its quest to have the internal draft declared illegal. In February 1991, Mr. Justice Hill of the Federal Court of Australia, found the internal draft, in what he described as 'a borderline case', not to be an unreasonable restraint of trade.[56]

In September 1991, a Full Bench of the Federal Court, comprising Justices Sheppard, Wilcox, and Gummow, overturned Mr. Justice Hill's decision. Mr. Justice Wilcox, for example, said that:

> ...the right to choose between prospective
> employers is a fundamental element of a
> free society. It is the existence of that right

which separates the free person from the
serf.[57]

The New South Wales Rugby League, in October 1991, unsuccessfully sought
special leave from the High Court to appeal the decision of the Full Bench of
the Federal Court. The transcript of that hearing reveals the following statement
made by Mr. Conti, the New South Wales Rugby League's legal counsel:

> ...a restraint which deals with, or addresses,
> the right to choose one's prospective
> employer, as they [the Full Bench of the
> federal Court] put it, was if I could use the
> expression, inherently or almost inherently
> unreasonable. You could not jump, really,
> over that hurdle. That, of course, is terribly
> important to us because it means that if that
> principle is maintained, and it is doubtless
> as important for Australian rules, then any
> form of draft in the end is not just open to
> us.[58]

If the Rugby League Players' Union had been unsuccessful in the Adamson
case it is likely that the legal costs involved would have forced it to disband or,
at a minimum, be reduced to virtual impotence.[59] Adamson has not only stuck
an important blow against labor market controls,[60] but has also enhanced the
stature of the Rugby League Players' Union.

Since the draft case the Rugby League Players' Union has embarked on a campaign of obtaining an award for Rugby league players establishing various minimum terms and conditions of employment.[61] During January and February 1992
there was a degree of disquiet between the Union and the League and clubs,
concerning the playing of a 'World Sevens'[62] competition, as a pre-season promotion. The major issues of concern to the Union were payments to players and
possible problems associated with clubs terminating contracts for players
injured during the competition. Mr. Justice Hill (a different Mr. Justice Hill
from that of the Federal Court who initially heard the Adamson case), of the
Industrial Commission of New South Wales, directed the parties to resolve such
issues via negotiations. Eventually, the clubs agreed to provide indemnities for
players if they were injured during the 'Sevens' and, with some minor exceptions, to split prize money with players on a 50-50 basis.[63]

Again, following directions from the Industrial Commission of New South Wales, the Union and the League are in the process of negotiating a first award for players of professional team sports in Australia. For its part, the Australian Football League Players' Association is in the process of negotiating a new collective bargaining agreement with the Australian Football League. They are entering into such negotiations with the knowledge of the Adamson case having declared the external draft to be an unreasonable restraint of trade.

As a result of the Adamson case both the Rugby League Players' Union and the Australian Football League Players' Association may be on the verge of establishing a more significant role for themselves in the operation and governance of their respective sports. It will be interesting to observe how future events unfold.

Notes

---

[1]See Price, R. "Trade union membership." In Bean, R. (ed.), *International labour statistics: A handbook, guide and recent trends.* London: Routledge, 1989, pp.146-181, for comparative data on trade union membership for nations belonging to the Organization for Economic Co-operation and Development.

[2]The Australian Bureau of Statistics Survey of *Trade Union Members* for August 1990 provides the lower figure, while a survey of *Trade Unions* for June 1991 provides the higher figure.

[3]For further discussion concerning Australia's system of industrial relations, the role of industrial tribunals, and their relationship with unions see Dabscheck, B. and J. Niland, *Industrial Relations in Australia.* Sydney: George Allen and Unwin, 1981; McCallum, R.C., M.J. Pittard, and G.F.Smith, *Australian labour law: Cases and materials* (second edition). Sydney: Butterworths, 1990; and; Deery, S.J. and D.H. Plowman, *Australian industrial relations* (third edition). Melbourne: Mc Graw-Hill, 1991.

[4]It was originally called the Victorian Football League Players' Association. Prior to the 1990 season the Victorian Football League changed its name to the Australian Football League which resulted in a change of the name of the Players' Association.

[5]Its original title was the Association of Rugby League Professionals. The change of name occurred in 1991.

[6]For accounts of the activities of player associations in English soccer and North America see Dabscheck, B. "'Defensive Manchester': A history of the Professional Footballers' Association," In, Cashman, R. and M. McKernan, (eds.), *Sport in history: The making of modern sporting traditions.* St Lucia: University of Queensland Press, 1979, pp. 227-257; Dabscheck, B. "Beating

the off-side trap: The case of the Professional Footballers' Association." *Industrial Relations Journal*, 17: 4 (1986), pp. 350-361; Dabscheck, B. "'A man or a puppet?': The Football Association's 1909 attempt to destroy the Association Football Players' Union." *The International Journal of the History of Sport*, 8: 2 (1991), pp. 221-238; Harding, J. *For the good of the game: The official history of the Professional Footballers' Association.* London: Robson, 1991; Scoville, J.G. "Labor relations in sports." In Noll, R.G. (ed.), *Government and the sports business.* Washington: Brookings, 1974, pp. 185-219; Dworkin, J.B. *Owners versus players: Baseball and collective bargaining.* Boston: Auburn House, 1981; Berry, R.C., and W.B. Gould, "A long deep drive to collective bargaining: Of players, owners, brawls and strikes." *Case Western Reserve Law Review*, 31: 4(1981), pp. 685-813; Berry, R.C., W.B. Gould and P.D. Staudohar, *Labor relations in professional sports.* Dover (Mass): Auburn House, 1986; Staudohar, P.D. *The sports industry and collective bargaining* (second edition). Ithaca: Industrial and Labor Relations Press, 1989; Miller, M. *A whole different ball game: The sport and business of baseball.* New York: Birch Lane Press, 1991; Voigt, D. Q. "Serfs versus magnates: A century of labor strife in major league baseball." In, Staudohar, P.D. and J.A. Mangan (eds.), *The business of professional sports.* Urbana: University of Illinois Press, 1991, pp. 95-114; Korr, C.P. "Marvin Miller and the new unionism in baseball." In, Staudohar, P.D. and J.A. Mangan, (eds.), *The business of professional sports.* Urbana: University of Illinois Press, 1991, pp. 115-134.

[7]See footnote 4.

[8]On some occasions the Australian Football League has allowed poor performing clubs several draft choices ahead of other clubs.

[9]See Dabscheck, B. "Sporting equality: Labour market vs product market control." *The Journal of Industrial Relations*, 17: 2 (1975), pp. 174-190, for a critical examination of the Australian (Victorian) Football League's zoning and transfer system.

[10]125 *Commonwealth Law Reports* p. 353.

[11]See footnote 5.

[12]Unreported. *Foschini vs VFL and South Melbourne* (Supreme Court of Victoria, 1982), No. 9868.

[13]Clubs could also trade such players at the end of the season for other players or external draft choices. Such trades are not allowed to be oiled by the exchange of money. The Australian Football League, following representations from the players' association, also has a mid-season voluntary draft for players who are cut from club lists during the season.

[14]For a detailed examination and critique of the draft see Dabscheck, B. "Abolishing transfer fees: The Victorian Football League's new employment

rules." *Sporting Traditions*, 6: 1 (1989), pp. 63-87.

[15]The various controls governing the recruitment and transfer of players have been a continuing source of litigation—though only the New South Wales Rugby League's draft has been challenged by a players' association. For reviews of the case law see Beiker, N. and P. Von Nessen, "Sports and restraint of trade: Playing the game the court's way," *Australian Business Law Review*, 13: 4 (1985), pp. 180-197; Dabscheck, B. "Sporting labour markets and the courts." *Sporting Traditions*, 2: 1 (1985), pp. 2-24; Kelly, G.M. *Sport and the law: An Australian perspective.* Sydney: Law Book Company, 1987; Owen-Conway, S. and L. Owen-Conway, "Sport and restraint of trade," *Australian Bar Review.* 5 (1989), pp. 208-224; Smith, G. and H. Opie, "The withering of individualism: Professional team sports and employment law." Paper presented at The Law of Professional Team Sports Conference, Melbourne, Victoria, May 1991; Ward, B. "The player contract - A comparative analysis." Paper presented at The Law of Professional Team Sports Conference, Melbourne, Victoria, May 1991; Love, C. "Drafts, salary caps and the New South Wales Rugby League case." Paper presented at The Law of Professional Team Sports Conference, Melbourne, Victoria, May 1991; McDonagh, M. "Restrictive provisions in player agreements." *Australian Journal of Labour Law.* 4: 2 (1991), pp. 126-150; Browne, J. "Playing contracts." In *Sports and the Law.* Business Law Education Centre, September 1991, pp. 43-88; Lindgren, K.E. "Sport and the law: The player's contract." *Journal of Contract Law*, 4: 2 (1991), pp. 135-145.

[16]For details concerning the negotiation and operation of the salary cap in North American basketball see Berry, R.C. and G.M. Wong, *Law and business of the sports industries, Volume I, Professional sports leagues.* Dover (Mass): Auburn House, 1986, pp. 165-169, and pp. 391-402; Berry, Gould, and Staudohar, pp. 181-188; and Staudohar, pp. 109-113.

[17]The Sydney Swans and Brisbane Bears are allowed 60-man rosters because of problems associated with being in non-traditional Australian football states. These clubs have also been provided with additional income to defray the costs involved with players moving interstate.

[18]Whether or not clubs spend all of the money they are entitled to under their salary caps, is dependent on the existence of drafts, the mix between guaranteed and performance based pay, and the success of the club on the field.

[19]Sandercock, L., and I. Turner. *Up where, Cazaly?: The great Australian game.* London: Granada, 1981, pp. 60, 121, and 123.

[20]This is the nickname given to teams which tour or play representative matches against overseas teams.

[21]Interview with Martin Gallagher, Official of the Rugby League Players' Union, Padstow, June 14, 1990.

[22]Football Times, mimeo, not dated. Information supplied by Bernard Whimpress, South Australian National Football League.

[23]*Rugby League Week,* August 24, 1974.

[24]*Daily Telegraph,* April 20, 1974.

[25]*The Australian,* August 11, 1978.

[26]*Minutes of Management Committee, Professional Footballers' Associations,* 14 February 1960.

[27]*The Australian,* April 7, 1989, December 21, 1989 and, January 11, 1990.

[28]Telephone interview with Glenn Bartlett, President, Western Australian Football League Players' Association, April 17, 1991.

[29]The Victorian Football Association was formed in 1877. At the end of the 1896 season, eight clubs broke away to form the Victorian Football League. As already mentioned the latter changed its name to the Australian Football League at the end of the 1990 season. The Association and the League have been rivals since 1896. For details concerning the breakaway see Sandercock & Turner, pp. 38-53.

[30]Quoted in Sandercock & Turner, p. 60.

[31]*84 Commonwealth Arbitration Reports 675.* For an account of the activities of the union see Dabscheck, B. "Out of bounds. The 1955 Australian Football Players' Union." *Journal of Australian Studies,* 27 (1990), pp. 32-39.

[32]For accounts of the developments of World Series Cricket see Forsyth, C. *The great cricket hijack.* Camberwell: Widescope, 1978; and McFarline, P. *A game divided.* London: Marlin, 1978. For an examination of the legal battles associated with World Series Cricket see Scott, J. *Caught in court.* London: Andre Deutsch, 1989, pp. 100-111.

[33]Most first class cricket matches are played over several days, with Test Matches currently running to five days. The apparent length of such games does not necessarily guarantee a result. Approximately thirty per cent of the Test Matches Australia has played in have resulted in a draw. One-day cricket is an attempt to produce a contest which guarantees a result. Such matches are looked on with disdain by purists.

[34]The Australian Cricket Board also organized domestic, or interstate, as well as international matches. The Cricketers' Association was seeking to enroll state players.

[35]David Richards, the Chief Executive of the Australian Cricket Board, regards it as "a very, very important committee, probably the most important committee the Board's got." Egan, J. *Extra cover.* Sydney: Pan, 1989, p. 331.

[36]For further details concerning the activities of the Cricketers' Associations see Dabscheck, B. "The Professional Cricketers' Association of Australia." *Sporting Traditions.* 8: 1 (1991), pp. 2-27.

[37]The information contained in this paragraph is based on a telephone interview with Eric Marocchi, Official of the Soccer Players' Association, April 24, 1992.

[38]For details concerning its formation see Dabscheck, B. "Industrial relations and professional team sports in Australia." *The Journal of Industrial Relations,* 18: 1 (1976), pp. 28-44. See also Stewart, B. *The Australian football business: A spectator's guide to the VFL.* Kenthurst: Kangaroo Press, 1983, pp. 91-96.

[39]*Inside Aussie Rules,* (Australian Football League Players' Association Members' Newsletter), December 1990.

[40]See *The Australian* May 18, 1978, July 20, 1978, August 1, 1978, March 28, 1979; *The Age* July 19, 1990 and; Halfpenny, K. "When good sports flex industrial muscle." *Workplace: The ACTU magazine,* (1991), pp. 6-9.

[41]Discretion exists for the registration of smaller unions; however, the status of such small unions is subjected to regular reviews. It is conceivable that if the Australian Football League Players' Association obtained support from the Australian Council of Trade Unions it could be successful in obtaining registration.

[42]For details see Dabscheck (1976), pp. 38-40.

[43]Interview with Peter Allen, Melbourne, July 9, 1990.

[44]For details of these negotiations see *The Australian* July 8, 1989, June 19, 1990, July 13 and 16, 1990; *The Sun* June 18, 19 and 29, 1990, and July 12 and 14, 1990; and *The Age* July 12, 14, 19 and 21, 1990. Ward claims that this contract is unfairly weighted against players. Browne (1991), the Australian Football League's solicitor, offers a contrary view, and claims that the League has made important concessions to the Players' Association.

[45]The Australian Football League was traditionally a twelve team competition based in Melbourne, with a regional team from Geelong. In 1982, South Melbourne moved north and became known as the Sydney Swans. In 1987, the competition was expanded to fourteen with clubs from Brisbane (even though it played most of its games on the Gold Coast) and Perth. In 1991, a team from Adelaide entered the League. The major motivation for transformation from a city to a national competition has been a desire for sponsorship and advertising revenue associated with exposure on national television. The New South Wales Rugby League has also expanded regionally and interstate, though so far only into Queensland and the Australian Capital Territory. It has been mooted that new teams may be located in other (Australian Rules football) states and New Zealand. Cricket has traditionally been an interstate competition. Both soccer and basketball are organized on a national basis, since 1977 and 1979 respectively.

[46]See Buti, T. "History of the WAFL players' association." *Papers in labour history,* No. 4, Perth Branch, Australian Society for the Study of Labour History, 1989, pp. 42-51, for an account of the association's activities up to this point.

[47]Telephone interviews with Glenn Bartlett, January 17, 1991, April 17, 1991, and April 9, 1992. Also see Industrial Relations Society of Western Australia, *Newsletter,* November 1990.

[48]*Industrial Commission of New South Wales,* Mr. Justice Bauer, No. 271/90 (Not reported).

[49]For details see Sydney daily newspapers in the period June to August 1990.

[50]*The Sydney Morning Herald,* March 29, 1990; *The Australian,* March 30, 1990; *Basketball Week,* April 24, 1991; Interview with Damien Keogh, Official of the Basketball Players' Association of Australia, Wollaware, May 2, 1990. Telephone Interviews, September 6, 1990, April 15, 1991 and April 9, 1992.

[51]*The Sydney Morning Herald,* February 22, 1992.

[52]Data based on AFL '92. *The Football Record,* May 7, 8, 9, 10, 1992 reports that there are only 11 players in the Australian Football League who first played in the 1970s.

[53]Adam, J. "Representing player interests in professional team sports." Paper presented at Sport and the Law workshop, Launceston, Tasmania, June 1989, p. 23. It should be noted that similar statements could be made by the great majority of union leaders.

[54]The Major League Baseball Players' Association has derived substantial income from such endorsements. See Miller, pp. 142-152. The Professional Footballers' Association derives much of its income from a share of television rights. In 1992 they were involved in a dispute, successful as it turned out over such shares, with the organizers of the new Premier League in English soccer.

[55]For example see "A Summary of Major Accomplishments by the VFLPA 1980-1988," *On The Ball,* VFLPA, April 12, 1988.

[56]*(1991) 27 Federal Court Reports 535.*

[57]Unreported. *Adamson and Ors vs New South Wales Rugby League and Ors.* (Full Bench of Federal Court of Australia, New South Wales Registry, 1991) No. G79. The quote comes from p. 45 of Mr. Justice Wilcox's decision.

[58]*Transcript, New South Wales Rugby League and Ors vs Adamson and Ors, High Court of Australia, Registry* Sydney, October 24, 1991, No. S127 of 1991, p.14.

[59]The Australian Football Players' Union disbanded after it failed to obtain registration before the Commonwealth Court of Conciliation and Arbitration. See Dabscheck (1990). The Professional Footballers' Association was reduced to

virtual impotence following an unfavorable decision in the 1912 Kingaby case (unreported). For details see Dabscheck (1979).

[60]In 1991 the Victorian Supreme Court declared qualifying periods for residential qualifications for cricketers to be an unreasonable restraint of trade. Unreported. *Nobes vs Australian Cricket Board* (Supreme Court of Victoria, 1991). No 13613. Also see 1982 Victorian Reports 64 which found the Australian Football League's zoning system to be an unreasonable restraint of trade.

[61]See *Industrial Commission of New South Wales*, No. 26 of 1992.

[62]Rugby League is played with 13 players a side. 'Sevens', a competition borrowed from the amateur Rugby Union code (Rugby League split from Rugby Union over the issue of payment to players for lost time from work and injuries) where seven players a side play a shortened game. 'Sevens' provides a free-flowing game with high scoring and has proved to be popular with spectators.

[63]For details see *Daily Telegraph Mirror*, January 17, 1992; *The Sydney Morning Herald* January 18, 1992, January 31, 1992, February 4, 1992, February 5, 1992, February 6, 1992, February 7, 1992, February 8, 1992; and *The Australian* February 6, 1992.

Chapter 8

Keeping Up with Europe: The Introduction of Professionalism into German Soccer in 1962/63

Siegfried Gehrmann

The current discussion on the unification of Europe is centered on politics in the widest sense. At the center of this interest are the proposed concepts and decisions of individual governments and parliaments with respect to economic and political integration. One question has received less attention, however: how far, in contrast to various spectacular plans and proposals, Europe actually has progressed on the way towards integration. That is, how far the everyday value systems and ways of life of the various national social groups in Europe have progressed towards assimilation and acceptance of each other and are thus on the way towards the formation of an homogeneous "European Society." In this context one must think of the whole field of pastime and leisure and, in this, of such important spheres as entertainment and sports. Concerning the last-mentioned paradigm one should not only ask to what extent certain sport disciplines share similar quantitative importance and a similar social profile in the different countries, but to what degree they could assume the same structure and organization after a temporary development of national characteristics. The theme discussed in this chapter, the decision of the German Soccer Association (Deutscher Fußball-Bund hereinafter referred to as DFB) to introduce professional soccer into Germany should be considered within the framework of these problems.

The Decision in Dortmund

On July 28, 1962, in Dortmund, Germany, the fifteenth post-World War II meeting of the German Soccer Association took place. The executive committee proposed to the assembled delegates the following two motions:

145

> 1. The delegation moves that as of August 1,
>   1963, a centralized national league under
>   the direction of the DFB be instituted
>
> 2. The delegation moves that this league be
>   constituted on a professional basis.[1]

Both motions were passed by a two-thirds majority. On the evening before this vote the *Sport-Beobachter*, one of the largest sports newspapers in West Germany, commented in a story headlined "The Fate of the DFB in Dortmund" as follows:

> If the national league becomes a unified
> German league, this will represent the most
> radical revolution in the history of the
> German Soccer Association.[2]

What the press at the time called a "soccer revolution" indeed represented a watershed in the history of German soccer. For the introduction of the Major League meant that in place of five regional upper leagues—north, west, south-west, and West Berlin—which included seventy-four teams, there was now only one league embracing sixteen teams for the entire Federal Republic of Germany (including West Berlin); and that the statute governing so-called contract players, introduced in 1949, was replaced by a new system of payment for major league players. While it gave them a higher earning potential, it simultaneously required them to pursue sport as a profession.

These two decisions put the top German soccer players on equal footing with those in other European countries, especially in England, Spain, France, and Italy. In discussing the circumstances that led to the introduction of the professional league in Germany, this author will examine why this step, relative to the rest of Europe, was taken so late and what specific resistance it had to overcome in Germany. The author is also interested in the league's new organization, its implementation, and its athletic as well as its social consequences.

Causes and Conditions

The decisions in Dortmund were taken in light of organizational, economic, and athletic problems already apparent in the early 1950s that in the meantime had become acute. One can examine them under the following four categories.

Firstly, the five regional upper leagues were a result of the post-war division of Germany into occupied zones which permitted only intra-regional expansion. The traditional federalistic structure of German sports, which may be traced back to the nineteenth century, also influenced this division. The consequence for the reorganization was that clubs had to be taken on in the higher divisions that could not—especially after the implementation of the statute governing contract players in 1949—support themselves financially. Such clubs could bear the financial burden even if with great difficulty, as long as they received considerable subsidies from the soccer pools which had been introduced in 1949 and as long as they had a stable group of spectators and therewith a continuously flowing source of income. Both conditions changed in the middle of the 1950s at the latest. Soccer pools got a dangerous rival with the Lotto which was gaining popularity. The soccer pools partly lost their market and their profits went down as well as the supplies with which the soccer clubs had been supported by then. The behavior of the spectators changed too. The influence of television on pastime was growing. More and more people who had gone to the games of "their club," even in the evening hours and in bad weather, now preferred staying at home or—and this was usual in those days—going to their pub which was equipped with a television set, in order to be entertained by the new medium. Both circumstances had a bad effect on the financial situation of many clubs,[3] which was bound to influence the sportive performance negatively. A great number of top players turned their backs on their clubs and went to those clubs offering higher sums. Thus, there developed almost immediately a two-class system whose differences became increasingly obvious in time: the economically sound clubs which competed for titles, and the poorer, mediocre clubs that fought year after year against relegation.

Second, the German national team won the World Cup in Switzerland in 1954, and four years later at the World Cup in Sweden it finished fourth. In striking contrast to these achievements, however, was the national eleven's chain of misadventures suffered elsewhere. For example, the team lost three of four games played in 1954 following the World Cup victory; in 1955 four of six games; and in 1956 five of eight. This obvious weakness of the national team was reflected in the modest achievements of German league teams on the international level. This was especially evident in the games for the European cup of the national champions, a competition which was introduced by the French journal L'Équipe in 1956 on the initiative of the well-known sport journalist Gabriel Hanot. In the first ten years of this competition only one German team was able to get to the final game. This was Eintracht Frankfurt, in May 1960. All the others were eliminated earlier. The games for the European Cup of the national champions were clearly dominated by clubs from Spain, Italy and

Portugal, like Real Madrid, CF Barcelona, Benfica Lisbon and International Milan. The weakness, both of the national team and the club teams, reflected the fact that in Germany—in contrast to the above mentioned countries—there was no elite league in which the best teams in the country were concentrated. Consequently, the diluted level of competition permitted the best players to "coast" from game to game. That is, because they were not required to extend themselves in order to win every game, they either grew soft or never achieved the mental and physical toughness demanded by international competition.

Third, the 1949 statute governing so-called contract players had long guaranteed that a player receive the maximum sum of DM 320 per month. Although, as suggested above, many clubs that followed this practice quickly reached their financial limits, a number of clubs in the upper leagues could afford to pay much more. Eager to win ever more games, these clubs quickly succumbed to the temptation to pay illegally high salaries for the best players. The functionaries appointed to root out such practices found it difficult to prove violations, for it was an open secret that many clubs had slush funds that never appeared in the books and made detection difficult. A common story: the ambition of petty functionaries to advance their clubs' fortunes struck an unholy alliance with the greed of many a player. The introduction of the statute of 1949 gave each player the chance to increase his income aboveboard. But this opportunity, as was quickly seen, carried its own burdens and risks. Since early in the 1950s the steadily increasing demands on players had unfortunate consequences on their earning power outside of soccer. *Kicker*, a popular sports magazine, described this problem as follows:

> Many a job and many a promising career
> suffered because a player had to be given
> time off for soccer. A star on the field,
> excellence in the office, this combination
> was unfortunately only rarely achieved.[4]

In the light of such circumstances it is no surprise that the players most in demand attempted, while at the peak of their careers, to cash in on their abilities above and beyond the limit set by statute. Already, by 1955, the number of such violations adjudicated by the German Soccer Association had drastically increased. As the gap between statutory regulation and actual practice widened, the "moral crisis" in German soccer became more apparent. All this merely exacerbated the dilemma facing the DFB. Had every violation committed by every player and every club been rigorously pursued, the danger that the guilty parties would have split off from the parent organization and formed their own body had to be countered. This implicit threat obviously restrained many a functionary: often a strict enforcement of the statutes was either foregone or selectively and arbitrarily applied. Such practices led in turn to a general sense of uncertainty and to an increasing loss of moral and practical authority on the part of the DFB.

Finally, as already implied, at the time of the modest beginnings of professional soccer in Germany, other European countries had already established such leagues. With the exception of England where, until 1962, certain restrictions were still in operation, this meant that the law of supply and demand governed the market for soccer players. From a German point of view the size of the resulting players' salaries, especially in Italy, and of the financial compensation to their former club assumed fantastic proportions.

In this context, what follows are some examples of the so-called transfer sums. These were sums which the new club of a player (changing his club) paid as a compensation to the club he had left and for which the statute for contract players of the German Football Association of 1949 prescribed 15,000 DM as a limit. In 1957 the Argentinian Omar Sivori from River Plate Buenos Aires changed to Juventus Turin for the transfer sum of 1,000,000 DM. In 1958 the Brazilian José Altafini from Palmeiras changed to AC Milan for 900,000 DM. In the same year Firmani from Sampdoria Genoa went to International Milan for 1,000,000 DM. In 1961 Dennis Law switched from Manchester United to AC Turin for 1,150,000 DM. Also in 1961, Luis Suarez from CF Barcelona went to International Milan for 1,650,000 DM, and in 1962 Luis del Sol from Real Madrid went to Juventus Turin for the record sum of 2,200,000 DM. The so-called handgelder, i.e. non-recurring and single payments, paid to the player joining the new club, were between 300,000 and 400,000 DM.[5] Considering these amounts it is not astonishing that German players also pushed into the Italian market. These players received "handgelder" amounts of five or six figures and their German clubs, which had been left, were able to fill their cashboxes with big transfer sums. Albert Brülls and Borussia Mönchengladbach, a club near Cologne in West Germany, held the record in this respect until 1962. This club got a transfer sum of 1,000,000,000 Lira from FC Modena, the club which Brülls joined. This was about 640,000 DM according to the exchange rate of that year. The player himself got a "handgeld" of 270,000 DM.[6]

The trend of a growing number of German superstars leaving their country for Italy (and to a lesser extent Spain) was regarded in German sports circles with rising alarm. The ghost of a "sellout" of German players and the resulting decay of sporting life haunted the scene.

Perspectives and Resistance

In light of these developments the general overhauling of "paid soccer" in Germany became a topic of discussion. For many experts it was axiomatic that the new organization must include a concentration of the top clubs in one league for example, the formation of an elite league embracing the Federal Republic and West Berlin and comprising sixteen to eighteen teams, and that this regrouping must be combined with a radical raise in players' salaries. In addition, it was recognized that increasing salaries would not only guarantee the players' and clubs' conformity with the statutes—thus "cleaning up" the game—but would also staunch the flow of top players abroad. It was perceived that an increase in pay was justified in consideration of the increasing demands that the new organization would make upon the players, for it was clear that the travel time required of the new teams would be drastically increased in comparison to the local schedules of regional leagues. Moreover, the concentration of the best teams in one league would require a higher level of performance from the players, which in turn would demand greater amounts of practice time that would preclude players from holding down jobs outside of soccer. Thus, professional soccer players would, by definition, make their livings chiefly by playing soccer, and the pay scale would have to reflect this fact, especially in providing players with a financial cushion while they made the transition from soccer to another career at the conclusion of their athletic life.

In almost direct proportion to the necessity, as perceived by many experts in Germany, of the reorganization of soccer along the lines just described, was the stubbornness of the lengthy resistance to these proposals. The nature of this resistance was chiefly ideological, the understanding of which requires a brief rolling back of the calendar. By the 1920s amateurism in Germany had assumed, both among the bourgeoisie and the working classes, a quasi-religious status. This cult of amateurism clashed so violently with professionalism that every form of professionalism was regarded as a manifestation of a decadent "Zeitgeist," a style of life derived from America that typified egoism, materialism, and greed. In contrast, amateur sport represented a kind of overall remedy against all the crimes of the modern age, beginning with alcohol and continuing through sexual promiscuity and including that threat to the young, the dancing mania.[7] It is not difficult to recognize how, in such a position, social criticism that was based on a large degree of cultural pessimism—both on the left and the right side of the political spectrum—was expressed. After it had entered even the sport ideology of National Socialism, it also survived the break of 1945. While the proponents of amateurism did not rely on the bizarre rhetoric of the early years, they continued to exercise their influence in many clubs.

Accordingly, professional sport was not recognized as traditional sport, but was merely tolerated as a necessary evil, as an unavoidable tribute that had to be paid to the spirit of the times.[8] If it could no longer be put aside—and on this point there was widespread agreement — then at least its further spread should be prevented as far as possible.

The Introduction of the Major Soccer League as Professional Sport

When the German Soccer Association, despite all the resistance and many unsuccessful attempts at reorganization, finally decided to establish a centralized league that guaranteed its players a higher income, it began immediately to implement the decision. By means of a complicated process that lasted many months, sixteen clubs chosen on the basis of athletic, financial and technical criteria constituted the new league. At the same time, a system regulating the modus of payment was developed. This work was carried out by a commission chosen by the board of the DFB. The commission determined that upper limits for monthly salaries, transfer sums, and bonuses payments should be set. Accordingly, a player who earned his living exclusively from soccer was entitled to earn 1,200 DM per month, whereas bonuses ("handgelder") and transfer sums were established at 10,000 or 50,000 DM respectively.[9] At the beginning of the 1970s all such restrictions were removed and the principle of free enterprise was introduced.

The introduction of the Major Soccer League ("Fußballbundesliga"), and of professionalism, had far-reaching consequences for the top players of German soccer. They affected the athletic level, the ability to compete internationally, and the social dimension. The games of the Major League met with high interest among the general public. "Major League Scores a Great Success," the *Sport-Beobachter* reported in a banner of its edition of January 5, 1964. Up to then, i.e., after the first half of the 1963/64 season, the Major League had already mobilized 3.4 million spectators. By the end of the season there were more than 6 millions. In the following year this number increased once more by about one million and games reached an average number of spectators of 24,000 to 26,000.[10] If these numbers already prove the great value of the Major League games for entertainment, their attractiveness can only be seen clearly, if one takes into consideration their role in a medium that had been gaining overwhelming importance in Germany since the 1950s, namely television. By way of example, one of the most popular telecasts of ARD (Allgemeine Rundfunkanstalten Deutschlands or General Broadcasting Stations of Germany) was the "Sportschau," telecast every Saturday from 6.05 pm to 7.00 pm. This telecast was mainly filled by reports on the games of the Major League.[11] A statistical inquiry made in the beginning of the 1980s showed that about a quarter of all registered television sets, which accounted for nearly six million, were regularly switched on for the "ARD-Sportschau."[12] Considering that a great number of them belonged to households with more than one person—nearly every household had a television set then[13]—one might most reasonably assume that the number of people watching the games by way of television was at least double the sum, so that a quarter or a third of the inhabitants of the Federal Republic of Germany saw this telecast.[14]

In spite of their great popularity, the high revenue gained by entrance fees, and the sums paid by the television stations, many clubs were soon deep in debt and were on the verge of ruin after some years. Critics of professionalism, who had prophesied such a development before the foundation of the Major League, saw their warnings now confirmed. How could this come about? In his informative study "Fußballprofis. Die Helden der Nation" ("Soccer Professionals. The Heroes of the Nation") Manfred Blödorn blames the egomania of honorary, i.e., unpaid, club functionaries. "Pursuing the aim of German championship," Blödorn writes, "they became agitated and were driven into risky financial maneuvers. Emotions conquered economic reason, and the temporary success justified everything... The fact astonishes," the author continues, "that business-men, so successful in industry, calculating every penny there, examining every investment twice or thrice, lost their brains in soccer..."[15] In order to pay the huge debts, amounting to several million marks for some clubs after only a few years of membership in the Major League, many boards capitalized on the opportunity to sell the grounds of the club to the towns, or to conclude advertis-ing treaties with firms. In these treaties the firm obliged itself to grant financial and other material support, for which it was entitled to use sports wear — above all that of the players—for advertising purposes. By the 1970s this sponsoring got more and more important and aroused the growing interest of authors.[16]

As already mentioned, the financial misery into which many clubs stumbled was due in large part to their exaggerated ambition, i.e., to the fact that they spent more money for employing top players than the club cash-box allowed. Therefore one must ask: What did the players earn in the first years of the Major League? and What can we know about the social background, i.e. the origins and the education of those players who had made sport their profession? No systematic inquiries over a longer period of time exist which might allow a sat-isfying answer to these questions. Therefore, once more, reference will be made to Manfred Blödorn, who offers some data which are at least a kind of a random sample. According to him, during the 1973/74 season the majority of the 370 Major League players had a yearly income between 60,000 and 70,000 DM.[17]

Taxes subtracted, this meant a net income of 45,000 to 50,000 DM. Compared to the average net income of those days from 14,000 to 18,000 DM this was certainly a salary most people could only dream of. But it could not be compared with the income of the top stars of the Major League. Players like Günter Netzer, Borussia Mönchengladbach, Wolfgang Overrath of FC Cologne, Franz Beckenbauer and Gerd Müller, Bavaria Munich, and Uwe Seeler of Sport Club Hamburg, secured yearly net incomes between 180.000 and 240.000 DM. Such chances of earning money could not completely stop the drain of German players to foreign clubs—this was, as described, one of the main aims of professionalism—but they affected a check on emigration which made itself felt. As Blödorn shows further the players analyzed by him came nearly without exception from the lower levels of the social pyramid, i.e., from the working class, artisans and clerks:

> 265 of the interrogated professionals of the Major League, [Blödorn says] stated the following jobs of their fathers: 41 workers, 57 artisans, 54 clerks, only 13 officials and 14 freelances, 46 did not answer the question. The professionals themselves had been trained in the following callings: 5 workers, 109 artisans, 112 clerks, and 8 officials; 20 were studying or had interrupted or broken off their studies, 7 had become professionals without being trained in a job.[18]

If one takes the height of salary as a standard, the professional Major League players were—taking into consideration their starting-point—social climbers. Further inquiries will have to show whether these players got into closer social contact with members of such professional groups who disposed of the same or similar incomes but had a different origin and education.

The social mobility of the players corresponded in some way to the mobility in space. A short comparison will show that: 135, that is 42%, of the 321 players who had a contract with one of the 16 clubs of the Major League for the season of 1963/64 came from the junior sections of their own clubs or had changed from clubs not far away, i.e. in every case from clubs within the same town in which the new club was situated.[19] The situation had fundamentally changed, for example, for the beginning of the season of 1990/91: the statement just made was only true for 39, that is 10%, of the 395 players engaged by the clubs of the Major League.[20] In other words: 90% of the players having a contract with the clubs of the Major League came from other localities. The causes of this change can easily be seen. First, it was important that the institution of the Major League started a process of selection that concentrated the top talent produced by the different regions of the Federal Republic of Germany on the few clubs of the league as a central playing class. An ambitious sportsman who commanded the necessary talents wanted, as a rule, to play in a club of the first class, wanted to be "first class." If a chance offered itself, he put up with the separation from his home and his club. Second, the prospect to earn much money within a short time under the conditions of professionalism, indeed considerably more than the old job could provide, caused many players to leave their surroundings. So on the one hand it is true that the introduction of professionalism led to greater social and spatial mobility. Thus, the top level of sport mirrored a change which possibly took place in greater parts of society and was only more conspicuous in professional sport. On the other hand the so-called social costs connected with this process cannot be neglected. These costs were felt in the club life and in the relation between club and adherents.

In a traditional club social life and comradeship were important.[21] Professionalism drastically changed this feature. Players began to compare performance and salaries, and the resulting envy and dissatisfaction often destroyed the relaxed and friendly atmosphere. Club life began to lose social density and warmth. Professionalism also introduced a note of coolness and distance between clubs and fans. During the period of amateurism, players were often deeply involved in the community life of the club. The fans who lived near the club saw a player as one of them and could easily identify with him. Professionalism meant that players from the top teams were no longer exponents of a certain social milieu. As new players, signed by these clubs, often came from different areas of the country (see above), they were often totally unknown to the supporters of the club. This situation created a process of estrangement between fan and club that was intensified by the player's higher income. An income gap quickly grew between player and supporter as well as a status problem that the players' private homes and expensive cars made apparent. Altogether this tendency meant that the many fans that had remained faithful to the club in hard times suddenly lost their readiness to tolerate bad play and their willingness to ride out lean years waned. Fans became consumers accustomed to measure a player only on his performance and his entertainment value. Soccer as a consumer item and circus act—this trail was first blazed in the Fall of 1963.

The foundation of the Major League, and the realization of professionalism, meant that German soccer developed a structure similar to that of soccer in other European countries in two decisive fields. How far this was also true for the social and economic frame and consequences would have to be ascertained in comparative inquiries. A short glance at recent studies on the history of soccer in England, Italy, and France shows, however, that conditions and trends were similar. In these countries professional players are recruited from members of the working and the lower middle classes and a kind of magic triangle of professional soccer, economy, and show business has developed.[22] But throughout discussion of these aspects, even if they are interesting phenomena of social history, one should not forget soccer itself. The foundation of the federal league brought about a considerable increase in sportive achievement among the leading clubs of West Germany. This can be deduced very easily from their successes in the games for diverse European cups (for example the European cup of the national champions or the European cup of the national cup winners). Clubs like Borussia Dortmund, Borussia Mönchengladbach, Sport Club Hamburg, Eintracht Frankfurt and, above all, Bavaria Munich won these cups repeatedly or got front places in the qualifying contests between sometimes more than 30 teams from the different European countries.[23] In the soccer metropolis of Europe, in London, Liverpool, Manchester and Glasgow, in Barcelona and Madrid, in Turin, Milan and Amsterdam, the teams of the German Major League impressed the spectators with their technical level and their achievement. They were described in detail to the public abroad in such well-known sports papers and magazines like *La Gazetta dello Sport, L'Equipe, Match* and *Football Monthly.* They experienced a new attention from the international sports public they had never sensed before. Aboveall, this meant that at least as far as soccer was concerned, German sport was "keeping up with Europe."

Notes

---

[1]Quoted from Dr. Walter Erbach, 65 Jahre Westdeutscher Fußballverband e. V., Duisburg 1965, p. 167

[2]*Sport-Beobachter*, July 26, 1992

[3]Cf. the corresponding petitions of the DFB to the Federal Secretary of Finance and to the Secretaries of Finance of the single states of the Federal Republic of Germany, 1962, February 23, concerning: Effects of the introduction of a top player class with better paid contract players on taxation, DFB-Archives, Frankfurt/Main

[4]N. N., Bundesliga-Probleme sind alle lösbar, in: *KICKER,* December 10, 1956, p. 6

[5]N. N., Ausverkauf deutscher Spieler geht weiter, in: *Sport-Beobachter*, July 11, 1962

[6]N. N., Modena bezahlt 640.000 DM für Albert Brülls, in: *Sport-Beobachter*, July 16, 1962

[7]Cf. Siegfried Gehrmann, Fußball - Vereine - Politik. Zur Sportgeschichte des Reviers 1900-1940, Essen 1988, pp. 24-7

[8]Ludwig Wolker, Um das Ethos im deutschen Sport. Referat auf der Zonensporttagung am 13. Juni 1947 in Köln, hrsg. vom Zonensportrat der Britischen Zone, o. O. o. J. (1947)

[9]Bundesliga-Statut. Beschlossen vom DFB-Beirat am 6. Oktober 1962, Kapitel 6, DFB-Archives, Frankfurt/Main

[10]*Sport-Beobachter*, June 14, 1973

[11]Burkhard Trapp, Angebot und Nutzung von Sportsendungen im Fernsehen (1976-1985), in: Josef Hackforth (ed.), Sportmedien & Mediensport. Wirkungen - Nutzung - Inhalte der Sportberichterstattung, Berlin, 1987, p. 332

[12]Ibid., p. 334

[13]Manfred Blödorn, Das Magische Dreieck: Sport - Fernsehen - Kommerz, in: Wolfgang Hoffmann-Riem (ed.), Neue Medienstrukturen - neue Sportberichterstattung?, Baden-Baden / Hamburg 1988, p. 101

[14]Considering the enormous social importance of television as a medium influencing public opinion it would be very interesting to inquire systematically what kind of influence the attractiveness of soccer had on the spread of television, i.e., to what degree is determined the individual decision to buy a television set. It is justified to suppose that this spread in the fifties and sixties would not have been so fast and so wide without the great popularity of this kind of sport. There exist informative indicators for this connection from the early history of television: When the games for the world-championship took place in Switzerland in 1954 the number of television owners in the Federal Republic increased eightfold in the same year, namely from 11.658 in January to 84.278 in December. - Cf. Lothar Mikos, Unterhaltung pur. Kulturelle Aspekte von Fußball und Fernsehen, in: medium, June 1982, p. 18

[15]Manfred Blödorn, *Fußballprofis. Die Helden der Nation*, Hamburg, 1974, p 41.

[16]Thomas Sutter, *Rechtsfragen des organisierten Sports,* Bern - Frankfurt - New York 1984; Pascal Biojout, *Le sponsoring*, Limoges, 1983

[17]Manfred Blödorn, *Fußballprofis,* p. 59.

[18]Ibid., p. 62.

[19]Calculated from the data in: Die Bundesliga 1963-1968. Eine Dokumentation in Zahlen. Zusammengestellt von Emil Dumser, Stuttgart, 1969, pp. 6-13.

[20]Calculated from the data in: Fußball-Sport. Bundesliga 90-91, Sonderausgabe, SH2, pp. 30-4.

[21]Siegfried Gehrmann, Fußball in einer Industrieregion. Das Beispiel FC Schalke 04, in: Fabrik - Familie - Feierabend. Beiträge zur Sozialgeschichte des Alltags im Industriezeitalter, hrsg. von Jürgen Reulecke und Wolfhard

Weber, Wuppertal 1978, S. 51 ff.; Siegfried Gehrmann, Fritz Szepan und Ernst Kuzorra - zwei Fußballidole des Ruhrgebiets, in: Sozial- und Zeitgeschichte des Sports 1988, 3, pp. 64-8.

[22]Cf. for England: Tony Mason, "Football," in: *Sport in Britain. A Social History*, ed. by Tony Mason, Cambridge 1989, pp. 146-186; A. J. Arnold, *'A Game That Would Pay': A Business History of Professional Football in Bradford*, London 1988; Peter J. Sloane, "The Labour Market in Professional Football," in: *British Journal of Industrial Relations*, 7 (1969), pp. 181-199; Richard Cashman and Michael McKernan (eds.), *Sport. Money, Morality and the Media*, Kensington 1981; Stephen Wagg, *The Football World. A Contemporary Social History*, Brighton 1984; cf. for France: Alfred Wahl, *Le balle au pied, histoire du football*, Paris 1990; Alfred Wahl, *Les Archives du Football: Sport et société en France (1880-1980)*, Paris 1989; Pierre Delaunay u. a., *100 ans de football en France*, Paris 1986; Richard Holt, *Sport and Society in Modern France*, London 1981. Cf. for Italy: Gianni Brera, *Storia critica del calcio italiano*, Milano 1978; Vittorio. Caminiti, *Il romanzo del calcio italiano*, Bologna 1980; G. P. Ormezzano, *Storia del calcio*, Milano 1985; Antonio Ghirelli, *Storia del calcio in Italia*, Torino 1990.

[23]The beginning of this series of successes beginning now was made by Borussia Dortmund. The Dortmundians defeated the English cup winner FC Liverpool in the final for the European cup on May 5th, 1966, in Glasgow, Scotland, by 2:1. The most spectacular successes were won by Bavaria Munich, which was cup winner of champions of the single European countries in 1974, 1975 and 1976.

Part 4: Sport and the South African Question

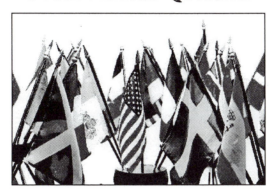

Part 4: Sport and the South African Question

During a lecture to a group of white physical education students at a South African university, in August 1991, I observed that the Springbok emblem, the flag and the anthem of the Republic would have to be replaced if South Africa were to be readmitted to the world of international sport, since they are symbols of political oppression for the majority of South Africans. This remark set off a storm of protest and debate culminating in the announcement by one student that she did not understand what all the fuss was about since sport had nothing to do with politics. The incident was symbolic of the apolitical stance taken by many of the (predominantly white) sports administrators and students during the lecture tour (see Craig and Rees, this section). Of course, sports practitioners in South Africa and abroad are not the only ones to have overlooked the political significance of sport. Until recently, scholars interested in explaining social behavior would have dismissed sport as an activity with no social or political importance. The following chapters should be required reading for all who share this view.

The chapters in this section document the role played by sport in the profound changes currently taking place in South African society. They show how sport has been used in the struggle to support and to undermine apartheid. They chart the development of the non-racial sports movement, and the lifting of the international moratorium against sport competition with South Africa. They also show how sport can symbolize future social relations in South Africa, and further, how it is indicative of broader social changes in the global village.

These chapters are symbolic, on another level, since they contain contributions by South African scholars (Hendricks and Baxter) who were invited to present their views on sport in South Africa at the 1992 Conference of the International Society for Comparative Physical Education and Sport. Were the international moratorium still in place at that time such scholarly interaction could have been more difficult.

The international boycott in sports, particularly the case of South Africa versus New Zealand in Rugby, is the subject of the chapter written by historians John Nauright and David Black. In it they argue that Rugby is an essential element of the cultural identity of dominant groups in both countries, and show how the issue of race, specifically the question of whether or not to include Maoris in New Zealand teams playing against South Africa, led to political tensions in both countries. The Rugby boycott was particularly significant because it symbolized the isolation of white South African males from similar groups in New Zealand and Britain, groups which would be seen as least likely to perceive sport as a legitimate arena for protest against apartheid.

Sociologist Denver Hendricks presents a provocative analysis of the recent changes in South African sport. Using Eliasian terminology he suggests that, in the long run, these changes are part of the process of "functional democratization" by which power inequalities between "insiders" (the white establishment) and "outsiders" (the non-white majority) are reduced. Over the short run, however, ending the sports boycott has reduced the power of the outsiders. Hendricks describes the current situation in sport as an alliance between the insiders and a majority of outsiders which leaves the majority worse off than they were before. What has been a race struggle in South African sport is now becoming a class struggle.

In the third chapter, sociologists Peter Craig and Roger Rees draw on the work of Anthony Giddens. They present sport as a cultural construction which can be used as an example of how institutions change as the world moves from the era of "modernity" to "postmodernity." Following Giddens they argue that sport, like other institutions, is reflexive, fluid, and unpredictable, but has the potential to become a "social movement" which can provide guidelines to significant social transformations. Craig and Rees cite the development of the non-racial sports movement and the use of South African cricket in support of the "Yes" vote in the 1992 referendum as examples of this movement.

Finally, John Baxter, Head of Sports Administration at the University of the Witwatersrand, Johannesburg, provides an inside view of events behind the recent changes in South African sport. As a significant "player" in these events, he gives a first-hand account of the birth of the non-racial sports movement, the political struggle between the NOSC and SACOS, and the lifting of the international sports ban. He sees potential for the non-racial sports movement to provide a positive vision of the future in South Africa, but also fears that the movement will look like a "sellout" if power sharing between the white and non-white community on a wider political level does not keep pace with the changes in sport.

Although they differ in their interpretation of the future of sport in South Africa, the authors of these chapters remove the analysis of sport from a political vacuum, and place it within a broader political and social context. They also symbolize the future for the study of sport in the global village. On the micro level sport can be investigated as a significant force in peoples' lives which, following Eric Hobsbawm, "invents" their social traditions. On the macro level sport can be analyzed as an element of wider social change, from a number of sociological perspectives including those of Elias and Giddens. In short, these papers demonstrate that the study of sport in the global village has great theoretical and practical significance.

C. Roger Rees

Chapter 9

It's Rugby That Really Matters: New Zealand-South Africa Rugby Relations and the Moves to Isolate South Africa, 1956-1992

John Nauright and David Black[1]

This study is part of a much larger project of the same name which investigates links between South Africa and New Zealand within the sport of Rugby football. In both countries, Rugby has been called a "secular religion" and it has been central in creating and sustaining a cultural identity among the dominant power groups of white men in each society. The significance of sport to white South Africans is undeniable as seen by the use of South Africa's return to international cricket and impending return to international Rugby in the recent white referendum on reform. While South Africa's success in the cricket World Cup during the campaign was crucial, the possibility of a return to the world Rugby stage also played a key role. The Pretoria Afrikaans newspaper *Beeld* front-page headline of March 5, 1992, "All Blacks op Loftus" reveals this.

This chapter demonstrates the vital role played by international Rugby in the creation of predominantly male and white defined national identities in both New Zealand and South Africa, and its prominent role in the national and international politics of each. On the basis of this analysis, the authors then argue that the psychological and political impact of the international sports boycott, and more particularly the Rugby boycott of recent years, on white South Africans, has been an important source of pressure to dismantle apartheid.

Rugby and the Construction of "National Identity" in South Africa and New Zealand

Rugby was first played in South Africa in the late 1860s and in New Zealand in 1870. By the 1890s, Rugby was played by most white males, and some males from the indigenous populations in both countries. The central position of Rugby within both societies was ensured by successes in their nation's first official international tours of the British Isles, New Zealand in 1905 and South Africa in 1906. Both tours came close on the heels of crises in emerging national identity.[2] Immediate comparisons between the Rugby teams of both countries were made in the British press following the early British Isles tours. However, South Africa and New Zealand were not able to play against each other before World War I. Since then, New Zealand and South Africa have played Rugby test series against each other in 1921, 1928, 1937, 1949, 1956, 1960, 1965, 1970, 1976, and 1981 (planned series were canceled in 1967, 1973, and 1985). The first two series ended in ties, and South Africa won five and New Zealand won three of the remaining series.

New Zealand sociologist and activist Richard Thompson sums up the passion for Rugby in both South Africa and New Zealand. South Africa and New Zealand, he asserts, share "not merely a passion for Rugby, but a similar approach to the game, and the Rugby rivalry is felt to be distinctive...[In both countries] Rugby is a man's game, not a game for girls and sissies, and to play it the hard way is to play it the man's way." He continues, "[A] defeat reflects unfavorably on the quality of New Zealand manhood and its way of life."[3] The famous late South African author and former Liberal Party leader, Alan Paton, stated that "white South Africans are madly enthusiastic about Rugby, and especially about playing New Zealand."[4] In addition to these testimonials concerning the role of Rugby in South Africa and New Zealand, one must remember that for much of this century Rugby was compulsory for white boys in South African schools and also in some New Zealand schools. In other New Zealand schools, Rugby was often the only winter sport offered until the 1970s. This has meant most members of the dominant group in both societies shared a common cultural practice, Rugby.

While officials in both countries have attempted to downplay links between Rugby and politics, it is clear that the two were closely intertwined from the early twentieth century. In 1905, New Zealand Prime Minister, Richard Seddon was labeled "Minister of Football" after the press revealed he had match reports sent out as government messages.[5] In both countries, many international and first class Rugby players have attained positions of power within government.

In South Africa there have been close links between Springbok captains, the ruling National Party (NP), and the secret Afrikaner Broederbond, formed in 1918
by Afrikaner nationalists, whose members have dominated many positions of
power in post-World War II South African society. Since the NP came to
power, in 1948, all Springbok captains except one have been NP members, or
members of both the NP and the Broederbond. The manager of the 1965 tour to
New Zealand, Kobus Louw, a Broeder, was a Secretary in the Department of
Coloured Affairs, and later became a Cabinet minister, as did tour Captain
Dawid de Villiers, also a member of the Broederbond. Significantly, Piet
Koornhof and Gerrit Viljoen, Ministers of Sport in the late 1970s and early
1980s have been Secretary and President of the Broederbond respectively. They
have also been key players in the current initiative for constitutional change.[6]

International Rugby and Mounting Political Controversy

Rugby relations between South Africa and New Zealand since the 1920s have
been a persistent source of debate, especially in New Zealand. The origins of
these debates are rooted in the two countries' differing experiences of race relations. New Zealand's general policy approach, since the Treaty of Waitangi of
1841, attempted to include Maoris within a wider, albeit white-defined society,
while South African racial policies in the twentieth century have been based on
principles of racial segregation and white domination. In 1921 the Springboks
played the Maori All Blacks and won by a point. The emerging difference in
racial attitudes was summed up after the match by a South African reporter
named Blackett, who was "sickened" at the sight of white New Zealanders
cheering for Maoris against members of their own race.[7] However, the best New
Zealand Rugby player of the 1920s, if not of alltime, George Nepia, was
excluded from selection from the 1928 All Black tour of South Africa because
he was Maori.

Exclusion of Maoris from tours of South Africa sparked little controversy in
New Zealand before the Second World War. After the South African National
Party came to power in 1948, and soon began implementing their apartheid
policies, sporting contacts began to be questioned by a few New Zealanders.
This took several years to develop as there was no protest during the 1956
Springbok tour of New Zealand. It seemed as if the whole country united
behind the single goal of defeating South Africa to gain revenge for losing so
badly to them in 1949. In the days before television and close links between
New Zealand and the outside world, the awareness of South Africa was limited
to its status as a Rugby power and ally in the British Commonwealth and during
World War II.[8] When debate developed in 1957, it centered on the exclusion of

Maoris from trials for the proposed 1960 All Black tour of South Africa and the New Zealand Rugby Football Union's (NZRFU) complicity with South African requests that they be excluded, rather than on the internal racial policies of the South African government. The slogan protesters developed was "No Maoris, no tour" and anti-tour petition drives were organized in New Zealand by the Citizens All Black Tour Association (CABTA) and by groups within South Africa including the South African Sports Association (SASA), which organized and promoted non-racial sport in South Africa. Thousands of South Africans and New Zealanders petitioned the New Zealand government to cancel the tour. Still, New Zealand Prime Minister Walter Nash decided not to interfere with the decision of the NZRFU on the tour, which confirmed his National Party's policy of "non-interference" with sporting bodies.

Despite the domestic protests and emerging international opposition resulting from the Sharpsville Massacre of peaceful black protesters on March 21, 1960, the NZRFU went ahead with the 1960 tour. The depth of The National Party's commitment to challenge South Africa after Sharpsville was reflected in parliamentary statements made by W.S. Goosman, M.P. for Paiko. He stated that he was "for the whites" in South Africa. He justified his position by arguing, "imagine what the position would be in this country if we had four coloureds to every white person!"[9] Goosman's statements were suggestive of a strong undercurrent in the National caucus who were clearly sympathetic to white South Africa if not openly pro-apartheid.

"Like Fleas on a Dog." The Beginning of Real Conflict: The 1965 Springbok Tour and New Zealand Politics, 1965-67

The New Zealand parliament is dominated by the conservative National Party and the more liberal Labour Party. During most of the 1960s, the National Party, under Sir Keith Holyoake, was in power. National's policy regarding sporting contact with South Africa was that there should be no interference with the right of New Zealand sports people to participate with whomever they pleased. In general, National's policy on South Africa in the 1960s rejected sanctions or other formal protest actions.

The National government of the 1960s and early 1970s had little sympathy for those who protested against sporting contacts with South Africa. J.A. Hanan, in his capacity as Minister of Maori Affairs, spoke at a reception for the Springboks at Gisborne which was attended by many Maoris. He complained about "a minority of people with 'peculiar ideas'" who he said were not making the Springboks welcome. Hanan sparked a controversy when he stated, "I have said in the past that in a democracy you have to have these people. Well, I suppose you do—in the sense that a dog has fleas." Hanan defended himself by arguing that the welcome given to the Springboks would have greater impact than "all the placard carriers, than all the protest meetings, than all the exhortations of some trade unions that their members should not attend the games." Hanan made his, and his party's view clear as he continued, "What a monstrous thing, to attempt to deny the right of a citizen of this country to go to a football match, to exhort him to boycott a football match."[10]

During the 1965 tour, the question arose as to whether Maoris would be allowed into South Africa as members of an All Black side for the proposed 1967 tour of South Africa. Maoris had not been chosen to go in 1960 despite the protests of thousands of petitioners. Both political parties agreed, however, that Maoris should not be excluded from future tours as it was not New Zealand's practice to openly discriminate on racial grounds. Dr. Danie Craven, head of the South African Rugby Board (SARB), assured NZRFU officials and the government that Maoris would be allowed. Prime Minister Hendrick Verwoerd, the architect of apartheid, chose to keep quiet before the 1965 Springbok tour of New Zealand, refusing to comment on whether Maoris would be excluded from future tours to South Africa. But just prior to the last international match in 1965, he stated that all future teams touring South Africa would have to abide by South Africa's "local custom." It was clear to New Zealanders that this meant no Maoris. Prime Minister Holyoake subsequently announced the Government's view in Parliament by saying that "as we are one people we cannot be fully and truly represented by a team chosen on racial lines."[11] In order to avoid Government embarrassment, the NZRFU postponed the proposed All Black tour of 1967.

International Pressure and South African Politics, 1966-70

Verwoerd was assassinated in 1966 and the more reformist, or *verligte* (enlightened) John Vorster became Prime Minister of South Africa. In 1968, Vorster made a dramatic decision allowing the NZRFU to send Maoris on upcoming tours. Behind the scenes, however, it was intimated to the NZRFU that there should not be too many Maoris and that they should not be too dark![12] This move by Vorster was the first real attempt by the South African government to alleviate international pressure in the sports arena, and heralded a myriad of reformist measures over the next twenty years. It was clear that future cancellation of New Zealand Rugby tours was too high a price to pay for the continuation of total Apartheid in sport. Vorster's decision to allow Maoris into South Africa as members of an All Black team contributed to a split in the NP and the

Broederbond. Several members of parliament in the Party would not tolerate what they saw as the erosion of apartheid.[13]

Both the NP and the opposition United Party viewed the campaign to isolate South Africa in international sport and the controversies over the admission of Maoris and the Basil D'Oliveira affair as different matters.[14] United Party member of parliament, D.J. Marais, pointed out that the international campaign to isolate South Africa in sport had been led by "the Afro-Asian and communist countries."[15] What both parties really wanted to avoid was a full-scale onslaught by traditional sporting allies. Marais warned the government that total isolation was possible unless the government acted. In 1969, South Africa Minister of Transport, Ben Schoeman, affirmed the government's intention to concentrate on the maintenance of traditional sporting ties with New Zealand, Britain, Australia, and France.[16]

In order to prevent mass opposition, and to promote South Africa and its policies of separate development, Vorster sent one of his most senior diplomats, P.H. Philip, to New Zealand to serve as Council-General in 1969. Philip distributed much pro-apartheid information on South Africa, wrote numerous letters to newspapers, and spoke to countless groups during his tenure, which lasted until 1976. He also held numerous parties and dinners to which many All Blacks and National Party members of parliament and Cabinet ministers were invited. Commentators at the time pointed out that he was a very senior diplomat to be sent to such an unimportant country as New Zealand, with whom South Africa's economic relations (and strategic ties) were "insignificant."[17] However, Vorster's government clearly thought the maintenance of Rugby (and other sports) links with New Zealand was important both for white support at home, and from the standpoint of international relations and attempts to combat growing sanctions movements. Vorster's plan was successful initially, as sporting contact between South Africa and New Zealand actually increased between 1968 and 1972. South Africa was pushed out of many international competitions and organizations during these years.

Sport and the South African Question in New Zealand, 1976-70

Once Vorster cleared the way for Maori participation, the SARB invited the NZRFU to tour in 1970. The NZRFU eventually sent a team which included two Maoris and one Polynesian. Despite Vorster's concession to New Zealand, protests against the 1970 tour continued. Members of the groups, Citizens' Association for Racial Equality (CARE) and Halt All Racist Tours (HART), raised the stakes and worked for the elimination of all sporting contact with

South Africa so long as it practiced apartheid in sport. Both groups harnessed support from academics, trade union leaders, and church officials in the main cities (and Rugby test match venues) of Auckland, Wellington, Christchurch, and Dunedin.

The origins of CARE were rooted in the controversy surrounding the 1960 tour of South Africa. The 1959-60 protests raised awareness of racial issues among a number of white New Zealanders. In 1964, a small group of Aucklanders held meetings which led to the formation of CARE that October.[18] CARE became involved in domestic and international racial issues, but the media chose to focus on its protests against playing Rugby with South Africa. HART was an organization formed in the late 1960s to stop New Zealand sporting contests with South Africa, but as an organization, did not involve itself in wider issues taken up by CARE. Although CARE and HART launched a campaign to prevent the proposed 1970 tour of South Africa, the Holyoake government was satisfied that once Maoris had been accepted by the South African government, then it would not prevent the tour from taking place. The print media were divided on the issue with some, like the *Dominion* in Wellington, supporting tours based on merit selection. Others, like the *New Zealand Listener*, opposed tours with South Africa. In "Sport Within the Laager," the *Listener*, citing Vorster's political handling of the D'Oliveira affair, openly criticized any contact which would bolster the South African regime.[19]

Rugby vs. the Commonwealth Games: New Zealand, 1970-74

Protests against the 1970 tour in New Zealand, and again against the proposed 1973 Springbok tour, were partly motivated by concerns that Christchurch might lose its bid to host the 1974 Commonwealth Games. New Zealand's record on U.N. resolutions against South Africa in the 1960s was regarded by non-white Commonwealth states, among others, as distinctly "unimpressive" as it voted against or abstained on nearly every resolution which condemned South Africa.[20] New Zealand also staunchly defended South Africa at the International Olympic Committee meeting which expelled it from the Olympic movement in 1970. In addition, African Commonwealth leaders used Australia's new tough stance on sporting contacts with South Africa to pressure the New Zealand government to take a similar stand not to compete with South Africa until it abolished racial discrimination in sport.[21]

In late 1972, New Zealanders elected a Labour Government, led by Kirk, with a large majority. During the election campaign, National tried to reverse their sagging position in the polls by capitalizing on Labour's opposition to Rugby links

with South Africa. Just prior to the election, the Party took out full-page advertisements under the banner headline: "National will not be blackmailed into
canceling the Springbok tour... Not by the Federation of Labour... Not by
HART and CARE."[22] National's last-minute strategy failed, but the Party was
right in its portrayal of connections between Labour Party leaders and anti-tour
groups. Three of Kirk's Cabinet members were also members of CARE. Kirk,
however, walked carefully around the issue of the proposed 1973 Springbok
tour. Before the election he stated several times that he opposed the tour, but
would not interfere with decisions of sporting bodies. After assuming power, he
commissioned reports from the Ministry of Foreign Affairs and the police on
possible consequences of a tour. The police reported that 10,000 demonstrators
could be mustered in the major centers of Auckland, Wellington, and
Christchurch and would "engender the greatest eruption of violence the country
has ever known."[23] This report, combined with threats from black
Commonwealth countries to boycott the 1974 Commonwealth Games in
Christchurch, eventually forced Kirk's hand. The organizers of the
Commonwealth Games warned National, before the election, that African and
some other Commonwealth countries would boycott the Games if the tour came
to pass. However, National did not make the report available to Labour or to the
public.[24] The NZRFU, for its part, left it to the Prime Minister to determine the
fate of the tour, calculating that he (and not they) would be stigmatized by a
decision to cancel. An attempt by the South African Rugby Board to include
token blacks in the tour party was exposed on the eve of the tour, and Kirk was
finally forced to call it off. Subsequently, in 1974, he stated that any team representative of any sporting organization which practiced apartheid at any level
would not be welcome in New Zealand. As a result of Kirk's action, an African-
led boycott of the 1974 Commonwealth Games was averted.

Muldoon, Rugby and International Sport, 1975-78

Politically, the cancellation of the Rugby tour proved damaging to the govern-
ment. The new populist NP leader, Robert Muldoon, made Rugby relations with
South Africa a central campaign issue in the 1975 election. A cartoon in the
New Zealand press during the campaign portrayed SARB President Danie
Craven as Muldoon's running mate. Rugby sources leaked a story that the
Springboks would come to New Zealand if National were elected and
National's election manifesto made it clear the South Africans would be made
welcome if they were invited.[25] The end result of the election was that National
reversed the outcome of 1972 and won a large majority.

Although the Springboks did not immediately come to New Zealand, the All Blacks toured South Africa in 1976. Muldoon stated clearly that his government would not interfere with sporting bodies who, he felt, should be free to decide their own sporting policies. As international outrage mounted over the juxtaposition of the All Black tour with the Soweto student uprisings, twenty-two African countries boycotted the 1976 Montreal Olympics due to New Zealand's participation. During that All Black tour of South Africa, Canterbury Rugby official B. Drake further displayed an undercurrent of attitudes in conservative New Zealand circles when he stated, "the sooner the people of Africa go back to the jungle the better."[26] In November 1976, the United Nations passed, by acclamation, a resolution calling for a sports boycott of South Africa. The pro-apartheid undercurrent in Rugby and National Party circles in New Zealand, matched with Muldoon's refusal to interfere with NZRFU decisions on Rugby relations with the SARB, meant that New Zealand faced increasing attacks from the world community.

In 1977, the effort to avoid a similar boycott of the 1978 Edmonton Commonwealth Games, again over New Zealand-South African Rugby links, led to the adoption by Commonwealth Heads of Government of the "Gleneagles Declaration on Apartheid and Sport." The Gleneagles Agreement called on all Commonwealth governments to discourage sporting contacts with South Africa.[27] Spearheaded by the Canadian government, and orchestrated by the Commonwealth Secretariat, it subsequently emerged as perhaps the most important international landmark in ratchetting up the comprehensiveness of sport sanctions. Muldoon's agreement to Gleneagles facilitated the success of the Edmonton Games, but the Agreement was framed in such broad principle that considerable room to maneuver remained for the obstinate New Zealand Prime Minister.

<u>South African Responses to Increased Isolation, 1970-81</u>

The history of South Africa's reforms in sport have been well documented. What is important to note here is how these changes related to the maintenance of Rugby ties with New Zealand and other countries. As suggested, the admission of Maori All Blacks was the first major concession made by the South African State which allowed them to resume regular sporting contact. This was short-lived, however, as the NP refused to make any further concessions until after the cancellation of the 1973 tour of New Zealand. It became clear, given the strongly anti-apartheid stance of the Australian and New Zealand Labour parties and the success of British protesters, that regular international Rugby contact in other sports would be virtually impossible without some concessions.

The issue came down to South Africa's willingness to maintain all the major aspects of apartheid versus increasing international condemnation of apartheid. Once the Vietnam War ended, much of the energy created in the war protests was redirected toward the anti-apartheid movement.

The 1981 Tour in New Zealand and South Africa

In 1981, New Zealand society was ripped at the seams over the Springbok Rugby tour.[28] Many New Zealanders questioned themselves, and debated and fought with others, including members of their own families, as massive demonstrations greeted each match and forced the cancellation of one. An opinion poll taken in New Zealand during the tour showed that forty-nine per cent opposed the Springbok presence, while forty-two per cent favored the tour, a striking contrast to the 1973 polls.[29] The NZRFU weighed the possible costs of the tour with benefits to Rugby and determined that the government could call off the tour, but they would not. Muldoon stated repeatedly that he would not force any sporting body to cancel matches with sports people from any country (despite behind-the-scenes threats to those wanting to go to Moscow in 1980).

On July 6, 1981, just two weeks before the scheduled Springbok arrival, Muldoon delivered a speech on national television. Muldoon defended his actions, stating they were in line with principles he had argued for in the Gleneagles Agreement. Muldoon reaffirmed that the vast majority of New Zealanders abhorred apartheid, but argued that people did not need to hate South Africans as individuals. Evoking powerful imagery, he referred to a recent visit he made to a Commonwealth war cemetery in Italy. About a dozen New Zealand graves were alongside South African ones.[30] This vision of fallen New Zealanders and South Africans lying side-by-side was aimed at a central core of New Zealand national (as defined by the white-male elite) identity. Thus, white South Africans were directly tied into the two main defining aspects of the "true" Kiwi man—war and Rugby.[31] In addition, Muldoon firmly defended New Zealand's human rights record and defied any country to insult New Zealand. Muldoon felt he had to take a tough stand as 1981 was also an election year. National had an eight-seat majority in the ninety-two seat parliament, but several members had very slim majorities. National faced a threat from the Social Credit League on the right which led Muldoon and National to continue playing the Rugby issue. It has been stated that several National members of parliament became very public Rugby supporters in 1981.[32]

The key crisis point in the tour was on July 25, when 4,000 protesters marched on the Rugby field in Hamilton. The police were forced to cancel the match after about 300 people invaded the ground and occupied the middle of the field. Some angry fans attacked protesters and HART and CARE leaders, John Minto and Tom Newnham, among many others were injured by the angry fans.[33] The police had to ask for the cancellation of the match because, in addition to the protesters on the field, a pilot had stolen a plane and threatened to fly it into the grandstand. South Africans viewed this incident live on television and many whites must have been rudely awakened to the depth of animosity felt by many New Zealanders toward their "boys." Images of the New Zealand police beating protesters, and fortress-like Rugby stadiums behind barbed wire, "shocked the nation" in South Africa.[34] Confronted with such dramatic levels of hostility for the first time, the Springboks returned from New Zealand with "more enlightened views on race" and began to question the necessity of many apartheid laws.[35] During the tour, Muldoon and his government bluntly defended a "minimalist" interpretation of the Gleneagles Agreement, clearly violating the spirit, if not the letter of the document.[36] At one point, Muldoon declared Gleneagles "a dead duck," and asserted that New Zealand was sure to pull out of it.[37] National, determined to avoid scenes like the one at Hamilton, gave the police license to use whatever force was necessary to prevent protesters occupying Rugby grounds.[38]

Since 1981, there have been no official Rugby tours between South Africa and New Zealand. The only international Rugby South Africa has played since then was at home against South America in 1982 and 1984, England in 1984, and the unofficial New Zealand "Cavaliers" in 1986. In 1982, the Commonwealth Games Federation adopted a Code of Conduct which gave the Gleneagles Agreement clear and tough guidelines in the context of the Commonwealth Games (New Zealand and Britain abstained from the code).[39] Subsequently, in 1985, the NZRFU announced plans to mount another All Black tour of South Africa. However this time, the recently elected Labour government of David Lange vigorously opposed the tour, which was finally canceled when New Zealand's High Court "granted an interim injunction arguing that... the tour would be contrary to the Rugby union's statutory commitment to promote and foster the game."[40]

Sanctions, Rugby, and Change in South Africa

Commentators have long noted the relative comprehensiveness of sport sanctions against South Africa. Thus, Bruce Kidd asserted, in 1988, that "In scope and enforcement, the sports boycott has been significantly more effective than any of the other international campaigns to quarantine the apartheid state."[41] However, while acknowledging sport sanctions' indisputable impact in terms of levering (often somewhat illusory) changes in sport policy and practice from the South African regime, many commentators have been reticent in claiming broader political influence for them. Anthony Payne's assessment of the influence of the Gleneagles Agreement is representative. Having noted the complex of internal and external factors precipitating the changes underway in South Africa since early 1990, he argues that:

> In the circumstances, it is wise to be cautious: Gleneagles was part of a broader demonstration of external opposition to apartheid which unquestionably had an effect on the political outlook of the Afrikaner political elite. But, of itself, the abrogation of sporting contacts between the Commonwealth and South Africa cannot be reckoned to have counted for much and, certainly, some of the wilder claims made both on behalf of and against the boycott should be discounted.[42]

It is the contention of the authors that, without resorting to "wild claims," an historically grounded understanding of the significance of Rugby in New Zealand and South African societies allows one to be both bolder and more precise in asserting a significant role for sport in helping to precipitate the current changes in South Africa.

Although all forms of international pressure and isolation had their supporters in the case of South Africa, sanctions advocates and analysts were overwhelmingly concerned with economic [trade and financial] sanctions.[43] This bias was reflected in the report of a "distinguished group of [sanctions] experts and researchers" to the Commonwealth Committee of Foreign Ministers on Southern Africa—*The Sanctions Report*—produced in mid-1989. The experts argued that:

> After a detailed study of the available data, we concluded that there is a threshold and that sanctions must be greater than that threshold if they are to have the required impact. We believe that a sustained cut in South African imports of 30 per cent is the minimum that would produce a fall in GDP that was significant to trigger an appropriate political response...[The report goes on] *to be politically effective, sanctions would need to cut world-wide purchases from South Africa by at least one quarter* [emphasis in original].[44]

Yet within months of this report's release, the present, now seemingly inexorable, process of change had begun. Clearly, with the wisdom of hindsight, its authors dramatically underestimated the importance of other sources of pressure for change or, perhaps more accurately, misunderstood the dynamics of this process.

Pressures and incentives from a variety of sources, as well as the bold and opportunistic political calculations of the NP government under F.W. de Klerk, can all be reckoned to have contributed to changes since 1989. Internal resistance, in particular, became a vital source of pressure. But, given the overwhelming power of the state's security apparatus and the very high, if stagnant, standard of living enjoyed by most whites, neither the limited external economic sanctions pressure nor the growing domestic unrest of the 1980s was sufficiently strong to force the government's hand in 1989. Bluntly stated, the majority of the Afrikaner and other white South Africans, through their state, simply did not manifest the stubborn determination to defend their apartheid-based "way of life" which most observers had anticipated. Their vaunted will to resist all forms of external and internal pressures was, or had become, weaker than thought; and their desire to be re-integrated into the mainstream of international culture and economic affairs was stronger than anticipated. It was in eroding "white South Africa's" will to resist exogenous pressure, and in heightening its longing to win re-acceptance into the international community, that sport sanctions in general, and Rugby sanctions in particular, made a vital contribution.

Clearly, the anti-apartheid sport boycott movement, in New Zealand and internationally, recognized the cultural and political significance of New Zealand-South Africa Rugby links. Following South Africa's expulsion from the Olympics, these links became the crucible of the sports sanctions struggle for both the boycott movement and South Africa. Robert Archer and Antoine Bouillon, having described the "constant skirmishing and subterfuges which [were] part of the modern South African [sporting] game" in the late 1970s and early 1980s, assert that "the real battle has been in Rugby—and the crucial battlefield New Zealand."[45] Starting in the mid-1970s, the effort to sever New Zealand-South Africa Rugby relations was the single-most important driving force behind the extension of sport sanctions internationally. The boycott of the 1976 Montreal Olympics, the adoption of the 1977 Gleneagles Agreement, the dramatic and widely reported events surrounding the 1981 Springbok tour of New Zealand, and the subsequent adoption, in 1982, of the Gleneagles Code of Conduct by the Commonwealth Games Federation, all originated in the controversy surrounding the struggle to stop Springbok-All Black Rugby. It is, thus, fair to suggest that this rivalry was one of the most important factors in the popularization and politicization of the apartheid issue internationally in this period.

It is not just in its catalytic impact on the international campaign for sport sanctions that the New Zealand-South Africa Rugby relationship contributed to external pressure for change, however. A distinction must be drawn between the impact of sport sanctions generally, and the loss of international (especially All Black) Rugby ties specifically. There is little question that sport sanctions of all kinds hurt sports-mad, white South Africans. However, it was relatively easy for them to rationalize, and deal with, their isolation from international table tennis, swimming, track and field, and even the Olympic Movement itself. For one thing these sports were governed by authorities in which Communist East Bloc and "radical" Third World national representatives could together muster solid majorities. Since these countries were, in South African government's world-view, part of the Moscow-orchestrated "total onslaught" against South Africa, it was comparatively easy to explain away isolation in such sports.[46] For another thing, white, and especially male and Afrikaner, South Africans simply did not care as much, or in the same way, about these sports as they did about Rugby.

Isolation from international Rugby was a different matter, on both scores. The dominant Rugby playing nations—South Africa's great rivals—were white, predominantly European in cultural origin, and thus "civilized" in white South African terms. They were the countries with which white South Africa's historical links were most intimate, and whose company they most wanted to keep. Cultural isolation from the British Isles, Australia, and New Zealand was much more keenly felt than isolation from "run-of-the-mill" African and Asian countries.

Furthermore, the loss of international Rugby links, in contrast with many other sporting rivalries, was bound to have deep repercussions among Afrikaners in particular, at both the "grass-roots" and elite levels. At the popular level, Rugby isolation was certain to shake the core Afrikaner electoral constituency of the NP. As of 1988, an Australian Foreign Affairs Department report noted:

> White teams and supporters nationwide, from major provincial organizations to the smallest hamlets, have seen the Rugby country they firmly believe to be the greatest in the world increasingly excluded from the international game and, in the eyes of many, denied their rightful place at the top of the world league.[47]

Beyond this, given the intimacy of the connections between South Africa's political elite, concentrated in the NP and the Broederbond, and the elite of South African Rugby, this particular sanction was especially likely to undermine the collective confidence of this crucial, dominant social group.[48]

It needs to be emphasized that the significance of these developments lay not simply in the fact of South Africa's isolation from the highest reaches of international Rugby, but also in the process of political controversy and struggle by which this outcome was achieved. In this respect, the New Zealand government of Robert Muldoon ironically made a key contribution to building international pressure for change in South Africa, not by its leadership, but by its obduracy in defending the autonomy of its sportsmen, and their right to compete against South Africa if they so wished. Every step forward in the extension of the boycott campaign from 1976 onward—the Gleneagles Agreement, the protests against the 1981 tour, the subsequent adoption of the Commonwealth Code of Conduct to clarify and police Gleneagles—was, in the proverbial phrase, like pulling teeth from Muldoon and his government. This is not the place for an analysis of Muldoon's motives in taking the stubborn stand that he did: suffice it to say that, as implied earlier, they had a good deal to do with domestic political calculations. However, each time Muldoon and his cohorts were forced to concede a round, the sport boycott movement in New Zealand and beyond, as well as the allied South African non-racial sport movement, heightened their profile, their degree of politicization and their determination to push on towards the complete dismantling of apartheid, as the necessary prerequisite for the elimination of racism in sport.

Thus, the spectacle of New Zealand society cleaved by the 1981 South African tour, and the resulting sense that no further tours could be safely mounted, had a significantly greater impact internationally, and on South Africa, than a quiet shelving of the tour would have had. Furthermore, the impact of the severing of New Zealand-South African Rugby links specifically, and the momentum of the sport sanctions movement generally, was sharply stimulated not because of, but rather in spite of, the actions of the New Zealand government. Conversely, the initiative in extending international pressure for change through action to end Springbok-All Black Rugby fell largely to the highly motivated, broadly based, and zealous domestic tour opponents in that country.

Conclusion

The importance of sport in general, and Rugby in particular, in precipitating political change in South Africa should not be overstated. The effect of the loss of Rugby links with New Zealand was, as these authors argue, essentially indirect and longer-term in nature, enhancing the sense of international isolation felt by white (particularly Afrikaner) South Africans, and weakening their resolve to defend their "way of life." However, it is the contention of the authors that the generally unexpected decision of the de Klerk government to launch the current process of change cannot be understood without an appreciation of the corrosive societal and psychological effects of steadily expanding cultural sanctions. Of these, the loss of international Rugby links, above all with New Zealand, were the most potent.

The skeptic will argue that, even if the foregoing analysis is correct in its assessment of the significance of Rugby in promoting change in South Africa, this is a special, or aberrant, case. No other society, it may be asserted, has been as widely and popularly disparaged as "white South Africa"; and no other society (save New Zealand and perhaps Wales) has shared the same passionate love for, and devotion to, its Rugby. In a sense it is obviously true that South Africa is unique. It is almost inconceivable that anything closely resembling the particular conditions which have prevailed there will arise elsewhere. In a more general sense, however, aspects of the South Africa case are less unique than has often been assumed—something which is becoming more apparent as the specter of apartheid fades. Gross and systematic human rights violations in other countries are receiving more attention than ever before, and the use of international sanctions is increasing, as evidenced in the recent decision to impose sanctions, including sport sanctions against the Serbian government in Belgrade. South Africa's deep passion for Rugby may be very nearly unique, but other countries have relied heavily on other sports in building national cultural identity, and share a comparably strong attachment to "their game."[49] Other examples of sport playing a crucial role in national consciousness and political life come readily to mind: cricket in the West Indies, and soccer in a number of Latin American countries. In addition, television interviews showed that the sanctions most affecting "men in the street" in Belgrade was the ban on the Yugoslavian team's participation in the European soccer championships of 1992. Furthermore, where sport does not have comparable significance, other dominant cultural practices may have a similar degree of political salience. Thus, the lessons of this distinctive case are likely to resonate elsewhere. Small societies with distinctive strengths will periodically find themselves at the center of important international political developments; sanctions involving dominant cultural practices—notably sport—need to be treated more seriously as a source of international influence; and dominant and traditional lobbies and social movements are likely to "intrude" even more regularly into international affairs.

Notes

[1]The authors wish to thank Sue Nauright who provided research assistance for this study, and John Nauright wishes to thank several of his recent students at Queen's University, Canada; Karla Bethune, Kate Collins, Jackie Gljuscic, James Keast, and James Ware, who all worked on the South African sport sanctions issue and sifted through some of the material used for this chapter. We would also like to thank Don McIntosh, who provided initial encouragement and comments on early drafts of this work. John Nauright also thanks the University of Otago, which provided funds to enable him to participate in the "Sport in the Global Village," conference.

[2]Laubscher, L., & G. Nieman. *The Carolin papers: A diary of the 1906–07 Springbok tour*. Pretoria: Rugbyana Publishers, 1990; Nauright, John. "Images of colonial manhood in the British mind: Colonial sporting tours to Britain, 1878–1912," *Canadian Journal of History of Sport*. 23: 2 (December 1992), pp. 54-71; Nauright, John. "Sport, manhood and empire: British responses to the 1905 New Zealand Rugby tour," *International Journal of the History of Sport*. 8:2 (1991), pp. 239–255.

[3]Thompson, Richard. *Retreat from apartheid: New Zealand's sporting contacts with South Africa*. Auckland: Oxford University Press, 1975, p. 2.

[4]Paton quoted in Woods, Donald. *Black and white*. Dublin: Ward River Press, 1981, p. 43.

[5]Nauright. "Sport, manhood and empire: British responses to the 1905 New Zealand rugby tour," pp. 239–255.

[6]Nauright, John, & David Black. "Much more than just a game: The role of rugby in the history and international relations of South Africa and New Zealand, 1921–1992," Unpublished paper, Queen's University, 1992; Wilkins, Ivor, & Hans Strydom. *The broederbond*. New York & London: Paddington Press, 1979.

[7]Blackett quoted in Nepia, George & Terry McLean. *I, George Nepia: The golden years of Rugby*. Auckland: A. H. & A. W. Reed, 1963.

[8]Pearson, M. N. "Heads in the sand: The 1956 Springbok tour to New Zealand in perspective," In Richard Cashman & Michael McKernan (Eds). *Sport in history: The making of modern sporting history*. St. Lucia: Queensland University Press, 1979; Phillips, Jock. "Rugby, war and the mythology of the New Zealand male," *New Zealand Journal of History*. 18:2 (1987), pp. 83–103; Roger, W. *Old heroes: The 1956 Springbok tour and the lives beyond*. Auckland: Hodder & Stoughton, 1991.

[9]*New Zealand Hansard*. (1960), p. 1136.

[10]Hanan quoted in *New Zealand Hansard*. (1960), pp. 964–968.

[11]*New Zealand Hansard.* (1965), p. 2527.

[12]Thompson. *Retreat from apartheid: New Zealand's sporting contacts with South Africa.* p. 2.

[13]Wilkins & Strydom. *The broederbond.*

[14]D'Oliveira, Basil. *The D'Oliveira affair.* London: Collins, 1969.

[15]Marais quoted in *South African Hansard.* (1976), p. 936.

[16]*Dominion,* 1969.

[17]Sorrenson, M. P. K. "Uneasy bedfellows: A survey of New Zealand's relations with South Africa," In *New Zealand, South Africa and sport: Background papers.* Wellington: New Zealand Institute of International Affairs, 1976.

[18]Citizen's association for racial equality (CARE). *Ten years of CARE.* Auckland: CARE, 1974.

[19]CARE. *Letters concerning proposed All Black tour.* Auckland: CARE, 1969.

[20]Sorrenson. "Uneasy bedfellows: A survey of New Zealand's relations with South Africa."

[21]*Rand Daily Mail.* (1973).

[22]Newman, Thomas. *Apartheid is not a game: The inside story of New Zealand's struggle against apartheid sport.* Auckland: Graphic Publications, 1975, p. 74.

[23]*New Zealand government white paper.* (1973), p. 5; Sorrenson. "Uneasy bedfellows: A survey of New Zealand's relations with South Africa."

[24]*Star.* Johannesburg, 1973.

[25]Trainor, L. "Sport and foreign policy," *New Zealand International Review.* (May/June 1976).

[26]Drake quoted in Halt all-racial tours movement (HART). *Information Sheet.* Christchurch: HART, 1976, p. 2.

[27]Macintosh, D., D. Greenhorn, & D. Black. "Canadian diplomacy and the 1978 Edmonton Commonwealth Games," *Journal of Sport History.*(in press); Payne, A. "The international politics of the Gleneagles agreement," In *The round table.* (1990), p. 320.

[28]Newnham, T. *Apartheid is not a game: The inside story of New Zealand's struggle against apartheid sport.*; Shears, Richard & Isabelle Gidley. *Storm out of Africa.* Auckland: Macmillan, 1981.

[29]*Eastern Province Herald.* (1981).

[30]*New Zealand Foreign Affairs Review.* (1981).

[31]Phillips. "Rugby, war and the mythology of the New Zealand male," pp. 83–103; Sinclair, Keith. *A destiny apart: New Zealand's search for national identity.* Wellington: Hodder & Stoughton, 1986.

[32]Shears & Gidley. *Storm out of Africa: The 1981 Springbok tour of New Zealand.*

[33]Shears & Gidley. *Storm out of Africa: The 1981 Springbok tour of New Zealand.*

[34]*Eastern Province Herald*. (1981).

[35]*Sunday Times*. (1981).

[36]*New Zealand foreign affairs review*. (1981); Payne. "The international politics of the Gleneagles agreement."

[37]*Rand Daily Mail*. (1981).

[38]*Rand Daily Mail*. (1981).

[39]Payne. "The international politics of the Gleneagles agreement."

[40]Payne. "The international politics of the Gleneagles agreement."

[41]Kidd, Bruce. "The campaign against sport in South Africa," *International Journal*. 43:4 (1988), pp. 643–664.

[42]Payne. "The international politics of the Gleneagles agreement."

[43]Anglin, 1990; Doxey, 1987.

[44]*South Africa: The Sanctions Report*. London: Penguin, 1989, pp. 114–115.

[45]Archer, Robert & Antoine Bouillon. *The South African game: Sport and racism*. London: Zed Press, 1982,p. 296.

[46]Davies, R. & D. O'Meara. "Total strategy in southwest Africa: An analysis of South African regional policy since 1978," *Journal of Southern African Studies*. 11:2 (1985).

[47]*Australian Department of foreign affairs and trade*. (1988), p. 140.

[48]Nauright, John & David Black. "Sport, power and society: A case study of the links between the Afrikaner Broederbond, the National party and South African Rugby administration in South Africa," (Working paper), (1993).

[49]Caldwell, Geoffrey. "International sport and national identity," *International Social Science Journal*. 34:2 (1982), pp. 173–184.

Chapter 10

Sport and Transformation: Observations and Projections on Developments in South Africa From an 'Eliasian' Perspective

Denver J. Hendricks

Limitations on space prevent a comprehensive exegesis of the problem being addressed. Eliasian sociology demands a developmental approach which, given the complexity of South African history, will (even in an extremely abridged form) consume many more pages than those permitted for this chapter. The problem is exacerbated by a similar incapacity to expand sufficiently upon aspects of the theoretical model[1] upon which the present thesis is predicated.

"Eliasian" (figurational) Sociology

Various aspects of the sociology of Norbert Elias and Eric Dunning underpin the arguments presented in this chapter. Elias conceives of societies as being comprised of aggregates of individuals and interest groups in dynamic interdependence with one another. A central characteristic of the "figuration"[2] formed by that interdependence concerns the inequality amongst individuals and groups with regard to the access which they have to power in it. Power, Elias believes, cannot be reduced to single "factors" such as the control over (scarce) economic resources, even though a thorough comprehension of that influence is indispensable to understanding disparity. Power is related, rather, to any resource which one group may monopolize at the expense of another. Resources may be so divergent as to include the need which an individual or group feels to belong to a wider figuration (of nations, for example, a significant aspect of this chapter). More specifically, Elias[3] relates social inequality to a complex interplay of access to resources, personality structures, styles of life, and cultural expression, the latter three which, amongst others, he designates the "social habitus" of the group. It impacts upon the relative "disgrace" and "charisma" of the competing groups, consequently, upon perceptions of their respective "levels of civilization"[4] and ultimately, upon disparate access to power. Elias has incorporated all of the above into his theory of "established-outsider," (or, in a sense, dominant-subservient) relations, which explicates social inequities. Elias proposes that there is a tendency in all figurations for inequalities to level out over time, through an unintentional process which he designates "functional democratization," the concomitant of a need for greater interdependence between individuals and groups which emerges as society becomes increasingly complex. That does not imply, however, that the established surrender their power and privilege to the ascending outsiders voluntarily; on the contrary, they persist in their efforts to perpetuate their vantage. They are reluctant to resort to violent means to achieve those ends given the repugnance associated with that strategy in modern societies. Alternative approaches have to be sought to procure those interests.

Violence and "Civilization"

The retreat from violence constitutes a central theme of "Eliasian" theories on the "civilizing process," the latter which constituted a major focus of his work. More significantly, Dunning[5] observes a strong relation between the growth of the phenomenon of sport (or "sportization"), and the decline of violence in society as it becomes increasingly complex (or "civilized"). It is important to note that neither Elias nor Dunning envisaged any of the processes described above as being linear. However, it seems reasonable to deduce that an association between a preponderance for violent behavior and low levels of sport participation (both qualitatively and quantitatively) is equivalent to a lower level of "civilization." Conversely, a predisposition toward restrained behavior along with higher levels of sport participation can be considered to be synonymous with higher levels of "civilization." The consequences of those perceptions for the habitus of outsider and established groups respectively have disparate outcomes for access to power within the figuration.

A Brief Overview of the History of South African Society

The history of South African society has been dominated by the systematic bonding of blacks, the "outsiders," into an interdependence of subservience with whites, the "established." That outcome can be attributed to a variety of controls, among which the monopolistic control of the established over the means of violence in the society is highly significant. That relationship has been entrenched through a variety of overt and covert strategies. The former relates to the (problematic) use of violence to secure conformity, while the latter refers to more sophisticated, subtle techniques to achieve the same end. The monopoly exercised by the established over education, politics, the law, the media, sport, and a host of other social institutions facilitates the latter handsomely. Through it they were able to undermine, in the most effective manner, the ability of outsiders to organize cohesively in order to challenge their inferior status. Rather, it exacerbated the lack of cohesion within that realm. The peculiar South African figuration epitomizes the Eliasian proposition[6] that often a cohesive, well organized minority is able to dominate a less well organized, divided majority.

Through the gradual process of "functional-democratization," characterized by a burgeoning degree of unity, the outsiders, who became cognizant of their common plight, were increasingly able to assert themselves against their oppression. In sport, their ability to rally under the banner of non-racialism[7] contributed to that unity. However, no single "factor" led to the decline of apartheid. Rather, the confluence of a variety of controls ultimately prompted the dramatic announcements by F.W. de Klerk, in February of 1990, of the commitment of the South African government to a program of reform which would eventually lead to the contemplated democratic society. Those controls included, amongst others:

1. the systematic exclusion of the society, and particularly of the established within it, from the international figuration of nations;

2. internal strife in South Africa on the labor, educational, religious, sports, and other fronts fostered by greater cohesion amongst the outsiders;

3. developments within the international figuration of nations, particularly the global demise of communism which, had the South African announcement of renewal not been forthcoming, would increasingly have focused the attention of the world upon the inequities of the apartheid system; and

4. internal and world-wide economic recession.

The decision to "abandon" apartheid was, therefore, not taken voluntarily, nor was it founded upon philanthropic considerations of the established. It was the logical precipitate of the confluence of a number of controls, some of which have been identified above. Developments within sport were interesting to the extent that it constituted one of the few domains over which outsiders were able to procure some form of monopoly. They were able to secure control over the access which the established had to international sporting arenas. That was not an insignificant monopoly either, given the passion[8] of the established for sport, their subsequent elaborate attempts to restore those links, and their efforts at undermining[9] that outsider power base in a number of ways. It manifested the desire and need of the established to be part of the international figuration of nations for, amongst others, it also provided them with significant exposure for similar quests for affiliation in other spheres as well. Moreover, it could have fulfilled a significant role in enhancing their esteem, and hence their morale and cohesion. Control over access to international sport was one of the first (if not the only) monopolies acquired by outsiders. The process through which it was attained was, however, a difficult one. The latter problem pertained to the reluctance of international sports federations, including the International Olympic Committee (IOC), to act decisively against the racism in sporting practice on the part of the established in South Africa. Only through persistent efforts and pressure from, amongst others, the African bloc, the communist countries, the United Nations, and sympathizers throughout the world was that actualized. All of the developments described above contributed conjointly to the announcement of the proposed renaissance of the South African social fabric by de Klerk in February 1990. That declaration facilitated South Africa's instantaneous readmission to the figuration of nations in virtually all spheres, including sport. Indeed, sport was one of the first domains into which South Africa was welcomed back. Again, the reasons for that were manifold. It related to:

1. the reluctance, in the first place, of international sports federations to exclude South Africa from that fraternity;

2. the pursuit of self-interest amongst key players in the politics of international sport, particularly that of the presidents of the IOC and of the International Amateur Athletics Federation (IAAF)[10]; and

3. the support from individuals and interest groups within the figuration of outsiders in South Africa for such readmission. Sport, and the readmission (of the established, primarily) to international competition, was used as a bargaining tool in the pursuit of political and personal interests by various individuals and groups in the country;

4. the support of the African bloc under the influence of the parties mentioned in 2 and 3 above, but also in pursuit of their own individual and national interests, particularly so in the light of the socioeconomic woes of the continent and the concomitant, forlorn hope for salvation through an association with South Africa.

South Africa's readmission to international sport effectively emasculated the outsiders with regard to the control which they had formerly wielded. That deprivation may have been a necessary outcome of the change which was supposed to have taken place in the society. The question which begs to be answered, however, is whether change has indeed taken place or, alternatively, whether conditions have "normalized" sufficiently to facilitate a just dispensation now, or in the foreseeable future. On the basis of available evidence, the prognosis would seem to suggest the obverse. Given the extent of the economic recession in South Africa, outsiders are probably worse off presently than they were at the height of the apartheid era. Inflation is rampant, between five and seven million people are jobless, and almost 75% of the population is either illiterate or semi-literate.[11] Outsiders constitute the major component of those statistics. In terms of the "access" which the outsiders have supposedly been afforded to sport, the situation is as precarious. Not only are blacks scantily represented on national teams (despite their numeric superiority in society) where they have been selected to represent South Africa (even at the Olympic Games in 1992), they compete without the recognition within their own country of being fully fledged citizens.

It may be argued, given the nature of the process of "functional democratization," that the process of "normalization" will be a slow one. Unfortunately, that constitutes the crux of the problem. Expectations among the outsiders about the imminence of their "liberation" (a perception attributable, in no small way, to the populist rhetoric of political and other players of various persuasions and with various agendas) have been elevated. However, the lack of tangible reformation has raised levels of frustration and anger. The latter is articulated in the intolerance and violence which preponderates in the country presently. Violence, in which people are being killed at the rate of between eight and ten a day, is directed at fellow outsiders. That phenomenon is popularly referred to as black-on-black violence. Apart from claims about the involvement of a "third force"[12] in the perpetuation of the violence, it is also a manifestation of the inability of outsiders to perpetrate such aggression against their oppressors, given the monopolistic control of the latter over the means of violence. Moreover, it is an articulation of the frustration experienced by outsider males, whose gender dominance within their own ranks is undermined by their emasculation in virtually every other sphere of social existence in the South African figuration. However, that constitutes a separate debate which will not be entertained here.

An "Eliasian" View and Diagnosis of the South African Figuration

The quest by outsiders for a more equitable distribution of power in the South African figuration is undermined by the fact that their (inter)dependence is economically founded. Their disadvantage in that regard is compounded by the magnitude of the economic recession currently mesmerizing the country. The statistics quoted earlier attest to that. The primary concern of the masses of outsiders is for survival. While their established counterparts are able to experiment with alternative styles of leisure, outsiders increasingly have to experiment with alternative styles of survival. It is reported[13] that five to seven million of South Africans (overwhelmingly blacks) live in "informal"[14] settlements, while one in four[15] finds employment in the "informal[16]" sector. Access to sport, or even political power (for that matter), is peripheral for the majority of outsiders. Only those with personal ambition or group interests actively participate in, or pursue power along, those lines. Their strategies to achieve those ends amount to little more than an exploitation of the aspirations and despair of those of greater disadvantage.

The established recognize the relative insignificance of change within the realm of sport (or even politics), hence their willingness to pursue a negotiated settlement in those spheres. Needless to say, the attempts at securing some degree of control over political reform (such as their requirement for a 75 percent majority vote to secure any form of constitutional reform) relate to concerns about the impact which a loss of that monopoly may have upon the associated monopoly which they enjoy over economic resources which, in the present figuration (and at the risk of a reductionist view), is seminal. A "settlement" of the sports question is even less problematic, for the impact thereof upon the outsider quest for power is even less significant. In fact, the consequence thereof from an established perspective may be quite the opposite, for, through it, they have managed to procure a coalition with a certain stratum of outsiders which has enabled them to undermine the leverage which the latter had acquired through their control over sport. It is not insignificant that substantial numbers of the more privileged strata of outsiders (from where black sportspersons derive primarily), who were formerly restricted from access to sport and other structures monopolized by the established, pursued those options vigorously when those curtailments were lifted. Earlier they had campaigned for such access through an affinity with the most deprived whose cause they were ostensibly facilitating through strategies such as self-imposed moratoria on sport and other forms of interaction which outlawed any form of alliance with what they labeled "racist structures." When restrictions were lifted, their interests were served, and that alliance was abandoned under the guise of the "unity" and "non-racialism" which had ostensibly been achieved in negotiations with the established. The latter development may, in fact, provide clues to emerging established-outsider relations which, in the "new South Africa," may run more closely along class lines.[17]

In capitalist countries such as South Africa, participation in sport is intimately connected to the socioeconomic circumstances of the individual. Access to, and excellence in, sport is delimited by the temporal, financial, and other resources which the individual is able to invest in it. Needless to say, the overwhelming majority of outsiders are unable to make that commitment. In striking a deal, outsiders have traded a commitment from the established to "development programmes"[18] for the disadvantaged, for their support for "South Africa's" readmission to international sport. "South African" sports teams have been readmitted to the international arenas of the world. "Development programmes" have yet to make their appearance. A report in the *Sunday Times* of June 7, 1992,[19] suggests that there are not going to be development programmes. It concludes that the burden would be the responsibility of the state. That notwithstanding, the concept of a "development programme" is a problematic one. It is another classic manifestation of an attempt to divorce sport from its social context, a tendency which outsiders resisted consistently at the height of their struggles in that sphere. A "development programme" can, at best, only be marginally successful. It amounts to little more than charity. It can never be sufficiently comprehensive to involve significant numbers of people, nor can it be sustained. Accordingly, very few people will benefit from it given the breadth and depth of the disadvantage suffered by outsiders. It is not sustainable, for those who might benefit from it lack the personal, familial, or communal support to facilitate continued participation. In any case, it can never facilitate equitable competition between outsiders and their established counterparts. That is not to say that no outsider will benefit. Rather, the level of intervention required to ensure equity is phenomenal. It will, at the very least, have to parallel the concessions and privileges afforded promising outsider athletes in the mines[20] and in the security forces, the two sources from which the majority of the limited number of successful, black sportspeople who have participated in the established ranks, have emerged. Even the proposal[21] of the National Olympic and Sports Congress (NOSC) to erect sports facilities in the enclaves to which outsiders have been confined will do little to rectify the situation. The availability of facilities in some of those areas for extended periods already has not impacted significantly upon participation or performance levels.

The advantages of a development program lie with the established. That benefit exceeds the cherished ideal of the readmission of South African sports teams to international competition, or even the benefit which that exposure holds for other aspects of interdependence within the figuration of nations of the world. It transcends the emasculation of outsiders whose monopoly over access to international sport allowed them some leverage in their quest for a more equitable distribution of power. The most significant consequence of the new arrangements relates to its impact upon the relative self- and group-esteem of outsiders and the established. The inability of outsiders to perform at comparable levels with the established, amicably illustrated by their low standards even in local league competitions, together with their dearth in representative, regional or national teams, contributes to the inculcation of inferiority complexes, and a concomitant disapprobation as individuals and as a group. At the same time it facilitates the approbation of the established. The former is encompassed in the internalization and admission by outsiders of their need to be "developed" (implicitly by the established). It represents a veiled affirmation of their inferiority. The latter is expedited by the superior performance levels of the established whose charisma is further enhanced by their apparent concern for the upliftment of outsider sport through their "development programs" in sport, their efforts at "civilizing"[22] the latter. The phenomenon of black athletes excelling once they join established sport to be guided under established supervision entrenches the relative "group disgrace" and "group charisma"[23] of outsiders and established respectively. The impact of the latter upon the "habitus" of the groups has been articulated above. It confirms the dependence of the outsiders upon the established. The repercussions thereof for access to power chances for the respective groups are clear-cut.

Conclusion

There is no urgent need for the established to pursue sophisticated strategies to preserve their power and privilege and, hence, the inequality of the South African figuration at this point in time. That may become necessary in the future as incongruities continue to level out. However, features of outsider sport, such as the low levels of participation both in terms of quantity and quality, do impact upon perceptions of the "level of civilization" attained by the group. That is amplified by their ostensible preponderance for violent behavior, a perception promoted significantly by the mainstream media through explicit depiction of the most savage scenes of black, internecine violence. It elicits sentiments of repugnance which impress upon the "disgrace" of the group, its habitus, perceptions of its "level of civilization" and, ultimately, upon its access to power. There is a prevailing sense, even among (more privileged) outsiders, that blacks are not "ready" to rule the country. It is that sensitivity which facilitates the ability of F.W. de Klerk to access the most impoverished outsider enclaves of the country where, often, he is received with the acclaim which befalls a hero.

Access to sport at every level is a right which all South Africans should enjoy. Accordingly, sport should be relieved of the constraints which inhibit such admission. However, within the context of the capitalist society, the circumscription of economic empowerment of outsiders places limitations upon that eventuality in both the short and longer terms. The authenticity of outsider emasculation is unquestionable. Their emancipation has been linked, inextricably, to the country's economic[24] growth. It places an even greater damper on prospects for upliftment and, hence, upon equity in access to sport, given the bleak projections of economic forecasters. In scenarios sketched by the latter,[25] the most promising prospect for economic growth in South Africa, which will facilitate indubitable, albeit slow, recovery and growth, is also the most unpopular option given the pervasiveness of populist rhetoric of "quick-fix" solutions to the hardships suffered by outsiders. The latter has come to characterize campaigns for political support. Through it outsider expectations have been elevated to the extent that a failure to "deliver the goods" is bound to have serious repercussions. That will be exacerbated by the disparities which outsiders encounter on a daily basis, also in sport, to which they will not have gained substantial access. All the symptoms of a potential inability to "deliver" are present, irrespective of the economic option which is selected. It is complicated by the time-frame within which outsiders expect such "delivery." Outsiders will have to be persuaded, difficult and painful though it may be, of the impracticality of their anticipations. That is the major challenge facing the society in the immediate future.

Dennis Brutus[26] intimated that it has never been the requirement of international sports federations that poverty should be eliminated from South African society before it could be readmitted to international sport. It can never be expected of sport to rectify those inconsistencies. In this chapter, it is not argued that sport should, or could, fulfill that role either. It simply cannot. The concerns articulated herein are, however, twofold. Firstly, the extent to which sport contributes to restrain the process of achieving a more equitable distribution of power in all realms of social interaction including that within the institution itself, as articulated above, is disconcerting. Secondly, the impact which that may have upon the frustration of outsiders who expect a swift transition to an equitable dispensation, if not one in which power changes hands completely may, potentially, destabilize the country even further.

The task of convincing outsiders to modify their expectations for short- and medium-term relief from their circumstance is a daunting one. It must be recognized that progress to equity will more likely require a time-frame of the order of generations. In the process new established-outsider relations will emerge which will bring along with it new inequalities most probably centered around the axis of social class.[27] That is not to say that those relations centered around the question of race will expire; it may merely recede from the prominence which it enjoys presently. Sport will reflect those developments and will continue to contribute to the struggle for power across the new divides which will emerge.

Established sport, or "neo-established," sport has been readmitted to the international arenas. A chapter on South African sport and social history has effectively been closed. The control and concomitant leverage which outsiders have monopolized within the realm of sport and, through it, over social developments, has been eradicated. The extent to which that leverage has been traded for political expediency will only be determined by time which, presently, is probably the society's most crucial commodity.

Notes

---

[1] The theoretical model employed in the present discussion comprises a combination of various aspects of the Sociology of Norbert Elias. A comprehensive summary of his work is contained in Mennel, S. *Norbert Elias: Civilization and the Human Self-Image*. Oxford: Basil Blackwell, 1989.

[2] Horne, J. and D. Jary, "The Figurational Sociology of Sport and Leisure of Elias and Dunning: An Exposition and Critique." In, Green, E. *Sport, Leisure,*

and Social Relations. London: Routledge and Kegan Paul, 1987.

[3]Elias, N. and J. Scotson, *The Established and the Outsiders: An Enquiry into Community Problems*. London: Frank Cass, 1965.

[4]Elias, N. *The Civilizing Process. Vol I: The History of Manners*. Oxford: Basil Blackwell, 1978.

[5]Elias, N. and E. Dunning, *Quest for Excitement: Sport and Leisure in the Civilizing Process*. Oxford: Basil Blackwell, 1986.

[6]Elias & Scotson.

[7]Archer, R. and A. Bouillon, *The South African Game: Sport and Racism*. London: Zed Press, 1982, p. 186.

[8]The passion of the established for sport is aptly described in Archer & Bouillon, p. 194.

[9]Archer & Bouillon, p. 194.

[10]See Robinson, A. "New Hope for SA Athletes." *The Argus*, (February 8, 1992).p. 18.

[11]Mxgashe, M. Interview: Barney Desai, Pan-Africanist Congress Press Secretary. *SASPOST*. 3: 3 (May 1992), p. 3 ; Agenda, *South African Broadcasting Corporation*.(May 5 1992); National Manpower Commission, May 14, 1992; *Radio Metro*. 7 o'clock news.

[12]The third force theory suggests that some covert agency with origins in the ranks of the established is responsible for inciting the violence referred to.

[13]Agenda.

[14]The term "informal" is a euphemism for the shack (squatter) dwellings erected, often illegally, by homeless people on vacant land.

[15]Agenda.

[16]"Informal" employment refers to the attempts by individuals to make a living outside of regular employment in the formal sector.

[17]See Esterhuyse, F. "Class War, not Race War the Next Step." *The Argus*, (August 1, 1992), p. 4.

[18]Development programs are strategies designed to uplift the quality of outsider sport to enable them to compete more equitably with their established counterparts.

[19]*Sunday Times* (June 7, 1992), p. 22.

[20]Mantashe, G. "Sport in South African Mines: An Area of Concern." Unpublished paper presented at SACOS Conference, December 1986.

[21]The NOSC proposal for the erection of 100 sports centers in black townships. See Roberts, C. *South Africa's Struggle for Olympic Legitimacy*. Cape Town: Township Publishing, 1991.

[22]Elias, 1978.

[23]Elias & Scotson.

[24]Standard Bank. "Die IMF se Perspektief op Ekonomiese Beleid vir 'n Nuwe Suid-Afrika." *Standard Bank Ekonomiese Oorsig*, (March 1992), p. 1.

[25]le Roux, P. du P. *The Mont Fleur Scenarios*. Bellville: University of the Western Cape, 1992.

[26]Dennis Brutus in an address to students at the University of the Western Cape, Bellville, June 1991.

[27]Mennel, p. 124; Esterhuyse.

Chapter 11

The Springbok Trials: Some Critical Reflections on South Africa's Unity Games

Peter G. Craig and C. Roger Rees

Introduction: "A World in Motion"

One of the most sanguine features of the geo-political changes that have occurred in an already remarkable decade has been that involving South Africa. With the establishment of the multi-party constitutional conference and the referendum of March 1992, the emergence in South Africa of a general political mandate for constitutional change appears to have been firmly established. The search for the means to politically, economically, and culturally emancipate the country from its legacies of colonialism and apartheid is a project that remains however fraught with difficulties. Not the least of these is the as yet undecided outcome of the constitutional conference and its attempts to establish some form of consensus which can direct South Africa's transition to non-racial government. This already difficult process, moreover, is having to take place within a context where the constant threat of large-scale civil violence from those who feel threatened or frustrated by the pace of change (or lack of it) is an everyday reality. On one side, there are right-wing extremists of 'Afrikaner Weerstandsbeweging' (A.W.B.), and their pressure for a separate "whites only" mini-state, while on the other, there are the warring political and tribal factions including the African National Congress (ANC) and Inkatha, which dominate life and death in the townships. As the decay from peaceful change into civil war in other parts of the world demonstrates, the threat posed by this violence should not be taken lightly.

However, despite the magnitude of these problems, the substantial changes that have already occurred and the sense of optimism and empowerment that they have created must be warmly welcomed. In particular, the recent and very public unification of South African sports organizations have been used by both the National Party and the ANC to provide the country, and the international community, with powerful ideological images of the developing discourse on the structure of South African society. What is probably most remarkable to those of us involved with sport is how, in a relatively short period of time, sport in South Africa appears to have undergone a startling transition from a social movement characterized by conflict and resistance[1] to one appearing to be characterized by compromise, integration and reconciliation. As a result, sport in recent months has found itself held out as one of the available sites of radical engagement between the different political, cultural and economic interests in South Africa. As such it has almost inevitably found itself presented by politicians, the media, and sports bodies with the daunting task of not only providing a vision of some possible future but also as acting as a potential vehicle for its realization. This role is vividly portrayed by Solomon Morewa, General Secretary of the recently unified governing body of soccer in South Africa (South African Football Association), who has been recently quoted as stating:

> We in sport see ourselves as transforming
> society: we are what society is. Soccer in
> South Africa has over one million affiliated
> players and is the most cross-cultural activi-
> ty in the country, embracing everybody
> including Zulus and Xhosas.[2]

The eloquence (and appeal) of this rhetoric aside, a number of important questions are clearly raised by this transformation. The first echoes that posed elsewhere by Critcher[3], in questioning how far cultural institutions such as sport are actually open to radical change. The second is whether the changes in the structure and organization of sport represented by the unification process can be accepted as evidence of substantial and meaningful change in the nature of South African society.

In endeavoring to answer these questions the presentation which follows will have two main themes. The first is to argue that to grasp the meaning of sport in South Africa, it must be primarily understood as a cultural construction whose continued production and reproduction is fundamentally structured by access to power and patterned social relations (class, gender and ethnicity). In part, the conceptual framework adopted by this chapter is, therefore, firmly located in the established cultural analysis of sport detailed in the work of Hargreaves,[4] Gruneau,[5] Jarvis,[6] and Sage.[7] The second is grounded in the debate which, in recent years, has attained a prominent position in European and North American sociology. It is a debate which has set itself the task of understanding the nature and structure of the institutional transformations that now appear to be locally and globally an endemic part of modern social life. At the center of this debate is a discourse about whether the age of "modernity" has undergone a subtle but profound change that has led us into an era of "postmodernity."

While it is impossible for this paper to represent the complex and sometimes impenetrable discussions that have informed this debate, it is hoped that the brief discussion of the recent work of Giddens[8] will demonstrate that this work provides a significant and provocative theoretical statement that offers some important insights into the dynamics of social change.

With these discourses forming the core of the conceptual framework we are also concerned to extend the discussion into an examination of three issues that are pivotal to the reconstruction of sport in South Africa. These are 1. the rise of the National Olympic and Sports Congress (NOSC) and its chaperoning of the unification of South Africa's sports organizations; 2. the impact and the images of the rapid readmission of South Africa to the international sports arena; and 3. the problems and contradictions that for many are still a powerful element in their experience of "post-apartheid" sport.

A Personal Note

While this chapter is intended to add to the critical discourse on sport in South Africa, it is also informed by the authors' own experiences of current changes taking place in South Africa. These are based on a visit to South Africa during August 1991 when, as guests of Edumove Forum[9] we were involved with a 'roving conference' program which literally took us on a journey across the length and breadth of South Africa. Under the theme "Sociological perspectives of movement activity" the authors and other colleagues made a number of presentations which were then followed up by workshops in which small culturally mixed groups of delegates examined and debated the themes raised by the presentations. While in this current setting this may seem to be an unremarkable structure and process, as we discovered however, in the South African context, the interaction between the various cultural groups which it facilitated was a radical departure from the normality of segregation that still dominates life in South Africa. The potential and the problems encountered by the delegates as they created and experienced this "alternative reality" went far beyond the issues raised by the various conference papers. It is with this experience in mind, that the authors of this chapter, and the others in this section, can in their own small way be a part of the very processes of change that they attempt to describe and analyze.

Sport and Culture: Representation and Reproduction

> ...image is to narrative as surface is to depth,
> appearance to reality, shallowness to complex-
> ity.[10]

One of the problems faced by an analysis of sport is that, as with other cultural activities, for the vast majority of its participants its everyday experience and meaning appears to be simple and non-problematical, it is a pleasurable and harmless recreational activity. However as the statement by Morris[11] suggests an uncritical acceptance this image provides for only a superficial and limited understanding of sport. Sport, as the work of cultural theorists such as Hargreaves[12] and Gruneau[13] has detailed, is a complex cultural construction that cannot be separated from the wider context of power relations.

As even a cursory examination of this work demonstrates, in an attempt to elaborate on these relations particular emphasis has been placed on the concept of hegemony. Indeed its application of this concept allied with its revisions of various neo-Marxian and feminist notions (e.g., ideology, class conflict, and patriarchy), has been one of the hallmarks of this work. Another has been its detailing of the historic and contingent relationship that exists between sport, power, and culture. Furthermore, though this work clearly identifies how sport can be deeply patterned by specific hegemonic relations, the reality of "the conflicting and contradictory meanings signified by sport"[14] also demonstrates that the cultural ownership of sport is constantly being contested and resisted. The construction of sport cannot thereby be regarded as a static and deterministic process but rather one that is fundamentally reflexive in nature.

Albeit that this representation of the diversity and complexity of this work has been necessarily discursive, there are a number of conceptual propositions critically identified by this discourse that are salient to the analysis of sport.[15] Briefly articulated they are:

1. That people must be understood as being born into a world that is historically and materially constructed. For individuals and the social groups they are members of, this means that access to and control of resources is inevitably unequally distributed. Though this has specific implications for class relations, it is also an acknowledged factor informing the experience of gender and ethnicity.

2. That knowledge must also be recognized as culturally constructed, legitimated, and reproduced. The control of the cultural production of knowledge is a vital expression of the political and cultural power of the dominant social group. The changing meaning of sport which the unification of the sports bodies in South Africa seems to herald is therefore as fundamentally located in the system of political and cultural legitimation and sanction as those which preceded them.

3. That despite the power vested in some groups through their control of South Africa's institutional structures, it must also be recognized that people are conscious and knowledgeable agents who take an active role in accepting or rejecting the events which make up their everyday reality. Hence, once the social and cultural contradictions and inequalities within South African sport were recognized, it is not surprising that it emerged as a highly visible site of resistance.[16]

The strength of the cultural critique of sport represented by the work of Hargreaves and Gruneau[17] and, more specifically, in relation to South Africa by Jarvie[18] is that it has produced a coherent and powerful critique of modern sport. In so doing, it has demonstrated that the manifest inequalities experienced in South African sport cannot be explained as either a manifestation of "natural" social divisions or the mere consequence of racial prejudice.

This acknowledged, it has however failed to adequately articulate the location of sport within the wider dynamics of social change. Social change in South Africa, although doubtlessly uniquely flavored by its internal cultural realities, must also be regarded as being firmly located in what is a globalized process of change. In an attempt to understand the implications of this the discussion will now turn its attention to the recent work of Anthony Giddens.

Modernity and Social Change: Opportunities and Risks

In two of his most recent and far-reaching works Giddens[19] has offered a provocative and extensive interpretation of the nature of modern society. While, in many respects, these works must be seen as a detailed response to the current discourse on "Postmodernism" it is not the intent of this chapter to explore this aspect of his analysis. As suggested above, the particular interest of this chapter lies with the detailed analysis he provides in relation to the possibilities and problems of social change and how these, in turn, intersect with the institutional and behavioral characteristics of "late modernity."

Through the development of various critical perspectives that have been an axial feature of much of his previous work, Giddens[20] argues that the characteristic social forms and experiences of modernity (such as sport) have been fundamentally shaped by the institutional dimensions and power relations of capitalism, industrialization, military power, and the structures through which the control and development of knowledge are maintained. Moreover, as the structures of modernity have matured they have developed new and ultimately transcendent characteristics. Within the contemporary period these are the globalized nature of modernity; the reflexive character of its institutions; processes of rapid social change that are not only endemic to the system but which are also increasingly radical in nature.

The consequences of this mean that the modern world has become "double-edged phenomenon." On the positive side, in comparison with the pre-modern era its institutions offer a vastly increased range of experiences, opportunities, and commodities that enable many people in the world today to enjoy a secure and rewarding existence. Unfortunately the consequences of modernity can also be seen as having a darker side.

One of the most ubiquitous demands of modern society has been its seemingly unquenchable thirst for the commodities of industrial production. As Giddens and others[21] have argued, the inherent logic of capitalism and the economic necessity to earn a living has meant the acceptance of industrialized work practices that in many instances are de-skilling, exploitative (human and environmental), and conflictual. The class, gender and ethnic relations that emerged from this process still remain a potent cultural force, despite the emancipations of the last decade.

In taking up one of the pivotal themes of postmodernism[22] Giddens also details how "late modernity" is more than ever a world where our existential reality (be it in terms of sport or our local community) is increasingly representational and depthless. At the heart of this mediation lies a globalized electronic mass media industry.[23]

In light of these conditions, Giddens contends that two of the imperatives of the late modern environment are the fluidity and uncertainty of its future. The risks and opportunities afforded by these imperatives thus require individuals and groups (and thereby institutions such as sport) to be in a process of "active intervention and transformation."[24] In essence, the modern condition is one where choices between security and danger, and between trust and risk, are constantly present.

Two of the conclusions about the structure of modernity reached by Giddens, the authors would argue, are particularly important for the analysis of sport and social change in South Africa. The first is that an essential ingredient of modern social life is its reflexive character. The second is that while local conditions are an essential part of the dialectic of change the processes are also deeply imbedded in the global nature of modernity. Simply put, these mean the future of South Africa must be regarded as an as yet undecided project. To put it in Giddens' own terms, which are fairly apt given South Africa's history, the future has yet to be "colonized." Furthermore if Giddens' arguments about the institutional and personal reflexivity of modernity are accepted, it can be suggested the recent accommodation of the reform process will be very difficult to curtail without also attempting a profound deconstruction of South Africa's modern institutional order. Within the dynamics of the choices that are now becoming available to the people of South Africa, it is possible for the future structure of all South African institutions, including sport, to be opened to a radical appraisal that can provide the substance for the development of the new political, economic, and cultural structures which South Africa so obviously needs.

On a more sombre note, it must be also recognized that Giddens' analysis, allied with that of the cultural theorists discussed earlier, makes it equally clear that it is altogether likely that for many in South Africa the struggle between the ANC and the NP for political and cultural control of the reform process will be profoundly threatening. As Craig has noted:

> The reality of change at the almost intangi-
> ble level of economics and politics is that,
> while we can recognize their potential, we
> can likewise realize that there are also many

threatening possibilities imbedded in the
process. To many therefore the comfort and
familiarity of the old ways and the old systems still hold a powerful and deep-rooted
attraction.[25]

In closing this section it is clear that South Africa now finds itself at a "fateful
moment' in its own history. Sport, because of its salience to the white community in South Africa, has found itself deeply imbedded in the political and cultural processes that will decide this moment. The question yet to be answered,
however, is whether sport has transcended its meaning as a pleasant and harmless pastime and become what Giddens has termed a "social movement":

As modes of radical engagement having a
pervasive importance in modern social life,
social movements provide significant guidelines to potential future transformations.[26]

'Attacking Down the Middle': Changing Game Plays in South Africa's Unity Games

Kidd[27] has rightly pointed out that the speed of the political reforms in South
Africa has caught much of the international sporting world by surprise. For
almost three decades the sporting links between South Africa and the rest of the
world have been directed by a moratorium on all sporting contacts (however
much of its actual implementation was fragmented and illusory). It is a policy
that, because of the events of the last few years, no longer can now be argued as
having little real substance. The key that has been produced to unlock the door
to international sport, the establishment of unified and non-racial sports bodies,
is not however a new one.

The image of a South Africa symbolically unified through sport is one which, in
the recent past, both the Nationalist Government and radical sports bodies associated with the liberation movement have attempted to present as their own.
Jarvie has argued that politically these representations were very different. On
the one side, the Nationalist Government's pre-1990s liberalist reforms, in
attempting to present sport (once they had depoliticized and unified it) as "...an
essential key to the process of integration and bridge building..."[28] can be characterized as "attacking down the right." Not surprisingly, its critics argued that
this use of sport merely revealed changes which were intentionally "cosmetic,
ideological and indeed peripheral to the lives of the majority within South

Africa."[29] Given the overtly socialist position taken by those resisting any "normalization" of sport in South Africa, Jarvie usefully extends the analogy used above to characterize this position as "attacking down the left." It is a position that is probably still best summarized by the South African Council of Sport's (SACOS) often quoted contention that "one cannot have normal sport in an abnormal society."

Recent developments, however, would suggest that neither of these political strategies is now truly representative of the current position of the sports organizations chaperoning the unification of the various sports codes. If a political strategy can be said to be informing this process it would appear to be one of political pragmatism. Or, if we may be permitted to once more extend the analogy, to be one that is "attacking down the middle."

<u>South Africa United: A Profile of the Coaches</u>

While most of the practicalities of unification are being played out at the regional level, the policies directing these negotiations have been increasingly determined by two of South Africa's non-racial sports organizations, the National and Olympic Sports Congress (NOSC) and the National Olympic Committee of South Africa (NOCSA).

An understanding of the rise of the NOSC and the NOCSA to their current powerful positions must, as Rees[30] has noted, be firmly located in the context of the struggle by the liberation movement against the apartheid regime. As has already been discussed, sport, because of its importance to the white population, has proved to be an active site of conflict between the communities in South Africa. Attempts to legitimate white rule by taking South African sport onto the world stage, or more recently, as the moratorium against sporting links with South Africa took effect, by bringing world sport to South Africa, have been actively resisted. Prior to the creation of the NOSC, this resistance was largely directed internally by the South African Council on Sport (SACOS) and externally by the South African Non-Raclal Olympic Committee (SANROC). The alliance between these organizations proved to be very effective, particularly in respect to maintaining South Africa's exclusion from the Olympics.[31]

With its promises to dismantle the apartheid laws, F.W. de Klerk's presidential address, in early 1990, radically altered the ground on which the policies of resistance had been constructed. For SACOS, in particular, this caused a problem. As the various apartheid laws were removed from the statute books there was a groundswell of pressure from both black and white athletes on the anti-apartheid sports bodies to develop new policies whereby continued reform could be encouraged by enabling South Africa's gradual readmittance to international sport.[32] For SACOS, given that the repeals have as yet done little to alter the gross inequalities created by apartheid sport or more fundamentally to address the reality of the continued disenfranchisement of the majority of the population, the gradual normalization of sporting relations between South Africa and the rest of the world was something they considered at best premature and at worst a gross political miscalculation.[33]

Even though this may be regarded as a principled stand by SACOS, it was evident to many in the ANC and the Mass Democratic Movement (MDM) the changing political conditions required some form of positive response. In sport it was the NOSC (it should be noted that when it was initially founded its title did not include the word Olympic) that rose to become the primary organ of this response.

At its official launch in Johannesburg, in July 1989, delegates representing almost all walks of life in South Africa pledged themselves to the following aims:

> 1. to establish a single, unified, non-racial, democratic sports movement as part of the MDM.
>
> 2. to encourage codes of sport to establish single national bodies.
>
> 3. to investigate and assist the various communities to create sufficient facilities to enable every sportsperson to develop his or her talents fully.
>
> 4. to cooperate with the MDM in working towards an apartheid-free society.[34]

Since its inception, the NOSC has seized the initiative in the formation of unified non-racial sports codes and has achieved prominence through its proactive domestic strategies (e.g., leading the high profile and successful demonstrations against rebel sports tours) which has established, itself internally and internationally, as the main conduit for the negotiations surrounding South Africa's return to international sport.

Following the watershed of its recognition, at the 4th International Conference Against Apartheid in Sport held in Stockholm 1990, as the major anti-apartheid sports movement in South Africa[35] the NOSC has gone on to play a major role in the multiplicity of meetings with international and Olympic sports organizations that have prefaced South Africa's return to international sport.

Although they have been more often recognized for their conservative tendencies, as the gatekeepers controlling entry to the world sporting stage, the role played by the international sports bodies has been of major importance. Throughout 1991 and 1992 the International Olympic Committee (IOC), the Association of African National Olympic Committees (ANOCA), the International Amateur Athletic Federation (IAAF), the International Rugby Board (IRB), and the International Cricket Conference (ICC) have been active in negotiating with the NOSC or its affiliates for the minimal conditions required for re-entry into their major competitions (these being the Olympics, Athletic World Championships, Rugby World Cup, and The Cricket World Cup). By far the most important of these has been that only teams drawn from sports unified under a single non-racial governing body would be permitted to compete internationally.

With themselves as the main conduit for negotiations and the unification mandate laid down by the international sporting community, which is a process they are largely directing, the NOSC and its Olympic counterpart, the NOCSA, must now be recognized as having established a significant powerbase within sport in South Africa. To a certain degree, the initial battles over the cultural ownership and future shape of South Africa's sporting institutions have, for the moment, been decisively one in favor of the radical reformers. This said, it would be wrong to suggest that the old institutional order, especially in relation to the established 'white' sports such as Rugby, cricket and swimming, does not still have a potent and authoritative position.

South Africa United: Holding a Torch for the New South Africa

In respect to this latter point the impending return of South Africa to the Olympic stage is proving to be a major battleground to decide who is to control the shape of sport's political and cultural future. On the surface, the controversy surrounding the Nationalist Government has continued, but given ANOCA's position, superfluous support of the South African National Olympic Committee appears to be about concerns over how the NOCSA is structured and run. However, at the heart of this issue lie many more fundamental questions about power, the cultural construction of sport, and its symbolic representation. For many of the white sporting community these concerns, have been focused on two issues. The first is the President of the NOCSA, Sam Ramsamy. The second is the debate surrounding the cultural symbols which the South African Olympic team will use to represent their country.

As the Chairman of SAN-ROC Ramsamy was, for almost two decades, one of the most vociferous and prominent leaders of the anti-apartheid movement. Through his appointment to the Presidency of the newly formed NOCSA, his commitment to non-racial sport has now been located in one of the most powerful positions in South African sport. For many in the white establishment though, his status as a hate figure, symbolic of the isolation and sense of loss endured by their sports, has only been reinforced by his appointment to a position that directly influences the conditions for their return to international sport. In its attempt to resist a further eroding of their powerbase, the Government has refused to recognize the validity of the NOCSA and is blocking any financial support. How big an impact this will have is, as yet, unknown as it appears likely that business interests in South Africa may well step in to fill the gap.

Though they are being vehemently resisted, both the NOCSA and the NOSC are adamant that the old symbols of apartheid sport will not be seen at the Barcelona Games. In particular, they are insisting that the Springbok be replaced by the Proteus (the national flower of South Africa), that the flag of the Republic be replaced by the symbol of the Olympic wings, and that the current South African National anthem be replaced for all official purposes with "God Bless Africa," the anthem of the liberation movement. The media impact of this will be undeniably profound for Afrikaners. The Springbok, the National Flag, and the "Disteem" are symbols central to their cultural identity. Their loss will not be trivial. As President de Klerk stated, in voicing the position of most Afrikaners recently, "I am a Springbok man."[36]

South Africa United: On Tour

The results of South Africa's return to the international sporting world have, for the politicians and South Africa's sports public alike, been rapid and dramatic. The formation and unification of South Africa's divided cricket boards into the United Cricket Board of South Africa was not surprisingly (given the history of cricket in South Africa) quickly reciprocated by the I.C.C. through readmission to the conference and an invitation to take part in the 1992 Cricket World Cup. For the Nationalist Government and the ANC the euphoria and interest generated by cricket's return to the world stage could have hardly come at a better time for it meant that images of South Africa's return to international sport would coincide with the crucial March referendum for a continuation of the reform process. Two events which occurred during the World Cup provide obvious but powerful statements of how sport in South Africa has become symbolically linked to the reform process. The first was a saturation advertising campaign run on behalf of de Klerk's government. Its images of cricket and the slogan "Without reform South Africa hasn't got a sporting chance" hardly need any further comment. The second came when the team, despite remarkable success in reaching the semi-finals, threatened to withdraw from the World Cup if the government's policy on political reform was rejected in the referendum. The referendum's "Yes" vote, and the team's outstanding performance (they lost a very close game to England in rather bizarre circumstances) was transformed, upon their return, into a triumphant celebration of the success of both (unified) South African sport and the process of political reform. The euphoric statements which accompanied their ticker-tape reception in Johannesburg bear even stronger witness to the symbolic significance of sports unification to the 'New South Africa':

> "It's wonderful how the country got behind
> us. It just shows what we've been missing."
> —Dave Richards, Wicketkeeper.

> "Today I'm proud to be a South African."
> —Adrian Kuiper, Vice-Captain.

> "We have begun to heal our land."
> —Alan Jordaan, South African Team
> Manager, 1992 Cricket World Cup[37]

Conclusion

Whether by design or default, sport in South Africa can be seen to be one of the few areas where the emerging discourse on the political and cultural reconstruction of South Africa can be sited. In understanding the current reform process in South Africa, of which the unification of sport is but one element, these changes must be understood as a manifestation of both local and global processes. Social change, moreover, is not a linear event but rather a reflexive, multi-dimensional project that is as much a concern for the individual as it is for the institutional order. The cultural reconstruction of sport, which the "unity games" of the last few years represent, is not therefore a process that can be analyzed in isolation from the broader political, economic, and cultural issues that are affecting not only South Africa but the rest of the world.

Because of its specific history it has been argued that sport has become an important social movement informing the fateful decisions that all South Africans face as they try to construct a new South Africa. Given this position is becoming evermore significant as South African sport reenters the world stage of sport, it is hardly surprising that recent statements by Nelson Mandela and Thambo M'Bekei suggest that, for the ANC at least, sport in South Africa is providing the country with powerful ideological images reflecting the future of South Africa.[38]

Clearly, in a remarkably short space of time, organizations such as the NOSC and the NOCSA have moved the image of sport to one of unification and reconciliation rather than segregation and conflict. While this is something that the international sports community should welcome it should do so only with reservation. For those involved in sport at the community level this reconstruction remains a distant reality.

Notes

[1]Jarvie, G. (Ed.) *Sport Racism and Ethnicity*, London: The Falmer Press, 1991.

[2]Miller, D. "South Africa swept by the wind of change," *The Times* (London), (March 25, 1991).

[3]Critcher, Chas. "Radical theories of Sport: The state of play," *Sociology of Sport Journal*. 3: 4 (1986), pp. 333-343.

[4]Hargreaves, J. *Sport, Power and Culture.* Cambridge: Polity Press, 1986.

[5]Gruneau, R. *Popular Culture and Popular Practices.* Toronto: Garamond, 1988.

[6]Jarvie, G. *Class, Race, and Sport in South Africa's Political Economy.* London: Routledge and Kegan Paul, 1985; and Jarvie, G. *Sport, Racism and Ethnicity,* 1991.

[7]Sage, George. *Power and Ideology in American Sport.* Champaign, IL: Human Kinetics, 1990.

[8]Giddens, A. *The Consequences of Modernity.* Cambridge: Polity Press, 1990; and Giddens, A. *Modernity and Self-Identity.* Cambridge: Polity Press, 1991.

[9]Craig, P. "Physical education and social change: Some critical comments on theory and practice" in Katzenellenbogen E. H., and J. R. Potgeiter (Eds.). *Sociological Perspectives of Movement Activity.* Institute for Sport and Movement Studies, Stellenbosch University, South Africa, 1991.

[10]Morris, Meaghan. "The man in the mirror: David Harvey's 'Condition' of postmodernity," *Theory, Culture and Society.* 9 (1992), pp. 253-279.

[11]Morris, 1992.

[12]Hargreaves, 1986.

[13]Gruneau, 1988.

[14]Jarvie, 1991, p. 179.

[15]Craig, 1991.

[16]Craig, 1991.

[17]Hargreaves, 1986; and Gruneau, 1988.

[18]Jarvie, 1985; and Jarvie, 1991.

[19]Giddens, 1990; and, Giddens, 1991.

[20]Giddens, 1990.

[21]Giddens, 1991; and, Braverman, H. *Labour and Monopoly Capital: The Degradation of Work in the Twentieth Century.* London: Monthly Review Press, 1974.

[22]Giddens, 1990; and, Giddens, 1991.

[23]Very few of the people who enjoy football on a weekly basis actually see a live game and, even more significantly, one wonders how many people experienced the recent violence in Los Angeles, an event which itself partly owes its origins to scenes of racist violence whose transmission and representation were created and dependent on a video recording.

[24]Giddens, 1990; and, Giddens, 1991, p. 12.

[25]Craig, 1991, p. 17.

[26]Giddens, 1990, p. 158.

[27]Kidd, B. "From quarantine to cure: The new phase of the struggle against apartheid sport". *Sociology of Sport Journal* 8:1 (1991), pp. 33-46.

[28]Jarvie, 1990, p. 176.

[29]Jarvie, 1990, p. 176.

[30]Rees, C.R. "The NOSC and the Non-Racial Sports Movement: Towards Post-Apartheid Sport in South Africa." Invited Address at the International Symposium for Olympic Research, University of Western Ontario, Canada, February 1992.

[31]Rees, 1992.

[32]Kidd, 1991; and, Rees, 1992.

[33]Ebrahim; Camera 7, August 28, 1991.

[34]National Sports Congress Press Release, 1989

[35]Report on the 4th ICAAS: 1990)

[36]"Dispatches," Channel 4, May 1992.

[37]*The Independent,* "S Africa welcomes 'raining champs'" April 1992.

[38]"Dispatches," Channel 4, May 1992.

Chapter 12

Toward a New Sports Dispensation in South Africa; 1985-1992[1]

John Baxter

This chapter examines the relationship of South African sport to politics within the context of a society in transition. A specific focus in the chapter is the transformation process in sport as a function of changes taking place in the country at large. This transformation is such that a mutually beneficial relationship has been forged between extra-parliamentary organizations and sports bodies, enabling each to realize their own objectives, namely unity, democracy, non-racialism and non-sexism. The introduction to the chapter represents a brief explanation of the context in which the symbiosis between sport and politics grew. An analysis of the process of unity follows and *power* is seen as one of the key variables. This discussion centers on meetings between sports bodies and the ANC, key players in these meetings, pro-active 'sports' politics and the tactics and strategies used to facilitate the movement of sports bodies towards single, united sports bodies. The conclusion deals with the re-active processes which threaten the current state of sports unity. It also considers recent changes that have taken place and how balances have shifted in the changing South African sports scene.

One cannot live in South Africa today without encountering, in every walk of life, the economic, social and political problems of the country. It is also the case that a South African sportsperson cannot play a game without becoming involved, directly or indirectly, in politics. Bluntly stated, South African sport cannot remain politically neutral as the country moves towards a new socio-political dispensation. The present strides that we are witnessing in South Africa, toward a united non-racial sports body, are actually proactive movements that emerge from a symbiosis between sports and politics. At the outset, it is important to comment briefly on the context out of which this symbiosis grew, then highlight several key meetings between extra-parliamentary organizations and sports bodies that nurtured this symbiosis, and conclude by identifying a major threat to sports unity that, if not addressed carefully, might severely restrict the pro-active movement toward a new sports dispensation in South Africa.

From 1985 to 1989 groups of influential white South Africans began having extensive and varied contacts with the then banned African National Congress (ANC). Some seventy-five meetings were reported.[2] Now, against the background of the South African government's oppressive measures to crush liberation movements inside the country and to restrict any communication with exiled political groups, these meetings must be seen as very significant. A growing number of people from the business, political, religious and sport communities were willing to risk confrontation with the government with regard to their contacts and meetings with the ANC, because they were convinced that no solution to South Africa's problems could be found independent of extra-parliamentary organizations.[3] There is little doubt now that these meetings with the ANC outside the borders of South Africa were to be of great significance in the transformation process within South Africa. In fact, it can be said that these meetings set the context for mutually beneficial associations between the ANC and South African sports.[4]

The Symbiosis Between Sports and Politics

The first signal of such beneficial associations came in earnest in 1985 when the United Democratic Front (UDF) nominated one of its activists, Arnold Stofile, a member of the South African Rugby Union, to give evidence in a court case over the impending New Zealand All Blacks Rugby tour of South Africa.[5] Stofile's evidence, along with pressure from the New Zealand anti-apartheid movement, resulted in the tour being abandoned. The controversy created by the cancellation of the tour led the ANC and the UDF to organize a number of meetings in Lusaka in 1986 with a representative group of non-racial sportspersons from South Africa. It was at these meetings that the ANC decided, with the support of the sports delegates, to take a pro-active role in South African sports. The ANC felt that the lack of vision of the sports bodies at the time and the inability of sports bodies to address the issue of a single sports federation, as well as their failure to really understand the nature of the relationship between sport and politics in South Africa, required intervention. It was suggested at these meetings that an interim committee, to be known as the Interim Committee of the National Sports Congress (ICNSC), would be established. The mandate of this committee was to lead the progressive sports movement in the country to a single sports federation and single codes of sports.[6] In retrospect, these series of meetings stand out as the catalyst responsible for the dynamic changes we are presently witnessing in South African sport, and they proved to be of great significance for other meetings that followed.

Thus, it was in September 1987 when a second signal was conveyed that another non-racial sports movement might grow,[7] that a former Springbok rugby player, Tommy Bedford, was included in a small group of South Africans who met with representatives of the ANC in Zimbabwe.[8] This meeting was followed in October 1988 by delegations from the South African Rugby Board (predominantly white) under its president Dr. Danie Craven, and from the South African Rugby Union to discuss the sports boycott and the formation of a single controlling Rugby body in South Africa (unity in South African Rugby was achieved in March 1992). Later in the same month a delegation from the National Soccer League and the South African Soccer Association met with the ANC in Lusaka, Zambia. This was followed by the South African Soccer Federation (affiliated to SACOS) delegation.[9] What was important about all these talks was that not only did they take place at the height of the state of emergency in the country, but that they were also pathfinders to serious discussions about the role of sports in facilitating the transformation process in South Africa by sports bodies nurturing sports unity among themselves. The prevailing attitude with regard to the role of sport seems to have been that a united non-racial sports body could go a long way in symbolizing the kind of unity that ought to exist in a non-racial South Africa. However, pro-action would be required; for realizing sports unity would be no easy task, given the political barriers separating one sports body from the other. For example, while the meetings that have just been described were occurring outside our borders, inside South Africa we were seeing the establishment of the Interim Committee of the National Sports Congress (ICNSC) and the South African Tertiary Institutions Sports Council (SATISCO) in 1986. (SATISCO, in February 1991, united with the South African Tertiary Institutions Sports Association (SATISA), up until this point an affiliate of SACOS, to form the South African Tertiary Institution Sports Union, SATISU).[10] This took place between sports bodies associated with the non-racial movement. The ICNSC grew very slowly during this period, due to external and internal political problems and the need to consult as broadly as possible with individuals, organizations and federations. The ICNSC was to re-emerge in May 1988 as the Sports Desk for the Mass Democratic Movement (MDM).[11]

During 1988, the interim committee of the NSC met in Cape Town with the South African Council on Sport (SACOS), in April, and with SATISCO in June. At first, the two meetings with SATISCO were very cordial and subsequently led to SATISCO affiliating with the National Olympic and Sports Congress (NOSC) in 1990.[12] However, SACOS (April, 1988) during its meeting with the ICNSC expressed concern at splits occurring within the organization and its codes of sport. The second meeting between SACOS and ICNSC in East London, in December (1988), proved to be more tense. SACOS wished to restrict the interim committee of the NSC to working in the rural areas and townships whilst it took charge of the urban areas. In addition, SACOS strongly objected to its members sitting on the interim committee of the NSC. The third meeting between the two parties in September 1989 in Port Elizabeth, attended by political and community organizations, appeared to distance the two bodies still further from each other.[13] The meeting came to a deadlock when the interim committee of the NSC refused to acknowledge SACOS as " the authentic sports organization of the liberation struggle." In November, 1989 SACOS passed a resolution which labeled the ICNSC as a rival organization and stated that dual membership of both the ICNSC and SACOS would not be tolerated.[14] What was the source of this conflict and deadlock?

The two major differences which arose between SACOS and the ICNSC stood on separate bases of socio-political principles. The ICNSC believed the time had come to engage white establishment sports bodies in dialogue, leading to negotiation and unity in each code. In doing this the ICNSC saw the opportunity to implement a program of education. Firstly, the mass-based sports movement and its communities would be informed of the changes occurring in our society. Secondly, the white community, in particular the establishment sportspersons, would be made aware of, and hopefully, come to understand the feelings and aspirations of the majority of people in South Africa who were making the thrust towards a united, non-racial and democratic South Africa.

The second major difference concerned the timing of the *entry* of South Africa as a unified nation into the global arena of sport. SACOS believed that there should be no contact or participation and that the sports boycott be maintained and strengthened until a new government was in place. However, the ICNSC counter-argued that sport must get its house in order prior to a new government being installed. The ICNSC left the meeting on the note that its doors were open to further meetings if the purpose was unity and consolidation of the non-racial sports struggle. This was an important tactic in that it demonstrated ICNSC's willingness to accommodate all parties in the struggle towards a new dispensation in sport.

Based, as it was then, on the conviction to facilitate communication between all parties, the ICNSC moved assertively to extend its sphere of influence. On

Sunday May 28, 1989 the National Executive of the Interim Committee of the National Sports Congress met with the author for three hours on the campus of the University of the Witwatersrand. The talks, which were open and to the point, focused on the reasons for the establishment of the ICNSC, the Freedom Charter,[15] the Harare Declaration,[16] and the need to establish a mass-based, non-racial, united and democratic sports movement towards a post-apartheid South Africa. The Executive Committee members explained the importance of sport in the struggle towards a new dispensation in a future South Africa. They stated that it was essential to address the question of unity in sport prior to a political settlement taking place in South Africa. The reason for this was that the state of the economy would pre-set the priorities of any new government, and these would relate to the needs and demands of the people for education, housing, employment and health care. A unified, non-racial sports body could play an important role in stressing the importance of development and upliftment of the disadvantaged. The Executive Committee also reiterated its commitment to offering the disadvantaged sports sector support, particularly in the areas of administration, management, organization and coaching. The skills and expertise of the established sports bodies would put them in a position to play a major role in raising the level and standard of the disadvantaged sports community.

In discussing the effects of apartheid on sport in South Africa, and the influence it had on the disenfranchised people, the ICNSC expressed its willingness and commitment to engage the very forces which in the past had been reticent to enter into discussion. It stressed the importance of development and upliftment of the disadvantaged sportspersons as an essential factor in the process of unifying sport at all levels. The ICNSC stated that its approach differed from the stand taken by SACOS of "No Normal Sport in an Abnormal Society." Rather than reacting, the ICNSC decided to act positively in the belief that sport should be united prior to a new government being established.

It was with this background information that the ICNSC invited the author, as an independent, objective party, to assist with the organization of a "Sports Conference '89" at the University of the Witwatersrand, in July of that year. This conference was to be the first step in bringing together sportspersons from the disadvantaged community in order that they could discuss the future of sport in South Africa. Its aims were to:

> a) establish a single, unified non-racial
>   democratic sports movement which
>   would be part of the Mass Democratic
>   Movement;

        b) encourage the formation of a single
           national body for each sport;

        c) assist communities in creating sufficient
           sports facilities to enable each sportsper-
           son to develop his/her talents fully; and

        d) co-operate with the MDM in working for
           an apartheid-free society.[17]

Bearing in mind these aims of the conference, it is worth noting with regard to
SACOS that:

        a) since its formation SACOS had made lit-
           tle inroad into the townships and there-
           fore was not representative of the masses;

        b) SACOS over the years was made up pre-
           dominantly of Indians and Coloureds and
           therefore had an ethnically based repre-
           sentation;

        c) in terms of the distribution of its mem-
           bership SACOS was and is significantly
           concentrated, in specific areas of the
           country, such as the Western Province,
           Natal, and the East London and Port
           Elizabeth districts of Border and the
           Eastern Province.[18]

At the Conference, in 1989, the ICNSC stated that they did not wish to
"encroach on the terrain of SACOS" and gave credit to SACOS for the stand it
had taken both nationally and internationally in the struggle against racist
sport.[19] Those SACOS representatives who attended the conference allegedly
defied a decision taken by their executive for its affiliate bodies not to attend.
However they participated in approving a resolution that the ICNSC meet with
their executive to resolve areas of disagreement between the two organizations.
As indicated earlier this was to prove unsatisfactory.

The Conference at the University of the Witwatersrand, however, proved to be a
great success, with some 475 representatives, delegates from a wide range of
organizations of the Mass Democratic Movement (MDM) taking part.[20] It was at

this Conference that we saw the first signs of a united, democratic and non-racial sports movement come forward to challenge "establishment sport" and the policies and principles of the South African Council of Sport (SACOS). Important decisions and resolutions were taken at the conference which would lead to the establishment of the National Olympic and Sports Congress (NOSC).

However, the emergence of the NOSC, in June 1990, heightened the concerns of the white establishment sports organizations and sports administrators while at the same time increasing the complexity of the South African sports scenario.[21] For years white sports administrators had attempted to draw SACOS sports affiliates into joining their sports bodies, but they had been rejected on the basis of apartheid politics. Now, the appearance of the NOSC, with its emphasis on principles of unity, democracy and non-sexism in a united, non-racial, and democratic sports movement, had broken the deadlock between those whites who wanted to talk and those members of SACOS who originally believed that there should be no contact with the white establishment. What is interesting to note here is that the focus of attention of the international community, the international anti-apartheid sports movement, and the South African Non-Racial Olympic Committee (SANROC) has shifted since the 1989 conference from SACOS to the NOSC. This was clearly demonstrated by the support received at the conference in July 1989 from anti-apartheid movements around the world, and at the Fourth International Conference Against Apartheid in Sport held in Sweden in September 1990.[22] The cancellation of the Gatting cricket tour and the support of the International Olympic Committee (IOC) for the NOSC also demonstrated this.[23] In addition, world sports federations accepted only those sports bodies in South Africa which had achieved unity and had a development program in operation, thus endorsing the stand of the NOSC.

The complexity of the South African sports scenario is increased by the competing politics of the three bodies: the white establishment sports bodies are linked to government; allegedly the NOSC has links with the African National Congress; and SACOS, which claims to be non-aligned, has more recently demonstrated a close affinity with the New Unity Movement (Num) and the Pan-Africanist Congress (PAC) after its unbanning in February 1990. Here we can clearly see the symbiosis between sports and politics.

The intensification of the struggle by those in the now *progressive* sports movement in South Africa, the media focus on sport, President F.W. de Klerk's speech of February 2, 1990, the release of the ANC Deputy President, Nelson Mandela, on February 11, 1990, the unbanning of liberation/political organizations, the release of political prisoners and the removal of apartheid laws, in June 1990 from the statute books, were monumental shots in the arm to the disadvantaged people of South Africa.[24] These events were to be of tremendous significance in the forward momentum of the process of change, and the mobilization of the people towards a just society. The world focus on South Africa began to force white South Africans to sit up and recognize that change was necessary for South Africa's survival into the future. The imperative need for the transformation process in South Africa could no longer be ignored.

As the politics of the day continued to unfold, those in the non-racial sports movement became more confident that they were indeed vital to the process leading to social interaction and integration. For years this opportunity had been denied them due to enforced separation of groups on racial and ethnic grounds and to a continual emphasis on the differences between people.

Today, the reality is that South African sport and South Africa's socio-political structure is in the process of transformation. Each facilitates the other in a mutually beneficial association. Yet, it must be noted that the strength of this symbiosis between sports and politics is also its weakness. There is still fragmentation between political groups and thus between their affiliated sports bodies. This fragmentation is exaggerated even more by a fear that, if not addressed carefully, it might severely restrict the pro-active movement toward a new sports dispensation in South Africa.

The Context of the Fear

What is the context of this fear? Unfortunately, it is racial. One of the greatest fears amongst the black community in South Africa, in the broadest sense, is whether or not it can hold the National Party and the government to its word. Past experience on the political front has raised cause for concern. In part, the black leadership in the non-racial sports movement expressed its fear and concern as to the sincerity of its white counterpart in the negotiations leading to unity. The fear of being manipulated and used is real. Whether it is justified, only time will tell. One of the strategies adopted by the non-racial movements has been to ensure that the progress on both the political and the sports level is kept in tandem with one another. The fear today is that, as sport continues to gain momentum in establishing unity and in its development, and as it enters into the global world, a united non-racial sports body will leave the political developments behind as one deadlock after another appears on the political front. Arising from this fear are the question of empowerment and the need to ensure that the non-racial community is able to control its own destiny in the future South Africa. This can only be realized when this community can take its rightful place in the boardrooms and so realize its responsibility.

On the other hand, white sports administrators fear:

> a) that white administrators would lose their positions and their influence and would be forced out;
>
> b) that sport would become highly politicized and that the "new" government would do to sport what the Nationalist Party had done;
>
> c) that projects in operation would be discarded and the funds would go towards black development only;
>
> d) that financial management and control would cease to exist and responsibility and accountability would be acknowledged but not adhered to;
>
> e) that in those sports where black sportspersons had not previously participated and where they took control, they would soon lose interest and after a while would "drop out" and leave a vacuum.

This chapter is the author's practical interpretation of the new sports dispensation currently underway in South Africa. The author believes that this dispensation can continue to play a pro-active role in facilitating the transformation process in South Africa, especially with regard to non-racial sports teams' capability to symbolize unity at all levels of South African society. Whether this dispensation holds depends on two crucibles:

> a) whether the symbiosis between sports and politics holds and,
>
> b) whether the thrust of and the imperative need for further talks as stated by the

Convention for a Democratic South Africa
(CODESA) continues.[25]

Should the current breakdown in the CODESA talks remain and should the symbiosis between sports and politics hold, it is probable that sport will once again become a national and international pawn to further the purposes of the competing political parties and liberation groups. In this regard, South African sports would merely be a reflection of the struggle between, say the National Party and the ANC, for political representation and power. What is interesting to note here is that the very strides made towards sports unity would then be of greater value than before as an effective means to an end of the competing political and liberation groups. The problem for sport, however, would be that it no longer played a pro-active role in facilitating the transformation process in South Africa. At best, sports would be weapons in the arsenals of the rival groups.

The question that emerges here becomes: Is it possible for sport to articulate its intrinsic belief that racial groups must share power, whether or not such happens in the wider political sphere? Another way of phrasing this question is: Can sports unity survive a break in the symbiosis between sports and politics? If power sharing does not happen at the wider political level, would the non-racial sports movement in pursuit of sport for sport's sake, not look like a sellout? Regrettably, the answer is that sports unity in South Africa cannot survive a break in this symbiosis. The historical effectiveness of sports as an historically concrete representation of unity (or disunity) in the country is dependent on the political process. As indicated at the beginning of this chapter, it is the case that a South African sportsperson cannot play his/her sport without becoming involved, directly or indirectly, in the political problems of the country. The best one can hope for in this symbiosis between politics and sports, then, is that sportspersons enter the process of transformation in sport and society at large so that they are able to better understand the changing circumstances in which they find themselves and, in this way, commit themselves and their respective groups to working together with political and liberation groups to bring about a truly democratic structure and system in South Africa. Then and only then can we realistically expect a non-racial sports movement come into existence and be meaningful in a non-racial South Africa.

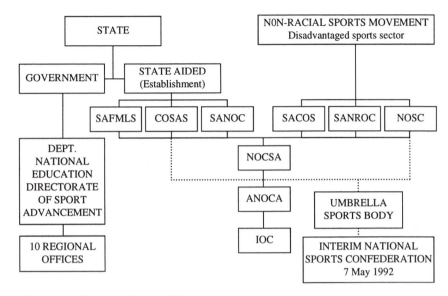

Figure 1—Sport in South Africa

List of Abbreviations

ANC–African National Congress *
ANOCA–Association of National Olympic Committees of Africa
CODESA–Convention for a Democratic South Africa
COSAS–Confederation of South African Sport
ICNSC–Interim Committee of the National Sports Congress
INOCSA–Interim National Olympic Committee of South Africa
IOC–International Olympic Committee
MDM–Mass Democratic Movement *
NOSC–National Olympic and Sports Congress
NSC–National Sports Congress
Num–New Unity Movement *
PAC–Pan Africanist Congress *
SACOS–South African Council of Sport
SAFMLS–South African Federation for Movement and Leisure Sciences
SANOC–South African National Olympic Committee
SANROC–South African Non-Racial Olympic Committee
SATISA–South African Tertiary Institutions Sports Association
SATISCO–South African Tertiary Institutions Sports Council
SATISU–South African Tertiary Institutions Sports Union
UDF–United Democratic Front *

* Political/Liberation Movements

Notes

[1] My thanks to Johan Barnard, Past-President of the South African Tennis Union and the Vice-President of Tennis South Africa, for his letter and comments on white fears. My thanks, also, to Vivian Reddiar, Sports Editor of the City Press, for comments and advice surrounding this chapter.

[2] Louw, R. (Ed). *Four Days in Lusaka: Whites in a changing society.* Five Freedoms Forum - African National Congress Conference, Lusaka, Zambia, June 29 - July 2, 1989.

[3] *Extra-Parliamentary Organisations.*
With the establishment of a formal parliamentary system in South Africa the majority of its people (African, Colored and Indian) were denied universal suffrage, i.e., one person one vote. From the onset, the disenfranchised people established extra-parliamentary organizations to address issues relevant to them. These organizations comprised the African National Congress, South African Communist Party, United Democratic Front, Azanian People's Organization, Non-European Unity Movement, and Pan African Congress, to name a few. More recently, organizations such as the Five Freedom's Forum (FFF) and Institute for a Democratic Alternative for South Africa (IDASA) have appeared. Over the years these organizations campaigned against the regime by various means, for a just and acceptable political and economical system in South Africa.

[4] Sport in South Africa has, historically, been divided on racial lines. It was boycotted from the 1950's to 1992 during which time it was used as a political weapon to pressurize the South African Government and the white community as a whole to accommodate black political aspirations.

[5] Roberts, C. (Ed) *South Africa's Struggle for Olympic Legitimacy. From Apartheid Sport to International Recognition.* Cape Town: Township Publishing Co-operative, 1991

[6] My thanks to Mr. Krish Naidoo, past General Secretary of the Interim Committee of the National Sports Congress, for information and comments with reference to a series of meetings between the ANC, UDF and representatives of the non-racial sports movement which took place during 1985 and 1986.

[7] It should be noted that until the Sports Conference in July 1989, the South African Council of Sport (SACOS) had, since 1973, along with the South African Non-Racial Olympic Committee (SANROC), been the sole non-racial sports body to challenge the white sports establishment and the racist policies of apartheid of the Nationalist Party Government. SACOS formulated an ideology of non-racial sport and campaigned for "No Normal Sport in an Abnormal

Society". Roberts, C. (Ed.). *Sport and transformation. Contemporary debates on South African sport.* Cape Town: Township Publishing Co-operative, 1989.

[8]Louw.

[9]Louw.

[10]The author attended the meeting at the Peninsula Technikon in Belleville where SATISCO and SATISA were unified.

[11]Mass Democratic Movement (MDM) arose from the banning of the UDF and was referred to as a loose alignment of organizations, bodies and groups, predominantly from the disadvantaged sector of the community, who aligned themselves with the ANC and the struggle towards a united, democratic and non-racial South Africa. The MDM comprised a broad-based alignment of political, labor, women's, church and civic groups to name a few.

[12]National Sports Congress, *Secretarial Report.* June 1, 1990, Cape Town.

[13]National Sports Congress, 1990.

[14]Roberts, C. (Ed.). *Challenges facing South African sport.* Cape Town: Township Publishing Co-operative, 1990.

[15]*Freedom Charter.*

This was adopted at the Congress of the People on June 26, 1955. It outlined the basic demands of the people of South Africa for a democratic state. The ANC formally adopted the Freedom Charter and its program for a liberated South Africa. It comprised political organizations such as the African National Congress, South African Indian Congress, Congress of Democrats and the Coloured People's Congress. The Freedom Charter was viewed by the disenfranchised as the first systematic statement in the history of this country of the political and constitutional vision of a free, democratic and non-racial South Africa. Williams, G., and B. Hackland. *The dictionary of contemporary politics of Southern Africa.* London: Routledge, 1988.

[16]*Harare Declaration:*

As a result of the unbanning of the African National Congress (ANC) and other liberation movements in February, 1990, certain basic conditions were drawn up and adopted by the ANC and its allies and supported by the Organization of African Unity and the United Nations. It was these conditions which formed the basis of the declaration. For further information on the Harare Declaration, Conference for a Democratic Future, *Report back*, 1989..

[17]South African Institute of Race Relations. *Race Relations Survey (1989/90).* Johannesburg: South African Institute of Race Relations, 1990.

[18]South African Institute of Race Relations, 1990.

[19]South African Institute of Race Relations, 1990.

[20]Roberts, 1990.

[21]The complexity of the South African sports scenario is clearly illustrated in the attached organogram.

[22]Roberts, 1990.

[23]*Gatting Cricket Tour:*

In July, 1989, at the request of Mr. Krish Naidoo, General Secretary of the ICNSC, the author met with Dr. Ali Bacher, Director of the South African Cricket Union, who was in the process of organizing two 'rebel' tours of South Africa in early 1990 and November of the same year. At this, the first of three meetings, the author's brief was to:

   a) advise and inform him of the National Sports Congress.
   b) appeal to him and the SACU to call off the planned tour.
   c) outline the possible role that he might play in cricket in the future.
   d) advise Dr. Bacher of the ICNSC's confidence in his ability to call off the
      tour.

This meeting took place at Dr. Bacher's home on the eve of his departure to England to continue with arrangements pertaining to the "rebel" tour. He also informed the author that he was to meet a member of the ANC in London. This meeting had been arranged by Dr. van Zyl Slabbert. The author's advice to Dr. Bacher was that he work through the ICNSC within the country as they were seen to be dealing with the sports issue at that time. At a subsequent meeting the author had with Dr. van Zyl Slabbert, it was suggested that cricket work through the ICNSC. After this initial meeting the author held informal talks with Mr. Joe Pamensky and with a number of major cricket sponsors appealing to them to assist in persuading Dr. Bacher and the SACU to call off the tour. This proved to be to no avail. The two final meetings that the author had with Dr. Bacher, at the request of Mr. K. Naidoo were to:

- appeal for its cancellation.
- advise him of the strategy and action which would be taken if the tour went
  ahead.
- give him a date by which time a letter should reach the ICNSC stating that
  the tour had been canceled.

A letter was sent by Dr. Bacher on September 11, 1989 to Mr. Naidoo requesting a meeting with him and the ICNSC "to discuss all aspects of the future of cricket in South Africa". The author then withdrew from talks with Dr. Bacher advising him that the ICNSC would continue its program to disrupt the tour. The unofficial/rebel English Cricket Team arrived in South Africa on January 19, 1990, to play eight games against a Springbok team and four games against other teams. The cost of the tour was estimated at R4m. Demonstrations began with the arrival of the team at Jan Smuts Airport and were to continue until February 14, 1990. On this date Dr. Bacher announced, after negotiations between the South African Cricket Union (SACU) and the ICNSC, that the SACU had decided to shorten the tour in support of the political changes underway as a result of Mr. de Klerk's announcements on February 2, 1990 in

Parliament. The SACU, after consultation with the ICNSC, agreed to cancel the second test match and reduce the number of limited-over games from seven to four. In addition, the second leg of the tour planned for November, 1990 was canceled; South African Institute of Race Relations, 1990.

[24]President F. W. de Klerk's speech of February 2, 1990 was seen as a watershed, opening the way for direct talks on the future of the country; South African Institute of Race Relations, 1990.

[25]The Convention for a Democratic South Africa (CODESA) was established at the end of November, 1991, where preparatory talks were held between some 19 participating parties. It was hoped that these talks would lead to serious negotiations. On December 20/21, 1991, the first plenary session (CODESA I) was held with the purpose of laying the foundation for the talks and setting up working groups. The second plenary session (CODESA II) took place on May 15/16, 1992, and talks continued for a month thereafter. Subsequently, the talks broke down altogether when the African National Congress withdrew from negotiations after the Boipatong incident.

Part 5: Sport in the New Europe

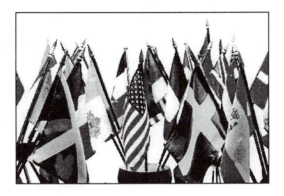

Part 5: Sport in the New Europe

Change is difficult. Even change of an evolutionary nature is difficult. When change is of a revolutionary nature, such as has been the case in Europe over the past five years, the problems which such change brings are often utterly disrupting of personal and social lives, and fragmenting of economic, political and cultural institutions. As an important social institution, sport is not immune to the effects of such change, as the chapters in this section aptly display.

Socio-historical analysis of change in sport has traditionally followed one of two paths. The first has been through the application of what has come to be known as the "modernization thesis," a thesis which, in the sporting literature, has been pioneered by writers such as Guttmann.[1] Among social scientists who take a more "critical" approach to the analysis of change, modernization is a framework which is considered too simplistic. Thus for scholars of sport such as Gruneau[2] and Hargreaves,[3] hegemony is a more useful organizing concept which can be more readily and usefully applied to change. "Markers" of the dominant, emergent and residual laments of sports practices, styles, traditions, beliefs and organization are, according to these scholars, more appropriately and fully described, analyzed and explained by employing a cultural approach.

In the chapters that follow, neither of these approaches is explicitly employed by any of the authors to a significant degree. Because of the newness of change, its revolutionary nature, and the lack of the necessary critical "distancing" from events, these chapters are largely first steps at description and analysis, conducted in a climate of uncertainty, ongoing rapid change and discontinuity. As such, the offerings are largely a-theoretical, and to this extent the reader is left with a degree of openness with regard to the interpretation of the events unfolding in Europe regarding sport.

The organization of the chapters follows a pattern in which Standeven (chapter 13), and Hartmann-Tews (chapter 14), raise general conceptual and methodological issues regarding the problems of implementing sport in the New Europe. Standeven argues the case for "the retention of diversity and distinctiveness in games." She fears that Europeanization offers the opportunity for cultural containment and neocolonialism through the threat of the rigidity of centralism, at the expense of both cultural innovation and the distinctiveness of localism in sport. Damkjaer also notes this concern in his chapter on Soviet and CIS sport (chapter 21). In her analysis of European sporting diversity, Hartmann-Tews highlights the fact that sources of data through which to guide policy are not readily comparable across (or even within) nations. In looking at sport in the New Europe, she suggests that cumulative European data cannot take full account of cross-national and cross-cultural differences, a problem of which comparative researchers should be fully aware.

The authors of chapters 15 through 19 look specifically at sport in the New Germany offering an in-depth study of such problems, and in particular the problems of high-level sport in the New Europe. There appears to be considerable agreement amongst the authors of these five chapters on Sport in the New Germany, that, in the post-Wall period, the GDR sports system has been dismantled, and that few of its elements have been incorporated into the unified German sport structure. As Vitelli and Semotiuk put it, "the West Germans simply imposed the existing sports structure, in the Federal Republic, on the athletes and territory of the former GDR." "Besserwessi" has meant that this has not been an equal union, and to the ideological victor have gone the administrative spoils. All the authors lament what appears to be a case of "throwing the baby out with the bath water," in the New Germany. In looking beyond Germany, Milshtein takes a more positive view of the progress being made at the structural level for the democratization of sport (Sport for All) throughout the New Europe in Chapter 20. He puts great stock in the Olympics. Damkjaer, by contrast, sees the effects of change as more negative with sport becoming increasingly commercialized.

In the final two chapters of this section Howell, and Sedlacek et. al., look at the influence of economic and political change on the organization of sport as a social and cultural institution in two areas perhaps less well known to many western sport scholars—Estonia and the former Czechoslovakia. These two case studies provide interesting insights into the extraordinary effects of the rapidly changing political order in the New Europe, stressing the fragility of political organization and the tenacity of cultural capital in these two areas.

The chapters in this section provide a unique look at the effects of geopolitical change on sport, and particularly high-level sport, in the New Europe. Such changes have affected and will continue to affect sport for all, as well as sport and physical education in schools in a Europe that is both a global market and global village.

Timothy J.L. Chandler

Notes

[1]Guttmann, A. *From Ritual to Record,* New York: Columbia University Press, 1974.
[2]Gruneau, R. *Class, Sports and Social Development*, Amherst: University of Massachusetts Press, 1983.
[3]Hargreaves J. *Sport, Power and Culture*, Cambridge: Cambridge University Press, 1986.

Chapter 13

Games, Culture and Europeanization

Joy Standeven

Games are, at one and the same time, products of culture and vehicles for the transmission of culture. Further, games as a cultural activity are a form of cultural expression. Throughout the world there are numerous examples of games that are culture-specific: in other words, they are unique to one culture. Yet, increasingly, games are shared by many cultural groups. Football, in its soccer form, and, to a lesser extent, basketball and hockey are now almost universal games, whilst noose-catch, liathroid laimhe and hu-tu-tu are less well known and rarely played outside their culture of origin. Whilst the origins of football go back many centuries, it was the codification of the rules of the game, more than a century ago, that was a significant factor increasing its popularity. Universities and schools developed and played football and other games more for their value as ways of establishing social control and training character than for their physical benefits. The values of games thus came to have a strong association with leadership, discipline, control, socialization, and rule-bound behavior; and they became a part of every missionary's armor as they dispersed throughout the empire, seeking to civilize and convert native peoples. In this way, alien games were imposed upon indigenous cultures. Socialization, through religion and education, led to the displacement of native activities and the subordination of indigenous cultures to dominant foreign powers.

Roberts' and Sutton-Smith's cross-cultural study of games in the 1950s and 1960s examined links between patterns of child-training and particular structures within games, linking the complexity and demands of a game to the culture of which it was a part. Sutton-Smith concluded that the thesis on the universality of forms of games and play with which he had started out was untenable.[1] Different cultures, he found, placed different demands on children in game-playing situations, and these could be directly linked to different emphases in the culture. There is, then, a sense in which games are a reflection of culture as well as a commentary upon it.

Games have been absorbed into the school curriculum of many cultures for different reasons. The new National Curriculum identifies the overall rationale in England and Wales in 1991, stating, "They are a part of our national heritage and offer a range of educational opportunities."[2] The legacy of the former public schools' stress on the values of games-playing is still to be found in the extent to which this part of the curriculum takes up more physical education time than any of the other five areas of activity (dance, gymnastics, outdoor activities, swimming, and track and field). The requirements of the National Curriculum ensure that games will continue to be taught to pupils in schools in England and Wales, because of what they mean as forms of human activity and expression. Whilst no reference is explicitly made to Europe, an appendix to the National Curriculum states:

> Recognition of the variety of cultural forms
> of sport and dance as expressions of her-
> itage, identity and achievement highlights
> the potential for understanding which stems
> from sharing and appreciating each other's
> experiences.[3]

Written specifically to respond to the principle of equal opportunity in the multi-cultural society, the document goes on to note that through learning a range of games (and dances) pupils "can recognize the richness and diversity of cultures other than their own."[4] Given this claim, it may be appropriate for schools to make particular attempts to introduce games from other European countries — for example, handball — into the curriculum. However, the need to treat different racial and ethnic groups equally, and to dispel myths and stereotypes, led the Working Group in England and Wales to state that "Reference to 'national games or dance' may be inappropriate."[5]

This chapter argues a case for the retention of diversity and distinctiveness in games, valuing and ennobling cultural heritage and differences. It sees in Europeanization — that is, the formulation of a European identity and citizenship — the opportunity for both 'cultural containment' and 'cultural innovation.' A parallel is drawn between the subordination of indigenous cultural activities that went with colonialism, and the innovatory cultural expression that can result from the transfer of activities from one culture to another. Which of these possibilities is realized is likely to depend upon socio-cultural relations of power.

Cheska's definition of a game as "organized play containing three essential elements"[6] is used in this chapter. She goes on:

> Without: (1) participants, opponents or
> sides; (2) organized procedure, a fixed
> sequence of action or plot; and (3) uncertain
> outcome, resolution or end result, a game
> cannot exist.

But games vary in their degree of complexity and the extent to which they emphasize participation as an expression of play, or achievement and a sense of competing to attain a recognized goal. Within this wide definition, a vast range of games can be identified in countries throughout the world.[7] But in this chapter, attention is focused on a selected number of examples: particular major or national games which have been exported from their culture of origin and have been taken up in other societies which do not share the same structures and values. Transported to new cultural milieus, some games took root within new contexts of tradition, values and lifestyles, and as a result can be seen to have undergone change. Alternatively, although the form of a game may have remained unchanged, the manner in which it is played has been modified to be compatible with different cultural traditions.

There have been many definitions of culture.[8] John Hargreaves states, "[Culture] ...is a lived practice formed by conscious human beings from their lived experiences and constituting for them a whole way of life."[9] And he goes on:

> There are two internally linked dimensions
> to this process of cultural formation: culture
> is both constituted by people consciously
> making choices and evaluations of their
> experience AND simultaneously, because it
> is also inherited from the choices and evalu-
> ations people have made in the past as tradi-
> tion it is also constitutive of choice and
> action...

Culture, then, can be innovatory and emancipatory; or, at the same or a different time, it may constrain and limit our experience. Raymond Williams[10] offers a model of three cultures which may co-exist at one time and in one place. The importance of his conception is the emphasis given to the way in which it is the 'dynamic inter-relations' of these cultural elements that show what a particular society is really like. The 'dominant' culture "holds sway over other elements at a given moment," and in the case of "a capitalist society will be the culture of the industrialist or entrepreneur";[11] whilst in colonial society it will almost certainly be the imperialistic foreign power. The 'residual' culture survives from the past to be "an effective element of the present, often in opposition to what the dominant culture represents."[12] Further, there is the 'emergent' culture, or "new meaning and values, new practices, new relationships and kinds of relationship [that] are continually being created."[13] The relation of the dominant culture to the residual or emergent cultures may be one of incorporation or, alternatively, an oppositional relation may be active. Tomlinson rejects the notion of culture as a shared way of life and states, "It is the relationship between... different clusters of values that must be probed if we are to understand the dynamics of a society and if we are to grasp the significance of everyday activities such as popular culture and sport."[14]

Turning now to a few selected examples of games as cultural experience, Riesman and Denny[15] trace the transformation of English Rugby into American football, identifying characteristics of American culture which influenced the change. In his comparative study of North American ball games with earlier forms of games in Europe and England, Finlay[16] argues that football has replaced baseball as the dominant game in North America because it is more attuned to a mature stage of capitalism. The fixed positional relationships of baseball are contrasted with the more fluid relations of American football and the "apocalyptic" meaning of the home-run compared with the averages that characterize football's statistics. Baseball is described as a "robber baron" game, its sports style giving way to the greater seriousness of football, which is projected as more compatible with the dominant culture of corporate capitalism.

Baseball was introduced to Japanese schools through their physical education programs in the 1870s and, by the 1950s, nearly 2000 high-school teams participated in the National High School tournament, and 2 professional leagues played events described as "on a par with their American equivalents."[17] But, although the game may have appeared to be the same as its American counterpart, Robert Whiting's probing analysis in *The Chrysanthemum and the Bat*[18] shows how, in contrast to the individualism of the American game, the Japanese game stresses the harmony of the team, reflecting the characteristic suppression of the individual for the group — a legacy of the residual culture and traditional social relations that pervade Japanese life.

Sutton-Smith[19] and Cheska[20] record the cultural disintegration and loss of traditional ethnic games that resulted from the imposition of colonial sports such as soccer and cricket within the schools and missionary activities in New Zealand and West Africa. But perhaps the most remarkable record and exposition of the subordination of indigenous culture and its replacement, albeit temporarily, by a colonial dominant culture — itself to become residual with the departure of the colonial power — is to be found in the work of Jerry Leach.[21]

The Reverend Gilmour introduced English cricket to the Trobriand Islands in 1903, when British colonialism arrived in New Guinea. The first players were converts to the Methodist church, where playing games was introduced as a substitution for native warfare, and the original rules closely resembled English rules — the mission converts, for example, used the white man's ball. In time, the Trobrianders transformed the game — an emergent culture, giving new meaning and new values, stirred. Since few people owned mission clothes, the islanders reverted to their former dress of war. Chants and dances were added; a smaller ball and a spear-throwing technique were adopted. The 1974 film made of this event is subtitled "An ingenious response to colonialism," and was produced to show "creative adaptation of tradition to contemporary circumstances."[22] Ingenuity was shown in the creativity of the players, the adaptation of rules and customs, the transformation of equipment, and the invention of new chants and social relations. Here then is a version of cricket barely recognizable to its originators. A cultural heritage has been transferred into a new cultural setting, and transformed into a new cultural experience; an emergent culture resisting and opposing a dominant culture; and with the withdrawal of the colonial power, the full release of ingenuity to 'rubbish' the white man's game and make it into 'our kind of cricket.' In this context, Trobriand traditions have been creatively adapted; for example, "rain magic has been given a new context for performance and belief," "dancing has been given a new context," and "cricket has given leaders a new domain."[23]

With this key example in mind, the question is raised as to the response that may be expected in the modern world to Europeanization. Will schools on the European mainland include cricket in their physical education curriculum? Will British schools introduce handball or pelota? If these games are transferred to new cultural milieus, will they be transformed? Will they look the same and mean the same? Or mean something different, even though they may look the same? Have our developed industrial economies lost the capacity for creativity? Will the learning of another culture's games become a resource for cultural innovation, or will our adherence to rule-boundness result in a loss of cultural expression? Will playing the games of another European nation facilitate cultural integration among the youth of the new community?

The European community is an outgrowth of the Second World War, a deliberate attempt to ensure peace in Europe and to guarantee democracy based upon economic treaties and political influence. The core of the EEC is a grouping of twelve Member States committed to economic, social and political integration. The origins of the community can be traced back to 1950 when France and Germany accepted the Schuman Plan, which set out to promote post-war economic recovery by combining the coal and steel industries of both countries. The 1951 Treaty of Paris established a European Coal and Steel Community (ESCS), placing under a combined authority the industries in six countries — France and Germany, Italy, Belgium, The Netherlands, and Luxembourg. In 1957 the same six countries set up the European Economic Community (EEC) through the Treaty of Rome. The implementation of the Treaty, the establishment of the Common Market, came into operation in 1958. Denmark, Ireland and the United Kingdom joined in 1973; Greece in 1981; Spain and Portugal in 1986. The Community, with a population of 344 million, next to China, is the world's largest trading entity and is growing in size and influence as further countries apply for membership.

The European Parliament came into being in 1979 with the direct election of 518 members by voters from the member states. The UK elects 81 MEPs every five years. The Council of Ministers consists of one Minister from each of the twelve Member States, with one member serving as President, on an alphabetical rotational basis, for six months. The period of the British presidency is just about to begin, and reference has already been publicly made to John Major's undisguised love of cricket. The European Commission, the EEC's equivalent of a Civil Service, and the European Court of Justice are the other two governing institutions of the Community, the latter exercising power over the Member States.

The end of 1992 has been set as the date for the establishment of the single market. The 1986 Single European Act has committed Member States to open their internal frontiers to permit the free movement of goods, persons, services, and capital between them. The Community, it is said, is not intended to create a 'monolithic' European state. It operates in nine official languages, and it claims to encourage 'national and regional cultural identities.' Nevertheless, there is a European flag and a European anthem, a European passport and a European driving license, which are said to promote a 'common European identity' and to be 'reminders of common European citizenship.'

What is the role of sport — and more particularly of games — in this tension between centrality, harmonization, and closer union among the peoples of Europe, and the need for a strong sense of cultural identity which corresponds to natural, historical communities, such as ethnic groups or countries?

In the final analysis, relations between nations, as between social groups, are culturally constituted. Cultural relations inevitably imply cultural power. John Hargreaves states:

> Cultures_ are profound sources of power, reproducing social division here, challenging and rebelling against them there, while in many ways accommodating subordinate groups to the social order.[24]

Physical education, of which games are an important element within a fully developed education for leisure in the new Europe, may achieve again the influence it had a century ago within the public schools and colonial cultures of Britain. As a socializing medium its role can be significant. As a bearer of cultural meaning it can limit both choice and action, but most importantly, it can liberate creative potential. New games, learned and played at school, imbued as they are with meanings and values, could be a resource for cultural innovation, an ingenious response by youth to the new European Community. But cultural relations of power between nations, reproduced within the structures of education, could result in curricula that merely accommodate and incorporate differences to a hegemonic cultural core. Physical educators and sport pedagogues need to be aware of the forces of cultural expression within games to ennoble cultural differences and encourage cultural innovation, rather than allowing their rule-bound form to result in cultural containment.

Notes

[1] Sutton-Smith, B. *The Folkgames of Children,* Austin: University of Texas Press, 1972.

[2] Department of Education and Science and the Welsh Office. *Physical Education for Ages 5 to 16*, London: HMSO, 1991.

[3] Department of Education and Science and the Welsh Office. *Physical Education for Ages 5 to 16*, p. 59, paragraph 43.

[4] Department of Education and Science and the Welsh Office. *Physical Education for Ages 5 to 16*, p. 59, paragraph 44.

[5] Department of Education and Science and the Welsh Office. *Physical Education for Ages 5 to 16*, p. 59, paragraph 44.

[6] Cheska, A.T. *Traditional Games and Dances in West African Nations*, Schorndorf, Germany: Hofmann, 1987, p. 14.

[7]Cheska; Opie, I. & Opie, E. *Children's Games in Street and Playground,* Oxford: Clarendon Press, 1969; Brewster, P. "Some Nigerian Games with their Parallels and Analogues", *Journal de la Société Des Africanistes,* (1954), pp. 25–48; and Sutton-Smith, 1972.

[8]Kluckholn, C. *Culture and Behavior, The Study of Society,* New York: The Free Press of Glencoe, 1962; Geertz, C. *Interpretation of Cultures*, New York: Basic Books, Inc, 1973; Hargreaves, J. "Sport, Culture and Ideology", In J. Hargreaves (ed.) *Sport, Culture and Ideology,* London: Routledge & Kegan Paul, 1982; Williams, R. *The Long Revolution,* London: Pelican, 1961; and Williams, R. *Marxism and Literature,* Oxford: Oxford University Press, 1977.

[9]Hargreaves, 1982, p. 47.

[10]Williams, 1977.

[11]Tomlinson, A. "Cultural Experience", In *Sport and Recreation in the Socio-Cultural Environment*, Brighton Polytechnic: Chelsea School of Human Movement, c1983, p. 4.

[12]Tomlinson, p. 4.

[13]Williams, 1977, p. 123.

[14]Tomlinson, p. 3.

[15]Riesman, D., & Denny, R. "Football in America: A Study in Cultural Diffusion", *American Quarterly*, 3 (1951), pp. 309–319.

[16]Finlay, J. "Homo Ludens (Americanus)", in *Queens Quarterly* 78, Ontario, Canada: Queens University, 1971, pp. 353–364.

[17]Andreano, R. "Japanese Baseball", In J.T. Talmini & G. H. Page (eds.). *Sport and Society.* Boston: Little Brown & Co, 1973.

[18]Whiting, R. *The Chrysanthemum and the Bat,* Dodd Mead & Co, 1977.

[19]Sutton-Smith, B.. "The Meeting of Maori and European Cultures and its effects upon the unorganized games of Maori children", in *Journal of Polynesian Society* 60 (1951), pp. 93–107.

[20]Cheska, 1987.

[21]Leach, J. "The Structure of Trobriand Cricket", Notes written for the Symposium "Problems of Anthropological Filming" in Section H of the British Association for the Advancement of Science, University of Lancaster, September 1976.

[22]Leach, p. 8.

[23]Leach, p. 11.

[24]Hargreaves, J. *Sport, Power and Culture*, Cambridge: Polity Press, 1986, p. 9.

Chapter 14

European Diversity: A Case for Comparative Research

Ilse Hartmann-Tews

The European political and economic landscape has changed enormously in the last few decades. The disappearance of the East-West conflict, the fight for regional autonomy, and the prospect of the European Single Market are only some of the principal events. The consequences of these developments will be felt in all sectors of society, including culture and sport.

As far as sports policy is concerned, the emergence of a coherent European way has always been retarded by the diversity and division of European sports structures and by particularized interests of the member states. To improve coordination and collaboration between them, several initiatives have been launched, involving consultation structures and cross-national information. Political and consultory bodies were set up at the European level in order to fulfill the need for information, dialogue, and cooperation between various sports authorities. These bodies include AENOC (Association of European National Olympic Committees), ENGSO (European Non-Governmental Sports Organizations), and CDDS (Committee for the Development of Sport). Ongoing data has been collected in the European countries on sport organizations, participation rates, promotion and economic aspects, facilities, legislation, and other aspects that are regularly documented in the *Sports Information Bulletin* provided by the Council of Europe.

The first question that arises from these initiatives and documents is which Europe are we talking about? The Europe of twelve or the former Western Europe? European sports policy at the governmental level consists of two organizations comprising a different number of member states, pursuing different objectives, and following different routes to achieve their aims.

The basic initiative to collect and collate data stems from the Council of Europe which, founded in 1949, now includes 26 member states, representing approximately 460 million people. Its main aim is to "reinforce political, social, cultural, and legal collaboration between European democracies."[1]

The European Community was founded ten years later. It is now made up of 12 member states representing approximately 325 million people. As a supranational organization to which member states delegate part of their sovereignty, it pursues a different objective, that being, "to promote a political, monetary, and economic union" via the Single European Market.[2]

Recent developments in Europe have jeopardized a coherent European policy and a simplification of the global situation. Furthermore, they document how difficult it is to integrate nation states without putting national identity and culture at stake. These experiences in the field of European policy are of relevance for comparative sports science together with a sociological approach to the development of sport. They bring attention to the individual case and its specific socio-cultural shape and inheritance within the greater context of Western Europe, Europe of the twelve or twenty-four. They analyze sport as a subsystem of society and examine the similarities and differences between various countries ensuring the availability of comparative data. Currently, basic information is provided by the Council of Europe and by national studies of the member states that shed some light on the structures of sport in the European countries. But all of them have to be characterized as multinational area studies as there has been no analysis of sport from a strictly comparative point of view. This sort of data collection raises some difficulties and risks not being able to grasp and identify differences and similarities. Two examples may serve to illustrate this point.

Structures of Sport

The term structure refers to the institutionalized framework of agencies and organizations promoting participation in sports and providing appropriate opportunities for facilities to take part in some sort of physical exercise. Thus, structure refers both to the governmental level of provision and responsibility, and to the non-governmental level of organizational units such as voluntary clubs, associations or federations, and commercially run sports clubs and centers.[3] The structures of sport in the European countries are characterized by variety, and diversity. Even at the governmental level one finds a wide range of different ministries, departments, or divisions responsible for sports matters.[4] The most widespread assignment of responsibility for sports policy matters in general can be found at the Ministry of Cultural Affairs (such as in Denmark, Greece, and Spain). Some states do have a specific Ministry of Physical Education and Sport (Luxembourg) or a Ministry of Education and Sports (France). But there are other ministries in charge of sports policy such as the Ministry of Education (Ireland), Health and Culture (Netherlands), Internal Affairs (Germany), as well as Tourism and Entertainment (Italy). Besides this responsibility for general sports matters at the very top level, regardless of the most subtle differentiations and administrative dependencies below, there is always a variety of different governmental units responsible for specific sports matters. Taking a diachronic perspective, structures become even more diverse as is the case with Great Britain. Before 1990 general sport matters were assigned to the Department of Environment and, in 1990, sport was briefly assigned to the Department of Education and Science. It is now the responsibility of a newly created ministerial department for The Arts and Sport. These different political placements for sport have to be closely analyzed as they depend not only on the political system but on the political culture as well. Obviously, it would be too easy to suppose a simple reflection of political embedding and relative importance of sport within general policy, but it is one indicator amongst others to evaluate different concepts of sport and sport policy.

Along with these different political embeddings of sport matters, the sports policy of the European countries varies as well. Italy and Denmark serve to illustrate this point. In Italy, the State (i.e., the Ministry of Tourism and Entertainment) is limited to a supervisory role in general sports matters. Sport policy in Italy is mainly driven by the National Olympic Committee (CONI), the umbrella organization and central administrative body of organized sport. Its sport policy has long been centered on promoting competitive sport at both professional and amateur levels. This preeminence of competitive sport, and the absence of sports activity in comprehensive educational programs, are two characteristics that seem to be obstructive to mass participation.[5] The state's role in general sports matters in Denmark is comparable to that found in Italy. The Ministry of Culture is in charge of general sport matters and has a supervisory role. Unlike Italy, there are several umbrella organizations for sport that establish a comparatively loosely knit forum of sports policy. Governmental and non-governmental organizations have a long tradition of cooperation that is based on the consensus that physical activity and sport are predominantly a means to support a healthy lifestyle and should represent lifelong leisure activities. These values are well reflected in the implementation of physical education as an obligatory educational program (since 1984), together with participation rates in organized sport and in clubs.

This brief overview reveals considerable cross-national variety that could easily be illustrated with other examples. There are various ways of providing an organizational frame for sports activities, legal forms for the central organizational unit of sport (club/associations), financing and funding of membership regulations, and of organizational policies. Bearing in mind these different structures, and the effort to bring together different cultural and national identities, it is surprising that the data collected on a multinational level are often reduced to more general findings about recent developments in sports. Two of the generalizations illustrate the difficulties and risks of a comparative sociological analysis with multinational data.

Central Features of Sports Development

1. Trend of pluralization
Pluralization, in this context, refers both to the people who take part in physical activities and to the sports that are practiced. The basic findings supporting this thesis state that over the past two decades there has been an enormous growth in sport participation across all European countries. This steady growth of participation rates goes hand in hand with a diminishing significance of gender, age, and social position as discriminating factors of active participation in sport.[6] Indeed, male and female participation in sport has been rising all over Europe. However, the significance of gender in participation rates in sport suggests considerable contrasts across the European countries. Denmark and Germany, for instance, have a rather high proportion of women active in sports clubs (20-35%), whereas in Italy and Greece, participation rates are much more structured along the lines of traditional gender roles.[7] Without taking into account the cultural embedding of physical activity and gender roles any data suggesting change in participation rates are liable to interpretation that does not meet reality.

The more general findings of a trend of pluralization of sports participants is accompanied by the observation of a growing diversity in the sports practiced. Obviously this trend has been fostered by new products such as skateboards, or modified products like cycles and skis. This has occurred at a time when the leisure industry has been one of the most rapid growing segments of the economy.

However, natural conditions including climate and geographical aspects, cultural values such as achievement and competition, or social conditions like welfare and leisure time, certainly do have an influence on the development of different sports. There are physical activities and sports that are much more prominent in one country than in its neighbor country as for example 'boules' in France and Spain, darts in Great Britain, or hunting in Italy.

2. Trend of differentiation

The term differentiation refers to the development of clearer distinctions between different forms and ideological underpinnings of sport.[8] In general three types can be identified:

- elite sport or high performance sport, typically professional

- organized and institutionalized amateur sport within clubs and associations (generally competitive sport)

- semi-organized or unorganized amateur sport for all, and leisure sport (jogging, fitness activities, etc.)

Since the 1960s these three types of sport have been increasingly growing apart. Their ideological underpinning is becoming more separated and their institutional frameworks more independent. In accordance with this trend, the development of the 1980s is often characterized in terms of deformalization.[9] However, this process occurs at a different rate and in quite different forms. This model seems to be most suitable to describe the German case but less useful in describing the Spanish, French, or Greece models. In West Germany the profile of the sport system, a huge network of approximately 80 sports federations and 66,000 clubs, has long been and still is (in many sports) predominantly competitively driven. The growing interest of more and more people taking part in some sort of leisure-oriented physical activity is a big challenge for the clubs. Being confronted with consumer demands and commercially run sports centers, which are becoming more and more attractive for middle-aged people, obliges the clubs to reflect on their traditional structure. Spain, on the other hand, is characterized by a loose-knit network of clubs whose most common feature seems to be its heterogeneity. Rising interest in sport participation has led to an increase in the number of sports clubs (20% within three years), which presently have a membership rate of about 60.[10]

Between Generalization and the Analysis of the Individual Case

The Danish case of rejecting central European policy demonstrates how sensitive nations, societies, and people are to the process of integration. Societies are products of their own history, geographical conditions, social and cultural experiences, and identity. These social facts have to be taken into consideration when aiming at a common European policy and a sound piece of research. In comparative research in the social sciences, the most crucial question seems to be that of the quality of data and validity of comparative data.

The source of the data, the purpose for which they are gathered, and the method of collection do vary considerably from one country to another. In Great Britain information about leisure and sports behavior is derived from sources such as the General Household Surveys and the BBC's time budget work. The French, on the other hand, regularly carry out surveys on what is called cultural and leisure behavior and provide a wider and more reliable coverage. In Germany, there are detailed membership statistics of sports clubs and numerous small scale surveys on leisure activities and their relevance within lifestyles. Such surveys might be expected to accomplish a reliable and coherent impression of the development of physical activities and leisure behavior. But far from it. The participation rates look as if surveys produce as many different results as the number of surveys themselves. Also, there is no use in generalizing on multinational data when intra-national differences overcome international differences. Moreover, there are fundamental problems in regard to the validity of available indicators of the development of the sport system on a comparative basis that cannot be overcome that easily.

Besides this methodological note on data processing and interpretation, there is another important cultural dimension to be taken into account when conducting comparative research. Sporting culture (including all forms of culture) is created in the context of enabling and constraining structures.[11] Considering that sports are cultural performances and are legitimized by quite different values and ideas, from an historical and cross-national perspective, it has to be recognized that social action must be analyzed in terms of the reciprocal relationships between human actors and social and cultural constraints. Thus, it seems that comparative social science within sport still has to find the balance between excessive, inadequate generalization and individualized case study concreteness.

Notes

---

[1]Council of Europe (Eds.) *Sports Information Bulletin.* XXIX (1992), 2233f.
[2]Council of Europe.
[3]Hartmann-Tews, Ilse. "Sportstrukturen-Handlungsbedarf aus sportfachicher und sportolitischer Sicht, *Sport im zusammenwachsenden Europa.* Aachen: Meyer & Meyer.

[4]Remans, A. & M. Delforge. *The Sports Structures in the Countries of the Council of Europe*. Brussels: Clearing House, 1987.

[5]Belloni, M.C. "Trends in sports in Italy," *Trends in Sports - Multinational Perspective*. Enschede: Giordano Bruno Culemborg, 1989, p. 225.

[6]Kamphorst, T. & K. Roberts (Eds.) *Trends in Sports - Multinational Perspective*. Enschede: Giordano Bruno Culemborg, 1989, 386f.

[7]Belloni; Harahousou-Kabitsi, Yvonne A. "Important reasons that inhibit Greek women's participation in physical recreation," *Journal of Comparative Physical Education and Sport*. XIII: 2 (1991), pp. 9-23.

[8]Kamphorst & Roberts.

[9]Digel, H. "Die Versportlichung unserer Kultur und deren Folgen Für den Beitrag zur Uneigentlichkeit des Sports," *Für Einen besseren Sport*. Schorndorf: Hofmann, (1990), pp. 73-96.

[10]Acthen, M. *Sportentwicklung in Spanien*. Koln: Deutsche Sporthochschule.

[11]Harvey, J., & H. Cantelon. *Not just a Game*. Ottawa: University Press, 1988.

Chapter 15

Unity of the Nation— Unity in Sports?

Wolf-Dietrich Brettschneider

In October 1990 the two German states merged together to become one. What is the significance of this date for sports in Germany? Two years have passed since the Unification Act. In what situation does sports find itself today? Did the Unification Act automatically produce a sports fusion? A small number of German 'sports officials' devoted themselves to such an illusion, and some still do. For them, it would be a dream come true if a sort of symbiosis could take place between the gold medal factory GDR and the F.R.G., where more than one-third of the overall population are members of sport clubs. Conversely, the image of a sports superpower, able to dominate the international sports arena, has worried more than a few non-German sports experts. These fears are unfounded. More fitting are the comments recently published in a German newsmagazine, "At the Winter Olympics East German athletes won Gold, Silver and Bronze whilst West German dignitaries counted the medals, celebrating them as a success of the unification."[1]

This author's thesis is more down to earth. It reads:

> The two opposing social systems have over the years developed sport systems that are worlds apart. The integration of these systems within the process of Germany's unification will not be completed for years to come by which time nothing will be left of the former GDR system.

In order to develop this thesis I will concentrate on some findings of a comparative study on the sports culture of children and youth in West and East Germany. As a kind of extended introduction I would like to give some information on how sport was experienced by the youth of the former GDR.

Elite Sport, and Recreational Sport in the GDR

That a small country of 17 million people could develop such a successful inter-national sports program was a source of pride among leaders of the GDR. It was also a source of wonder among international sports bodies such as the IOC, and among some countries which have replicated the GDR system. The leaders of the GDR hoped that success in international sport would divert the attention of the people away from their miserable existence under the socialist state. Male and female athletes embodied the "pretty face" of socialism; for example, Katarina Witt featured prominently in advertising, in the USA, during the 1992 Winter Olympics with the slogan "the two greatest things on ice—Katarina Witt and diet coke."

Since there are few, if any, published sources describing the development of the GDR sports "system" it is understandable that speculation was widespread. Today the process of reconstruction and critical reflection destroys the myths surround-ing the so-called secrets of GDR top-level sport, revealing a well-developed sys-tem. The integral system for seeking out and screening of talents included all chil-dren of the GDR and began as early as the first school year, sometimes as early as the kindergarten. It was repeated again in the third and sixth year. The children underwent anthropometric measurement and motor tests which were supposed to predict their body size, structure, and athletic ability at maturation. The judgment of sports instructors and trainers complemented the data, evaluated by a central research institute. These results formed the basis of decisions about who should be supported in what type of sport. In addition to the abovementioned active form of talent screening there was also another—more passive—form of searching for sporting talent. This occurred during competitions, which took place at different levels of performance in different kinds of sports. The best example of this were the Spartakiade Games, held each Summer and Winter in all districts. These results too were evaluated centrally by experts in the "Institute for Sport Sciences" at Leipzig.[2]

The selected children were sent to local sports centers for an extensive basic train-ing concentrated on specific sports which acted as "feeder" systems to the 25 elit-ist sport schools (KJS). These special schools served as the nucleus for promoting sports talent in the GDR. About 10,000 children lived, trained, and were educated here. They formed the pool from which potential Olympic champions emerged. Learning conditions in these schools were exceptional. For example, at one of the most efficient KJS, in Berlin, the ratio of students to teachers was 2:1, while the overall average ratio was 3:1.[3] These schools were formally under control of the Ministry of Education, but in fact they were controlled by the sports federation, the daily regime and the curriculum being dependent on the development and the individual performance of the children and the demands of the training and competition cycle.[4]

Strict criteria formed the basis of admission to such elite schools. These included not only great sporting talent, and good health, but also membership in a communist youth club, and the political trustworthiness of the family. In the event that these elitist student-athletes could not cope with the enormous pressure of performing at the high standard expected from them, they were sent back to normal schools. This procedure, which occurred in the case of 70% of the students, was called "re-delegation."

Much less attention was paid to the sporting needs of the majority of GDR youth than to these elite performers. Nevertheless, sports was an important element in the normal biography of GDR youth with 90% of them finding membership in the so-called Pioneer organizations. The significance of sports can be seen in the pledge of one of these organizations, "We pioneers are keeping our bodies clean and healthy, do sports regularly and cheerfully." It clearly shows how indispensable the educational and social demand was to include sport in the existing world of the children and youth.

Of great importance were the sport societies supported by the schools or by the National Sports Federation. Out of 5,369 schools in the GDR, 5,222 (97%) were directly linked to those sports societies, where qualified sport instructors, teachers, parents and old students taught sports, preferably the 'traditional' sports such as athletics, handball, soccer, volleyball, and gymnastics. U.S.-imported outdoor activities such as skate-boarding, surfing, mountain biking, or the various Eastern movement forms, so popular in West Germany, hardly existed in the East. Either ideological barriers or lack of equipment hindered their development.

Physical Education was compulsory and, more or less, identical throughout the whole country, since it was based on a central curriculum. Its dominant characters were effectiveness and intensity. Progress in performance was constantly recorded and evaluated according to set standards. The facilities were miserable. Only 52% of the schools had their own gyms with a size exceeding 250 m^2. The equipment too, compared to Western standards, was very poor.

Similarities and Differences

The interesting question now is whether the characteristics of the GDR sport system have left their traces, as far as sport involvement and sport concepts of young people are concerned. Two representative analyses—comparing East and West German youth—form the basis for answering these questions.[5] The findings of this study focus on 14-19-year-old boys and girls. This age group deserves our attention for two reasons:

1) For the GDR this age group was the most important with respect to establishing its sports system.

2) This age group is most directly involved in sports and therefore plays a decisive role in the present transformation process. It will be these youths, as the bearers of cultural and social change, who will determine the direction and speed of sport reform.

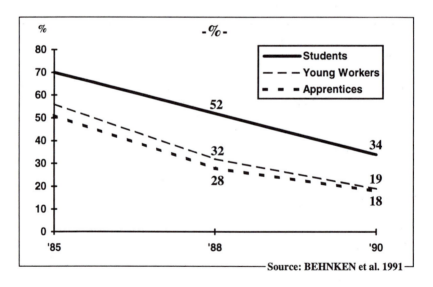

Figure 1—Identification of Adolescents and Young Adults with the GDR

It is worth mentioning that, since the mid-1980s, the solidarity between GDR youth and the government had been declining.[6] Long before the disintegration of the GDR, a revolution had already taken place in the minds of the younger generation. Unnoticed by the public, partly due to the influence of Western tele-

vision, the lifestyle and attitude towards life (of the GDR youth) had been continuously changing over the last decade. The extent of "Westernization" is
clearly seen by the fact that youth in both East and West treasured the individuality of their lifestyles and followed equal patterns of orientation (see Table 1).
However, it is also clear that youth in the East have a lot of catching up to do,
given the significance that certain areas of life have for them.

Table 1—Importance of Different Spheres of Life (14-19 year olds)

-%-	Total		Male		Female		Age: 14-19	
	East	West	East	West	East	West	East	West
Sport	39	27	45	35	32	20	65	48
Fashion	35	26	28	20	41	33	59	48
Health	96	92	95	91	98	94	98	88
Leisure	75	68	77	75	73	62	97	87
Fitness	55	44	63	48	48	39	79	62
Friends	79	75	77	78	80	84	94	94
Family	92	81	88	79	96	81	74	72

Source: EMNID 1991

Ninety-seven percent of the youth claimed, leisure time is very important—
compared with only 87% for the Western youth. Fashion also played a more
significant role in the East than it did for the West: 59% East to 48% West. For
almost all in the East, good health was a precious asset, just as it was for the
majority in the West—the percentage here, however, being slightly smaller.
Similar results were obtained for the question of personal fitness 79% to 62%.[7]

Now to the sport involvement. Since in the GDR almost everything was organized, informal sports activities were less popular among Eastern than Western
youth. Twenty-two percent of the youth in the West jogged regularly, in the
East only 15%. For aerobics, and the various forms of dance, the ratio was 14%
West to 6% East. The ratio was 31% to 17% in swimming and 14% to 9% in
table tennis. However, the findings referring to informal activities mark a total
contrast to those in institutionalized sports. Here, the level of participation of
the East German youth in sports such as athletics, handball, and volleyball was
2 to 3 times more than it was in the West.

The attention paid to sports among West German youth is far less than it is in
the East. An analysis of the significance of sports shows how big the differences

are. Two-thirds of the East German youth attach great importance to sports, compared to half of the West German youth.[8] Interestingly, this finding is reversed when considering active sport participation during leisure time. Here only 67% of East German youth include sport as part of their leisure time participation compared to 80% in the West.[9] Such differences may seem strange until the limitations of sport as a leisure time activity for GDR youth are taken into account. Leisure time for them was controlled and organized, and opportunities for sport participation were largely controlled by the State. In the West, the diversity of sports makes them a more recreational choice.

Table 2—Subjective Meanings of Sport

-%-	Total		Gender				Age: 14-19	
			Male		Female			
	East	West	East	West	East	West	East	West
Achievement	13	24	15	26	11	22	31	18
Fun	78	67	77	65	79	69	65	71
Effort	24	29	26	30	23	28	48	32
Relaxation	66	63	67	61	65	64	48	56
Competition	6	12	6	11	6	13	13	12
Social Experience	85	78	86	80	84	76	86	81
Fight	14	17	14	18	10	15	27	19
Play	78	74	76	72	79	75	69	77

Source: EMNID 1991

Similar differences occur over the question of what youth are actually seeking in sport. These results show that gratification and motives such as performance, effort, and competition find much more approval with the East German youth than with their peers in the West. On the other hand, West German youth put more emphasis on well-being, relaxing, and having fun. It would be easy to interpret these empirical results on the basis of modernization theories, emphasizing tendencies towards hedonism and individualism in our society.

There is a clear difference between what sport means for East and West youth. For East German youth sport is, above all, a summation of the different forms of institutionalized sport. Their sports activity underlies a pattern which is strongly oriented towards performance, effort and competition.[10] The West German youth take this traditional sports concept much more lightly, although they do accept institutionalized sports, as well as performance and competitive sports. However, they have hedonistic tendencies and an individualized value system, which are also characteristic for other areas of social life.[11] We may say that we are, at present, witnessing a kind of cultural reformulation of sport in West Germany. As to the youth in East Germany their sport concept reveals those characteristics typical for West Germany in the 1960s and 1970s. Presumably there will be a swift adjustment in sport as in leisure, and in recreation in general between East and West.

What Will Remain of the GDR Sport and How Will the German Sports of the 1990s Develop?

This section of the chapter is more speculative since it cannot be based on empirical data. Nevertheless, the following scenarios are offered:

1. Elite Performance Sport in the former GDR. The promotion structures of performance sport are no longer under the central political control of the communist party. Sport is now independent. The athlete, not the state, is now responsible for performance sport engagement. The enormous army of personnel consisting of 6,000 highly qualified trainers, and all the scientists and officials who attended to the athletes in all the 19 sports at the Winter and Summer Olympics are no longer needed. The efficient nationwide talent spotting program does not exist any more.[12] The promotion of talent is no more the result of exact analyzing and planning but as in the former FRG, left to personal engagement. The most important training centers have disappeared. The main items of the performance sport development of the GDR child and youth sport schools still exist on paper, but are now integrated in the normal school system losing their special status. The relationship between teacher and pupil has normalized, and the number of trainers reduced. Entering these schools is no longer restricted, but open to everyone. As a result the KJS have lost their reputation as elite schools and "medal factories."

2. Mass Sport: The above conditions apply to the mass sport as well. The former organization structure was an indispensable authority for socialization of the GDR youth. The membership in political organization, just like the member-

ship in sports organizations, was part of their normal biography. Membership in one of these sport organizations was not voluntary but obligatory. The pressure to perform well and be very disciplined prevailed. After the unification and the cancellation of all government subsidies many of these organizations ceased to exist causing a dramatic exodus (estimated at 77%) from the sport clubs by 14-18-year-olds. The reasons for this exodus are political and economic. The ideological basis for these clubs no longer exists, and the lack of government funding means that today, in East Germany, club membership means paying fees. The youth needs this money for other essential things.

Conclusions

The structures of the old GDR, which made the top-level sport so dominant, no longer exist. The organizations that had supported the mass sports have dissolved and are presently undergoing a metamorphosis. Sport is now playing a more subordinate role. German top-level sport is currently profiting from the effects of the long-term planning of the former GDR. Albertville has confirmed this. At the Olympic Games in Barcelona this 'bonus' was felt, probably for the last time. As to organized or informal leisure activities the former "wonderland of sport" is now showing the characteristic features of a developing country. Restoring an attractive sports system is dependent on an improved economic situation. In the course of the unification process, GDR sport will slowly be transformed into a West German form.

Some people complain about this situation and wonder why the Germans would want to change a system that was so successful. These critics see the danger of the baby being thrown out with the bath water.[13] The often uncritical adoption or imposing of West German values and norms on the East may lead to such an interpretation. But it is important to remember that, particularly, the elite sport system was established at the cost of the rest of the population. Finally, it is not easy to be free from prejudice when taking a closer look at German sports and its development. It is necessary to tear down the wall that still exists in the heads of many people—in the East as well as in the West.

Notes

[1]*Der Spiegel*, 1992.

[2]Bräuer, B. "Abschied von der Kinder- und Jugendsportschule?" *Sportpädagogik* 14:3 (1990), pp. 5-9; and, Wokalel, A. *Zum Transformationsprozeß des Sports in der DDR.* Gesamtdeutsches Institut: Analysen und Berichte, 1991.

[3]Wokalel.

[4]Rott, J. "Die Schulen der Olympia-Sieger". *Olympische Jugend,* 10 (1991) p. 11

[5]Behnken, J. et al. *Schülerstudie '90. Jugendliche im Prozeß der Vereinigung.* München: Juventa, 1991; and Emnid, *Sport- und Freizeitverhalten - ein Ost-West-Vergleich.* Bielefeld: Emnid, 1991.

[6]Behnken.

[7]Emnid, 1991.

[8]Emnid.

[9]Emnid.

[10]Pfister, G. "Zum Stellenwert des sportlichen Leistens bei Jugendlichen in der Bundesrepublik und in der DDR." *Sportwissenschaft* 16:1 (1986), pp. 61-75.

[11]Beck, 1986.

[12]Naul, R. "Elite Sport in Germany: The 1990s". ICHPER (Ed.), 2: 28 (1992).

[13]Hardman, K. "Physical Education in the Former German Democratic Republic." ICHPER (Ed.), 2:28 (1992).

Chapter 16

The Unification of the German Sports Systems

Soeren Damkjaer

The unification of the sports systems of the two Germanies was initiated even before the formal unification of the two states. After October 1990 the stipulations of the Unification Treaty meant that the sports structure of the Federal Republic was taken over by the five new regional states in the former GDR. In late 1991, a crisis developed caused by the doping scandals and new information on the extent of infiltration in elite sport in the GDR by the Ministry of State Security. The Winter and Summer events of the Olympic Games were to measure some aspects of the unification process. Despite the ideals of the sports community, a crisis developed for both elite sport and sport for all.

The Unification of the German Sport Systems

The relationship between sport and the political system is a classical one in the sociology of sport. The recent unification of the sports systems of the German Democratic Republic and the Federal Republic of Germany is a demonstration of the relevance of this form of analysis, illuminating the position of elite sport and sport for all in a situation of rapid social and political change.

One could debate the applicability of the terms unification or reunification. As the process has already proven, the two German states had indeed become quite different. Unification seems therefore to be the most appropriate concept as most GDR institutions were dismantled and the remnants were incorporated into the institutional structure of FRG. In the area of elite sport, however, the term reunification could be pertinent as the two Germanies formed a unified team until the late 1960s. Details of the historical development will be omitted, and the focus will be on the state of affairs in the late 1980s prior to the fall of the Berlin Wall and the subsequent development. Undoubtedly, a revision of the history of sport in the GDR shall be needed on the basis of what has been disclosed recently on the workings of the system and on the basis of fresh evidence and sources from archival material.

The construction of the GDR elite-model had progressed since the late 1950s. When the GDR was recognized as an independent sport nation, the results were outstanding. The political importance given to elite sport by the SED, the implementation by the State Committee on Sport and the DTSB as a mass organization, had resulted in a particularly efficient system of recruitment, research, and training. This was supported by the centralized organization and considerable enthusiasm in all parts of the sports organization. Manfred Ewald, as member of the politburo, was the party official responsible for this implementation of the will of the party.[1] In retrospect, it seems as if new attitudes were present in 1987-88. Elite sport had served its purpose for the state of the GDR and should be continued, but not necessarily on the same level and at the same costs. Among the top level of the party elite and the sports bureaucracy there was a recognition of the deplorable situation of sport for all in terms of participation, facilities, and support among workers and peasants. Manfred Ewald was demoted. This was the situation in the GDR up to November 1989.

Sports in the Federal Republic of Germany

In the FRG the sports system had been constructed on different principles. The competition between East and West, and the competition with the socialist GDR, directly influenced the construction of an elite model founded on support from the Federal level, from gifts, and sponsorships from the commercial sector. Organized by the Federal Committee on Elite Sport (BAL), and the DSB, this model followed the structure of the German Federal Republic. Elite sport was organized on the Federal level, sport for all in the regional states. The late 1980s witnessed a lively debate on the future perspectives on elite sport and sport for all. The proliferation of non-sportive forms of sport together with competition from commercialized forms of sport was seen as a challenge to the voluntary associations and their unpaid leadership. New motives of enjoyment and pleasure seemed to supplant the traditional functional values of sport for all.[2]

The sport systems of the GDR and the FRG were indeed very different. In the GDR sport of all kinds were embedded in the instrumental ideology of party policies on the working capacity and defense attitudes of the population. In the FRG, the DSB was defining new activities and new values in sport for all. In 1989 nobody imagined the revolutionary change of the party state in the GDR until it actually happened in November. The SED leadership under Honecker was unaffected by the signals, since 1985, from the Soviet Union of glasnost and perestroika. The dominant ideology was that such reforms were relevant in the USSR, but were unnecessary in the model state of the GDR. The power and authority of the SED regime seemed to have been consolidated since the recognition by the international community and by the FRG in the early seventies. Elite sport had played an important role in this consolidation.

The Year of Revolution

The revolution of November 1989 was followed by the interlude of Krenz and the provisional government of Modrow. A provisional leadership was elected in DTSB, and the top leadership directly associated with the SED regime was ousted. Plans were made for democratic elections in DTSB in March 1990 and a hectic period of blueprints for a reform of the whole sports system followed in the beginning of 1990. Reform, self-critique, reorientation and democratization were the catchwords of these months. In particular, the elite system was to undergo a total reconstruction as far as priorities and methods were concerned. Deep resentment and hostile attitudes, across the population, to elite sport and the former privileges of athletes were prevalent. The General Election, in March 1990, led to the government of De Maizier and pointed to an acceleration of the process of unification. What resulted in the DTSB and the world of sport was confusion. Plans were made for cooperation with the West German sports organizations, but became obsolete as quickly as they were agreed upon. They were overtaken by the political development. Cordela Schubert, the Minister of Sport in the GDR in the De Maizier government, was determined to purge elite sport of its SED past. The slimming of the organizational structure of DTSB led to the firing of officers and trainers. Financial cuts left the House of Sport in East Berlin half-empty by May 1990. The currency reform of July undermined the whole financial foundation of sport in the GDR.

Unification

The process of unification accelerated at an unexpected pace from August. The Unification Treaty dissolved the GDR into five regional states that joined the Federal Republic. In the paragraphs on culture and sport it was stated that the structure of the FRG would be extended to the new regional states. Sport for all was to be based on voluntary associations, democratic elections and unpaid officers, like the West German counterparts within the Ministry of Culture and Education of the regional state. Elite sport was to be administered using the existing structure of the Federal system, BAL and DSB. After extensive lobbying by influential parties, specific provisions were made for some major institutions that had been crucial in the former GDR system. The Research Institute on

Sport and Physical Culture in Leipzig (FKS), the Research Institute on Equipment (FES) in Berlin, and the Doping Test Laboratory in Kreishau were specifically mentioned in the text of the Treaty. The fate of the German Higher Institution of Physical Culture and Sport in Leipzig, effectively a Sport University producing highly qualified trainers, was undecided. The institutes of physical culture and sport in the universities, which incidentally had done almost no research, were subjected to the same screening procedures of the future staff as in other institutes and departments. The sports federations now merged with their Western counterparts. In December 1990, DTSB was dissolved. What was retained in the unified Germany of the elite structures were the following elements. The GDR elite, if it could and would continue under the new conditions. The aforementioned institutions of research and development, although with new functions and on a reduced scale in terms of personnel and on a reduced budget. A few trainers found employment in clubs and training centers. The elite sport schools for children and youth (KJS) were retained, but their budgets were reduced and their future was yet to be decided. The whole staff of the DTSB was fired. None was to be employed in the offices of DSB in Frankfurt. Out of an estimated 15,000 full-time employees and trainers that had staffed the GDR sports system only a few were retained in the unified system.

Although sport for all had suffered under the GDR regime, no support was given by the federal government in Bonn, as sport for all was provided by the regional states. However, theaters, museums, and other cultural institutions received additional funding despite the fact that they also were under the administration of the regional states. This is one of the paradoxes of the unification in sport. The transformation of factory clubs of the GDR-variety to voluntary associations proved difficult. The call for financial support, to formulate a new structure of voluntary associations, by the DSB were in vain. The number of members of sport associations was, in 1992, on the level of 8% of the adult population, far below that of 33% in the West.

A Year of Crisis

The leaders of DSB had, with their President Hans Hansen as spokesman, seen the unification of the two sports systems in accordance with the high ideals typical of the ideology connected with sport. This meant that the unification in sport of the two Germanies should be an example to the nation. In fact unification, in the case of most of the federations, had been fairly smooth with the exception of swimming and athletics where friction was frequent. This was a remarkable feat considering the differences in sports culture, in living standards, and in culture in general, between the two Germanies. In 1991, one year after the unification, two problems were to emerge, the practice of doping in the former GDR and in the FRG, and the question of the infiltration of the GDR elite sport by formal and informal agents from the Ministry of Security. Disclosure of the systematic doping practices had followed the dissolution of the GDR immediately upon the collapse of the wall. In 1991 new disclosures created a scandal. Reluctantly, investigation committees were established. The quality of investigation and the proposals for a solution cast doubt on the ability of the world of sport to cope with this serious problem, however. The disclosures, by the Gauck Commission on Stasi infiltration of all spheres of life in the GDR, also led to disclosures in elite sport. This forced the DSB to formulate a policy on handling disclosures that affected GDR leaders and trainers employed in the unified system. Again, the policy was to be more lenient than was the case in other spheres of society. This idealistic policy by the DSB created a problem of credibility. Were the sports organizations able to handle problems of this scale of magnitude within their own system of jurisdiction? Much was at stake. The disclosures of extensive and systematic doping practices, of centralism in GDR sport, and of Stasi-infiltration tainted the image of elite sport in the united Germany. The disclosures affected the political will to finance elite sport in the future. The increasing professionalization and commercialization already tended to make politicians wary of footing the bill of elite sport. If the sports organizations were not themselves able to control unethical and illegal practices, the status of elite sport was degraded in public opinion and in the political system. The reactions of the mass media were of course crucial. This was the moment of truth for elite sport in Germany, right at the beginning of the Olympic Year. The combined effect of the scandals and the tendencies to excessive commercialization of elite sport created a crisis one year after the formal unification.

The Olympic Year

For Germany, the Olympic Games in Albertville and Barcelona were the major events following unification. In Albertville the German team did well, but most medals were won by athletes from the former GDR. Especially in speed skating the athletes from the East excelled. The new and freer conditions had led to better results. The doping scandal of Katrin Krabbe, and two other athletes accused of changing the test tubes in South Africa, marred the triumphant mood. Also the Stasi-infiltration and cooperation was disclosed up to the events. The Krabbe affair was to continue. She was acquitted by the doping committee of Athletics Federation and later on technical grounds by the International Athletics Federation. Then, in July, she was once more accused of using illegal substances. Expectations were high for the Summer Games. German experts predicted an unofficial first place for the US team, a second place for the

Unified Team, and a third place for the German team. There was even the hope that Germany might accomplish second place. The first week of the Games was a disappointment. However, after winning an unexpected medal in swimming Dagmar Haase attacked trainers and the leaders of the German Federation of Swimming in an emotional outburst transmitted by television. She accused the Federation of unprofessionally handling the preparations and of unjustly dealing with a doping affair involving a friend. She no doubt represented the resentment of many athletes from the former GDR team.

A Complex of Issues

There were a number of issues involved after two years of unification. In federations like swimming and athletics, the friction among athletes from the East and West had not subsided. So the question of the unification of East and West was very much alive. The feeling among citizens of the five new states of being second-rate in comparison to the West was transplanted to elite sport. The affairs involving athletes from the East were seen by the eastern population as a symbol of arrogance from the West. There was another level involved, the question of losers and winners. Some athletes from the East were winners on the playing fields, in the mass media, and in securing sponsorships like Heike Henkel. Others were losers in the process. Dagmar Haase spoke as a representative of the losers when winning gave her the right to voice the resentment felt by colleagues. A third level concerned the performance of the leadership in the united Germany. The athletes pointed to the incompetence of leaders and officials in West German federations and compared it to the professionalism and competence of the former GDR. The German performance in the Summer Games were satisfactory, but below expectations. The Unified Team, including the 11 members of CIS and Georgia, won unofficial first place with 45 gold medals, 38 silver and 29 bronze medals. The U.S. team came in second with a score of 37, 34, and 37, and Germany occupied third place with a score of 33, 21, and 28. In Seoul the GDR team alone had won 102 medals. A more successful performance could have glossed over the discontent of some athletes from the East and raised the status of German elite sport. Now the Summer Games demonstrated the still unfinished process of integration. The result of the Games was not bad, but the overall impression is that German elite sport after two years of unification is still in a state of crisis. What was, in 1989 and 1990, seen as a merger of two different, but powerful elite systems that would place a united Germany in first or second place turned out to produce a satisfactory result, and nothing more. That the Unified Team, against all odds of uncertainty, dissolution and financial crisis, came in first was the paradox of the games. The first and last show in history of the Unified Team was a triumph, reflecting the strength of the Big Red Machine even in acute crisis and on the verge of extinction. The merger of the two German machines produced a product of an ordinary size. With this paradox the Olympic Games of 1992 ended.

Theoretical Perspectives

From the viewpoint of a sociology of culture one can regard the GDR sport system as an example of the process of "Unfinished Modernization" in the socialist system of the former Soviet Union and Eastern Europe. In contradistinction to the moderate or inferior performance of the economy at large it could, within the limited field of elite sport, produce extraordinary results although the costs were high. In sport for all, the old-fashioned content of the activities, the puritan ideology of work, and the militarization of the world of sport led to inferior results. Sport for all was simply not modern in any sense. The amalgamation of the two elite systems was, in fact, the incorporation of some parts of the former GDR system into the FRG model. The organizational principles of the FRG structure prevailed.

In retrospect, it is no wonder that the results reflected the strengths and weaknesses of the West German system. In sport for all, the success measured in terms of mass participation, diversity of activities etc., is much harder to evaluate. Sport for all is influenced by a number of cultural factors from tradition, subtle socialization processes, and consumer culture. It is hardly surprising that the quasi-modern sports culture of the former GDR could not easily be transformed into the modern or even postmodern tendencies in the FRG. Within the perspective of comparative physical education and sport the unification of the two Germanies offers a case for comparison of the actual sports cultures in a socialist country and within the mixed economy of the FRG. The unique historical situation, where one system is dismantled and the remnants are reintegrated into the structure of another, is an invitation to study the factors of body culture in its relationship with quasi-modern and even postmodern forms of sport. Although the conclusions over such a short time perspective must necessarily be tentative they can, hopefully, be regarded as hypotheses to further research. The Federal Republic, prior to 1989, represented an example of the tendencies in Europe of the development of elite sport, and sport for all, where elite sport was moving into a process of extensive commercialization and professionalization. This questioned the cultural significance of elite sport and the political commitment to support it. The Systemkonkurrenz, however, overshadowed all such considerations. The contest was between the State professionals of the East and the Professionals of the mixed economies of sport in the West. Ethical considerations of the exploitation of the athletes' body were non-existent within the political instrumentalization of the socialist countries and marginal in the West. In the West functionalist ideologies of sport for all, whether in the sociological or the biological sense, were on the wane. Body culture was now more in accordance with the tendencies of modern and postmodern consumer culture leading to new motives and new aestheticized forms of sport, some of which acquired new qualities as in the new non-sportive movement cultures.

The GDR was an example of the total instrumentalization of movement culture to the interest of the party state. This worked well as far as elite sport was concerned as the planning procedures and the planning bureaucracy could handle the limited parameters of success, given the excessive political and economic support by the SED. But sport for all could not be instrumentalized to the same extent, nor planned with the same results. Militarization was met with apathy, mobilization campaigns with retreat into the private world. In elite sport the unification has led to a crisis, despite all bland assertions after the Olympic Games. It has led to a complex situation of Ossies and Wessies, of winners and losers, of the confrontation of different cultures of sport and of different cultures in a wider sense.

Notes

[1]Wonneberger, G. (Ed.). *Körperkultur und Sport in der DDR*, Berlin, 1982; *DDR-handbuch*, Band 2, third edition, Cologne, 1985; Riordan, J. *Sport, Politics, and Communism,* 1991.
[2]Heinemann, K. & H. Becker, (Eds.).*Die Zukunft des Sports,* 1986

Chapter 17

German Unification and the Disintegration of the GDR Sport System

Victor Zilberman

The German Democratic Republic (GDR), which ceased functioning as an independent country at midnight, October 2, 1990, reunited with West Germany to again become a dominant state in the international community. In its 45 years of existence, the GDR became renowned for its international sport accomplishments. Under the terms of the 1990 unification, the GDR transformed its socialist political structure to western democracy and its economy to the free market. The GDR was to become an integral part of West Germany, with similar educational and sport structures. That complex transformation process not only involved the dismantling of the GDR political, economical, and sport system, but it also significantly changed the perception and attitude of the East German population toward high performance sport and its champion athletes.

<u>International Recognition of GDR Sport</u>

Unification, which was intended to be a positive experience for the East Germans, brought poor economic conditions, unemployment, uneasy relationships with their West German compatriots, and a media backlash toward the former GDR. Extensively criticized by the media were the former Communist government; social, economic, and environmental policies; as well as high performance sport and accomplished athletes. Particularly condemned were the high cost of elite sport, government secrecy, the privileged status of top athletes, drugs in sport, and athletes serving as informers for the GDR internal police (Stasi).

Prior to unification and negative revelations, for two decades East Germany was regarded as one of the leading sport nations based on its accomplishments in various World Championships and Olympic Games. A high degree of professionalism and close cooperation between coaches and scientists produced remarkable and consistent sport performances throughout the 1970s and 1980s. According to I. Jurkov, senior member of the USSR Research Institute of Sport, in contrast to other countries, the scientific contribution was regarded by the sport organizations and coaches in the GDR, as valuable and applicable.[1]

East Germany's sport accomplishments were magnified by its small population in comparison to the Soviet Union and the United States. From 1956 to 1988, East German athletes won three gold medals at the Winter Olympics in comparison to 25 won by the United States, which is a country 15 times larger.[2] At the Montreal Olympics, the East Germans produced one gold medal for every 188,000 citizens; the Soviets, one for every 425,000; and third place USA, one for every 6,327,000.[3]

The most impressive international performances, however, were obtained by the GDR women, who won more medals at the Montreal Olympics than the women from all of the other countries combined.[4] In figure skating, G. Zifert, A. Petch, and K. Witt, products of the highly successful coach Utta Muller, won more medals at the World Championships and Olympics than single women figure skaters of any other nation in the last decade. Their speed skating performances were as impressive with J. Boerner winning East Germany's ninth consecutive all-round World Championship title in 1990.

Unparalleled performances were displayed over the last two decades by the GDR's women swimmers who, since the 1976 Olympics, won the majority of events they entered. The results of the 1983 European Championships, where they won all gold and silver medals, and in 1985 when they won 12 out of 14 finals, exemplify their superior international performances.[5] At the Seoul Olympics, the GDR swimmers achieved their best performances in 73% of the events (the highest of all nations).[6] In fact, describing their superiority, Canadian National Coach, D. Johnson, stated that at the 1986 World Championship, there were the East Germans and then there were the world class swimmers.[7] In contrast, nearly a year after unification in August 1991, the German women returned from the European Championship in Athens with only two gold medals.[8]

It is clear to sport professionals that today's preparation of top athletes is highly complex, consisting of a combination of numerous methods, conditions, and factors, most of which were met by the GDR sport organization. East Germany's superior and consistent international sport performances are largely attributed to special training programs, nutritional diets, coaching, selection, use of stimulants, and financial rewards, to name a few. State-supported sport schools, most of which have now been closed, played a major role in the development of world class athletes. According to the President of the German National Olympic Committee, Willi Daume, parents are still interested in sending their children to sport schools which provide good education; however, due to increased costs, they are now unaffordable to the average person.[9]

Organization and Financing

The reorganization of East German sport began in 1989 prior to unification. The transformation of the GDR structure to the western sport model coincided with frequent changes in its leadership, financial cuts, and a modification of its goals and policies. The intent of the new leadership was to find a balance between mass participation and high performance sport as well as to move toward decentralization, elimination of secrecy, and abolition of performance-enhancing drugs. The organizational change also resulted in massive cutbacks of administrative jobs, which were reduced by over 80%; from over 12,000 employees prior to unification to 1,500 by 1991.[10] The doors were opened to the use of private sponsors and the professionalization of athletes, which is largely attributed to the change in sport federation policies, a new administrative style, and the consistent decrease in government funding. The transition to a more mass participation approach to sport was manifested in the use of sport facilities which, in 1990, became accessible to the general population. The emphasis for state support has been returned to sports for all, the original intent of the system. The days when officials would close the ice rink after Katrina Witt finished practice were over.[11]

The Olympic Committees amalgamated in order to speed up the unification process among the two sport systems. The GDR's high performance athletes were encouraged to train with the West German teams, and the number of sport meets between East and West Germany were increased from 130 in 1989, to 910 in 1990.[12] The ideological tool and effective promoter of high performance sport, the East German daily newspaper, *Doyches Shportaho*, widely read by the general population, folded in 1991 after 43 years of existence. Overstaffed and subsidized by its former government, the specialized daily sport newspaper could not financially survive in the free market economy.[13]

The breakdown of the efficient and successful sport system was not welcomed by the GDR sport specialists who were concerned with losing sport autonomy and wanting to see unification as an equal union rather than becoming West

Germany's twelfth province. Back in 1990, top coaches Y. Tanneburg (swim-ming), A. Munda (rowing), and others predicted the end of East German sport glory and diminished achievements of its athletes.[14] According to the Editor-in-Chief of the *Doyches Shportaho* sport newspaper, Klaus Kimmel, reduced financing of sport after unification led to the significant deterioration of the feeder system, causing the disintegration of the best European sport system. The results of such short-term vision, as predicted by Kimmel, will affect the future German performance at the Olympic Games.[15]

Following unification, the East German system of control, training, education, and research has broken down. Since October 3, 1990, DTSB and the office of General Secretary of Physical Culture and Sport have been abolished. For all of the former GDR sport associations, unification meant giving up their indepen-dence and joining their West German counterparts. In brief, most of their elite sport system was dismantled in the first six months of the unification process.[16]

The breakdown of East German sport coincided with the disintegration of the top clubs and teams. One year after unification the renowned sport club, Dynamo Berlin (prior to 1990 had a membership of 1,800), is at the point of folding. Similarly, the Boxing Motor Club of Magdeburg (six-time national champions) canceled its boxing program in 1990.[17]

Extensive migration to West Germany, which amounted to 700,000 in 1990, had a negative effect on the already troubled East German sport.[18] For example, in 1990, East Germany was unable to field a boxing team for a dual meet with West Germany, while at their previous meet in 1987, the GDR won with a score of 20 to 4. At the beginning of 1990, 50 of East Germany's best boxers were competing in the West German amateur league.[19] Similar events occurred in volleyball and basketball. Prior to the opening of the 1991 season, approximate-ly 30 former members of the GDR National Basketball Team moved to West Germany. Included were well-known players Y. Zonnefled, S. Lahe, L. Grosser, O. Ploman, and U. Zidel. The departure of top athletes to better economic con-ditions has also been damaging to the previously powerful East German swim program. World class swimmers who left Leipzig for different cities were R. Ferber to Offenbach, C. Zivert to Vuppertal, S. Shultse to Kanshtadt, and K. Yeke to Bughauzen. The most devastating effects of the athletic migration, however, were experienced in soccer. Players already competing for the United German National team were among the first wave lured to the West by high salaries. Among those were such stars as R. Shtiman, H. Fuks and T. Fogel. The only sport where athletes have not been enticed to Western Germany is ice hockey.[20]

The massive departure of top athletes and coaches, a decrease in the participation and organization of international and domestic competitions, and athletic assistance have been attributed predominantly to the inadequate financing of East German sport. Even though the German budget has been significantly increased (by 44% from 1990 to 1992) to absorb new territories, East German athletes, coaches and administrators assess the new financing of sport as insufficient to sustain former sport supremacy. Prior to unification the GDR, with a population of 17 million, had an annual sport budget of approximately $700 million U.S., whereas the all German budget in 1991, for a population of 81 million, amounted to $270 million U.S. (355 million DM).[21] The *Noyes Doychland* newspaper, estimated that maintenance of the existing East German sport facilities alone requires an annual cost of three billion DM.[22] According to Olympic Swimming Champion Michael Gross, the effects of drastic financial cutbacks threaten to eliminate what was known as the East German sport system. The GDR's exorbitant sport subsidies, however, are unrealistic in the Western economy.[23] The long-term success of the East German sport model has been predetermined by government emphasis on the preparation of the best athletes for the 1992 Albertville and Barcelona Olympics. Financial assistance for coaches, athlete development, facilities, and support staff have been vastly neglected.

Athletes

Poor economic conditions and broad social changes negatively affected high performance athletes' involvement in sport. East German sport participants must not only contend with the collapse of their government, but with the dismantling of their highly successful, if largely discredited, sports machine. After unification, athletes were left to train on their own, or with their personal coaches, but without state support which included monthly stipends, equipment, instant access to sport facilities, and travel expenses for competitions.[24] In welcoming political changes in Germany, Heike Drechsler, 1983 World Champion and 1988 silver medalist in the Seoul Olympics in the long jump, admitted that the loss of government support negatively affected her sport participation.[25]

Produced by one of the most successful and highly subsidized sport programs in the world, the GDR athletes were compelled to adapt to a new environment where amateur sport is not a profession and only a select few end up financially successful. As the state took less and less responsibility, high performance athletes began adapting to a new lifestyle by developing different careers, seeking stable employment, and taking personal responsibility for their future.

The unification and social reforms altered the population's perception toward high performance sport and top athletes who, to the East Germans, are a reminder of the old communist system. With so many problems in the country, the sport system became an easy target. In scattered incidents, elite athletes were scorned in public and their property vandalized.[26] People questioned the expenditure of millions by plants and enterprises to support secondary soccer teams rather than utilizing those funds to improve the population's fitness and health.[27]

Government and media deliberation about the GDR's sport began in the early stages of unification, in the fall of 1989. Highly criticized were the privileged status of amateur athletes, neglect of mass sport participation, and excessive financing of high performance, and drugs in sport.[28] According to the *Der Spiegel* magazine, the East German government annually spent the same amount on performance-enhancing drug research as on the professional development of teachers: five million DM. The practical application of those drugs cost the government another ten million DM.[29] The extensive reward program for sport performance was concealed from the general population. It was only after the 1989 political change, that people were informed about the price of producing sport superstars which amounted to one million DM for each Olympic gold medal.[30] In Germany, as in much of Eastern Europe, the once revered athletes are now seen as symbols of the misplaced priorities of the tainted former regime.

After unification, wide media and public criticism centered on the former communist government's use of their athletes' international accomplishments to propagate and justify the GDR's political goals. They backed up words with money, too, establishing a network of elite sport school which formed the backbone of the GDR sport system. The system employed a tremendous number of personnel to provide professional assistance to high performance athletes. According to Rainer Hageholz, director of the Dynamo Sport Society, "Each high performance athlete had a coach, doctor, masseuse, psychologist and sport conceptualizer to plan his program."[31]

In the past, each sport victory was proof, as Party General Secretary Erich Honecker put it, of "their better socialist system."[32] After unification, athletes began to realize why high performance sport was of such importance in the GDR. In the opinion of Olympic Champion Ulf Timmermann, the state used superior sport performances to overshadow the problems of East German society.[33] Two-time Olympic Figure Skating Champion Katarina Witt stated, "Now it is clear to me why athletes were so furthered; because we were our Republic's

only showcases, because our economy, unfortunately, was on the floor."
Furthermore, Witt, whose charm and brilliance put a human face on her country's communist regime, felt that the authorities misused her by displaying her
as a shining symbol of their system.[34] The general population's negative attitude
toward high performance sport was a disappointment to the East German athletes who have found it difficult to accept the fact that these same people not
long ago admired their international sport performances. According to Olympic
Champion runner Marita Koch, who broke 16 World records, people forgot how
proud they were of sport accomplishments of East German athletes.[35] Katarina
Witt, labeled by the media as a fanatical communist, was glad to be working
with the professional ice show in North America, "At least here, no one will
give me a hard time for being born in a country whose existence came to an
end," said Witt. "The audience is interested in my proficiency as a figure skater
and applaud if my performance is to their satisfaction."[36] Responding to persistent allegations, Witt stressed that, as with other top athletes, her life was figure
skating and she had no interest or time for politics, "I was proud to stand on the
pedestal when our national anthem played and our flag was raised."[37]

Haunted by a legacy of widespread steroid abuse, revelations of athletes cooper-
ating with the secret police, social changes, a poor economy, and the population
and media's negative attitude toward elite sport East German participants are
finding their involvement in sport less glamorous. In the past, the leading GDR
athletes had little to worry about beyond their performance. They now have to
seek sponsors, organize training, and plan their future, or drop out of sport altogether.[38]

Coaching

In the last two decades sport became a reputable profession in East German
society, resulting in a large number of scientists, coaches, and administrators
obtaining secure employment. Under unification, the field of sport has been
diminished to an amateur status where the majority of people involved are vol-
unteers. Highly qualified East German coaches have been subjected to massive
layoffs which are expected to continue after the 1992 Olympics. In skiing, 50
full-time coaching jobs were lost by September 1990; and in track and field,
only 72 out of 600 paid coaches were still employed as of February 1991.[39] In
rowing, the loss of full-time coaching jobs was as drastic. Prior to unification,
East Germany's eight rowing centers, which received 40 million DM annually,
employed 200 full-time coaches. In the United Germany, with significantly
lower subsidies, the number of full-time coaching positions is expected to
increase from three, prior to unification, to six.[40] In speed skating, the GDR

employed 200 coaches in comparison to 10 in West Germany. After unification, the East German coaching force was reduced to 25 by January 1992.[41]

In his interview with *Equip*, the French magazine, Willi Daume acknowledged high unemployment among East German coaches, stating that job retraining programs were created for them by the government. In his opinion, the former GDR had too many coaches and the United Germany could not employ all of them.[42] Even though the German Sport Association allocated 7.7 million DM in 1990-91 for coaching salaries, a considerable number of East German coaches, realizing the lack of employment opportunities in the United Germany, either quit coaching or began searching for positions abroad.[43]

In sports such as soccer, East German coaches had the hardest time competing for jobs with West German professionals. Only the top two East German Soccer League teams have been integrated to the West German Bundesleague. Even the highly qualified GDR national coach, Aduard Geyer, who lost his job upon the termination of the national team in 1990, had to take a coaching position in July 1991 with the Hungarian soccer team, Banyas (Shiofok).[44] A number of renowned East German coaches in cycling, track and field, and swimming took coaching jobs in South Korea, Austria, Italy, New Zealand, China, and elsewhere. As of 1991, out of 10,000 former GDR professional coaches, 500 remained employed in the Eastern part of Germany; 1,000 found coaching positions in Western Germany and abroad; 3,000 changed their profession; while the other 5,500 coaches became unemployed.[45]

Drastic cutbacks of coaches meant that the hierarchic and effective system for finding and training talent on different competitive levels across East Germany became nonexistent. In addition, there are no longer training centers for children, and former sport clubs have lost a great deal of financial support from the state to pay coaches.[46]

The integration of the GDR coaches into the German sport structure was painful and complex. The discrepant distribution of coaching jobs among West and East German sport specialists became a source of resentment and discontent. For example, out of 126 top skiers in the United Germany in 1990, half were from the former East Germany. Due to unification, the number of state-employed coaches increased from 12 to 18; however, only four of 18 coaches employed by 1990 were from the GDR.[47]

The Direction of German Sport

Adapting the GDR structure to the West German sport model, where high performance is of a lower stature, resulted in the rapid breakdown of the East German sport system. All the components that made it so superior (i.e., organization, finance, coaches, feeder system, support, and scientific staff) have deteriorated. According to M. Gross, the unification process occurred so fast that the positive features of the GDR sport system were destroyed, while the West German shortcomings remain in place.[48] The promises of Chancellor Helmut Kohl to maintain the high standards of East German sport could not be kept. The GDR's sport was rapidly disintegrating as the financial and organizational objectives of the German sport bureaucracy focused on supporting top athletes and teams. Meanwhile, according to Thomas Munkelt, 1980 Olympic champion in the 110 meter hurdles, "The basic training of young athletes which comprise the highly rated East German feeder system has been neglected and destroyed."[49]

During the unification process West German sport leaders, as well as star athletes, were consistent in predicting that western countries cannot match the financial commitment of the former GDR. In addition, it was stated time after time that Germany was not a dominant sport country in the past and it did not intend to become one. Witnessing German unification, the world sport community waited in anticipation to see how sport in Germany would evolve. Media speculations and predictions about the future of German sport were often simplistic and unfounded. For example, if the GDR, with a small population, was second to the USSR in the Olympics, then 17 to 64 million should logically produce a new world superpower. The *Sovietsky Sport* newspaper predicted the future of German sport dominance by adding up the strengths of both countries. Combine West German soccer, alpine skiing, equestrian, rowing, and tennis' B. Becker and S. Graff with East German swimmers, track and field, biathlon, bobsled, figure skating, speed skating, rowing and kayak, cycling, boxing, shooting, and diving; and there will be a nation with hardly any weak teams.[50]

A mathematical approach, however, does not provide an accurate assessment of sport in the new Germany. The example which shows that the sum of two is not always better in sport could be seen in rowing. At the 1990 World Championship, the GDR finished first as a team, 11 medals in total (five gold, one silver, five bronze); West Germany placed second with seven medals in total (3-3-1). At the 1991 World Championship, the United German team won as a team; however the medal total was more modest, ten in total (6-1-3). Similarly in luge, the combined team, at the Albertville Olympics, was not nearly as strong as the East and West Germans were individually. Even though in some sports international results are impressive, in most cases the performance at the major events of the combined German team is lower than previously anticipated. At the 1992 Albertville Olympics, Germany won only one more medal than the GDR in 1988 (26 to 25). Meanwhile, the total number of medals of the two Germanies in Calgary was 33 (25 East; 8 West).[51]

As unification becomes more of an event of the past, the East German population, domestically, has been more concerned with their integration into a new society, as well as with the economy and unemployment (35% overall and 63% among women).[52] Internationally, the events in the former USSR, Yugoslavia and Iraq attract more attention than sport. Thus, the criticism of Daume, and the call for his resignation by the Christian Democratic Party based on the poor state of sport is not supported in Parliament and is of even less concern to the general population.[53]

German athletes, who grew up under different political systems and had competed against each other, became a part of the same team in Albertville. In a symbolic gesture, the German NOC chose former East German bobsledder, Wolfgang Hoppe, as the German flag bearer for the opening ceremonies.[54] In sport, as in other segments of German society, efforts are being made to bring the previously politically divided nation closer together.

Conclusions

The transition of the GDR's centralized sport structure to the western model resulted in the total disintegration of the East German "miracle machine." Their amalgamation has been marked by substantial financial cuts, massive layoffs in administrative and coaching jobs and a backlash from the media and general population toward high performance sport and top athletes. In addition, the much envied East German feeder system which provided long-range consistent international sport performance has been totally dismantled.

The training and living conditions of East Germany's high performance athletes have also deteriorated. Rather than solely focusing on training and competing, they have had to finance their existence as well as take personal responsibility for their training environment and future outside of sport. With reunification, East German athletes and coaches have now been placed at the level and status of western world sport participants. In short, the events of unification illustrated that the effective concepts of the GDR sport system, such as professional coaching, scientific support, extensive commitment to high performance, and comprehensive support for amateur athletes, could not be adapted and incorporated into the western sport model of the United Germany.

Notes

[1]*Sovietsky Sport.* (January 19, 1990).

[2]*Montreal Gazette.* (January 4, 1992).

[3]*Montreal Gazette.* (August 30, 1983).

[4]*Montreal Gazette.* (August 30, 1983).

[5]*Sovietsky Sport.* (December 17, 1985), *Sport Life of Russia.* I (1985).

[6]*Champion Magazine.* (June, 1989), p. 37.

[7]*Montreal Gazette.* (November 30, 1990).

[8]*Montreal Gazette.* (October 2, 1991).

[9]*Sovietsky Sport.* (August 14, 1991).

[10]*Physical Culture and Sport.* VI, (1990), pp. 30-31; *Montreal Gazette.* (February 17, 1991).

[11]Janofsky, M. "In East Germany, Trauma Between Two Eras," *New York Times.* (April 15, 1990).

[12]Janofsky. 1990.

[13]*Sovietsky Sport.* (April 17, 1991).

[14]*Sovietsky Sport.* (July 24. 1990); *Physical Culture and Sport.* VI, (1990), p. 31.

[15]*Sovietsky Sport.* (September 11, 1990).

[16]Naul, R. "Elite Sport in Germany: The 1990's," *ICHPER.* XXVIII: 2 (Winter 1992), pp. 7, 20, 21.

[17]*Sovietsky Sport.* (May 9, 1991; and, April 8, 1990).

[18]*Sovietsky Sport.* (May 21, 1991).

[19]*Sovietsky Sport.* (April 8, 1990).

[20]*Sovietsky Sport.* (May 21, 1991).

[21]*Sovietsky Sport.* (July 30, 1991); *Montreal Gazette.* (April 16, 1990).

[22]*Sovietsky Sport.* (May 21, 1991).

[23]*Montreal Gazette.* (November 3, 1990); *Sport Abroad.* (September 17, 1990), p. 16.

[24]Janofsky, M. (April 15, 1990).

[25]*Sport Abroad.* Moscow, XIV, (July 1990).

[26]Janofsky, M. (April 15, 1990).

[27]*Sovietsky Sport.* (April 16, 1991).

[28]*Sovietsky Sport.* (November 29, 1989).

[29]*Sovietsky Sport.* (March 14, 30, 1991), (April 16, 1991); Rosellini, L., John Marks. "The Sports Factories," *U.S. News and World Report.* (February 17, 1992), p. 58.

[30]*Physical Culture and Sport.* VI, (1990), p. 30.

[31]*U.S.. News and World Report.* (February 17, 1992), p. 53.

[32]*U.S. News and World Report.* (February 17, 1992), p. 51.

[33]Janofsky, M. (April 15, 1990).

[34]*Montreal Gazette.* (December 24, 1989).

[35]Zilberman, Victor. "German Unification and Its Effect on Sport," *ICHPER.* XXVIII: 2, (Winter, 1992), p. 12.

[36]*Sovietsky Sport.* (August 19, 1990).

[37]*Sovietsky Sport.* (August 19, 1990).

[38]*Montreal Gazette.* (February 18, 1992).

[39]*Sovietsky Sport.* (September 12, 1990); *Montreal Gazette.* (February 17, 1991).

[40]*Sovietsky Sport.* (July 24, 1990).

[41]*CNN Report.* (February 16, 1992); *Montreal Gazette.* (January 4, 1992).

[42]*Sovietsky Sport.* (August 14, 1991).

[43]Zilberman, V. (1992), p. 14.

[44]*Sovietsky Sport.* (September 19, 1990); (July 13, 1991).

[45]*Sovietsky Sport.* (August 3, 1991); *Montreal Gazette.* (December 23, 1991).

[46]Naul, R. (1992), p. 20.

[47]*Sovietsky Sport.* (September 12, 1990).

[48]*Sport Abroad.* (September 17, 1990), p. 16.

[49]*Sovietsky Sport.* (July 18, 1991); *Montreal Gazette,* (February 17, 1991).

[50]*Sovietsky Sport.* (September 16, 1990).

[51]Janofsky, M. (February 15, 1990).

[52]*Montreal Gazette.* (May 28, 1992).

[53]*Sovietsky Sport.* (May 25, 1991).

[54]Rosellini, L. (1992); *Montreal Gazette.* (February 18, 1992).

Chapter 18

German Unification: Decline or Regeneration in Physical Education and Sport Sciences?

Roland Naul

Since October 3, 1990, the day of German unification, the GDR no longer exists. The former elite sport system declined immediately and was dismantled within a few months after unification.[1] However, political changes and a discussion to reform physical education in GDR schools soon began after the Berlin Wall came down in November of 1989. This was the beginning of democratization in the GDR and led to a re-evaluation of the whole sport system. The re-evaluation focused on physical education in schools. Therefore two time periods must be distinguished when discussing the changes of physical education in the former GDR:

1. The period between November 1989 and October 1990, when the German Democratic Republic still existed, and internal reforms were demanded, leading to a new P.E. curriculum.

2. The period between German unification in October 1990 and today, after five new states of the Federal Republic of Germany were founded and the East German system of physical education dissolved gradually.

Since October 1990, the dismantling process of the GDR sport system has progressed to varying degrees. Most of the changes have been in competitive sports. The school system and physical education instruction are currently following more West German standards, including their trends of teaching. A similar trend has been seen in the training of physical education and sports science teachers at the university level.

Changes in Physical Education at School

After November 9, 1989, when the Berlin Wall came down, broad discussion about reforms in physical education began. This discussion criticized old sport instruction in the GDR and demanded democratic renewal. The stratified discussion in the former East German physical education journals can be summarized by the seven following points:[2]

1. All paramilitary training as preparation for military service should be omitted.

2. All students must be encouraged, not just elite athletes. In addition to the performance principle, other educational goals need to be realized.

3. No authoritative educational content guidelines for teachers and students.

4. Expansion of physical education toward modern sport education overcomes the under evaluation of health and leisure time education.

5. Reformation and expansion of content areas, with the goal of introducing new types of sport and new teaching methods.

6. Three hours of sport per week, for all grades and six hours of sport per week, in the specialization courses of the last three grades in the grammar schools.

7. New curriculum and guidelines with new goals and contents, which yield more possibilities for teachers and students to cooperate and decide in sport instruction.

These suggestions and recommendations are the result of a one-year democratic reform discussion under the governments of Krenz/Modrow and de Maziere.

From October 1990 to the present, since the reunification of East and West Germany, there has been another development in physical education in the former GDR. The GDR was reorganized into five federal states: Mecklenburg-Vorpommern at the Baltic Sea, Brandenberg with the capital Potsdam surrounding the city of Berlin, Saxony-Anhalt, Saxony where the former Leipzig University of Physical Culture was located, and Thuringia with its well-known University of Jena. Each new state established its own school system, more or less modeling the West German school system. Each state also established working groups for preparing new curriculum in physical education to support the general developmental process. There are now partnerships between some West German states and the new states. For example, Lower Saxony is a partner of Saxony-Anhalt, and the author's home state, North-Rhine Westfalia, is a strong supporter of Brandenburg. Bavaria is in close connection with Saxony. Therefore, some trends toward establishing new curricula in the new states do exist. The state of Saxony-Anhalt already published its new physical education curricula in the spring of 1991,[3] duplicating the curriculum regulations of its partner, Lower Saxony.

These current developments are now examined carefully and critically. School and curriculum politics in the new states are largely controlled by West German administrators. For example, three governors of the five new states are former West German politicians. Their ideas may be valid but should only be used as guide for the new states to follow as they develop their own physical education curriculum. Unfortunately, some West German sport pedagogues support this trend without critical evaluation of the teaching styles coming in from the West. This then hampers our East German colleagues from continuing their own efforts to find democratic renewal in the curriculum commissions of physical education. The insensitive behavior of West German administrators and scientists has led to the new nickname "Besserwessi" (Besser = better, Wessi = West German), which intends to express that the West German knows everything better than the East German.[4] For the East German sport pedagogist this has created the impression that the old sport instruction in the former GDR was bad because it had high significance in socialist society. When East German colleagues observe sport instruction at West German schools, however, there is increasing doubt about whether the West is the only standard for renewing physical education.[5] Many physical education teachers and scholars from East Germany assume that order, discipline and a certain performance orientation in sport instruction are not specific elements related only to the socialist ideology.[6]

Due to the fact that these principles for physical education have been rejected by the West Germans, East Germany is now having a difficult time promoting any of the positive elements of its past sport instruction into today's H.P.E. curriculum.

From various visits in the last 18 months to physical education departments in Rostock, Potsdam, Halle and Leipzig, including conversations with students, physical education teachers and colleagues, this author presents the following picture regarding current physical education practiced in the schools:[7]

1. Many school directors have been dismissed and new directors view physical education more as a general relic of competitive sport in the GDR. In connection with the renewal of a humanistic general education in new school forms, physical education is now assessed as being less important and now only has minor significance in school education, compared to the former system.

2. Many physical education teachers and teachers of other subjects, have been dismissed on the basis of economic considerations. Due to the low number of generally available physical education teachers, more and more teachers from other subjects are having to teach physical education without qualified training.

3. Discipline, order, and the performance aspect have largely disappeared from sport instruction. Due to their unstable job situation and the changed status of physical education, the teachers have a tendency to let the students do whatever they want, rather than intervening and risking the accusation of being an authoritative ex-socialist; and

4. Boys tend to show more aggressive behavior during the lesson and girls are more likely to participate passively. New types of sport such as indoor hockey are introduced, but attempts to copy open instructional methods often turn into fights and brawls among the students.

Changes in Physical Education Teacher Training

The most important changes in physical education teacher-training, and in the structure of sport science institutes can be summarized in four points:

1. There are indications of a content renewal and expansion in the scientific training, especially in the subdisciplines of sport history, sport sociology, and sport pedagogy. Former courses in sport politics, like Marxism-Leninism and theory of physical culture have been eliminated. In the practical training, new types of sport, like tennis, and badminton are offered to expand the fixation on the six old basic sports of school like gymnastics, track and field, and so on. Unfortunately, the one-year internship for sport instruction, which many colleagues at East German institutes would have preferred to continue, has been discontinued due to lack of capacities and financial resources.

2. With the dissolving of the Academy of Pedagogic Sciences, the research center for physical education has been eliminated as the main coordination center for research on school sport in the former GDR. Various projects on sport instruction in grades five to ten in Greifswald and Zwickau, curriculum realization in Magdeburg and Halle, extracurricular sport in Rostock, and physical education in grades 11 and 12 in Potsdam have been discontinued due to the lack of funding and the unstable personnel situation at sport institutes.

3. The disastrous budget situation for research and scientific politics in the new states and the simultaneous criticism of the former GDR's high performance sport system leave no hope for financial support for sport scientific research on recreational and school sport in the near future. Unfortunately there is no research center for physical education in a West German state which could serve as an equivalent institution; and

4. So far very few sport scientists from the former GDR have lost their professional position based on political reasons. In the next few months, a drastic reduction of personnel will be enforced and more than 60% of the colleagues will lose their

jobs. The sections for sport science will lose their present academic status as a section within the universities and at some universities they will be integrated with other subjects, such as pedagogy and psychology, into one faculty. This follows the West German example. The structural fixation on teacher training and the administrative label as a subject of the humanities, will probably result in changed standards for teaching and research in the sport sciences. This action will probably lead to a rollback of the academic reputation of sport science and a lower ranking within the subjects of universities in the former GDR.

Facing the decline, an East German colleague expressed this to the author, "We have the impression that our sport sciences will soon be at an academic level similar to the one we were at during the 1960s."

Conclusions

What is the consequence of the documented and discussed development in the former GDR? Will it be decline or regeneration for physical education in schools, teaching physical education and research in the sport sciences at the universities? The answer is unclear. Unfortunately, many of the developmental trends identified clearly point toward the decline of a sport system and its infrastructure in schools and universities, especially in research. Some trends indicate a democratic renewal of contents in the communication between people involved in school sport and in training physical education teachers. However, Germans are obviously in a dilemma at present, a dilemma in several respects:

- The aimed for democratic renewal of school sport cannot lead to a socialist defamation of all former goals and objectives of sport instruction.

- The desired opening of contents and individualizing of physical education teacher-training cannot result in a collective blood-letting of sport scientific research.

This author believes that West Germans need to show more sensitivity toward their East German colleagues and offer them better ideas and concepts than the ones written down in the current structural plans, curricula and regulations for school sport and sport sciences in the new states. If we cannot offer new ideas for solutions together, and instead continue working with recommendations and criteria that were developed many years ago in the West, under totally different social conditions, there is a good chance East Germany will suffer more damage than benefit. Therefore changes in physical education must be summarized as follows:

- The West German curricula for physical education and new methods of open sport instruction are not a sufficient basis for a content and methodical renewal of physical education in the former GDR.

- The specifics of physical education in the former GDR require careful evaluation and testing for a new democratic beginning. By no means were all elements of former sport instruction only connected to a socialist educational ideal.

- A renewal of school sport in East Germany should improve the significance of school sport within the framework of a new general education in Germany.

There are definitely several features of physical education, physical education teacher training, and research on physical education that do not represent a product of socialism and are worth retaining. However, there is a very small number of people in West Germany who are willing to make differentiated efforts to save what some overzealous colleagues wish to reduce radically or even liquidate as Besserwessis. These colleagues will act as inquisitors of socialism and missionaries of unproven West German standards. They will suggest open strategies in physical education and sport science. Those few colleagues who want to prevent this development need intercultural support from other countries, from colleagues who follow these developments in Germany dispassionately and objectively and assess and evaluate the situation from a comparative and cross-cultural standpoint.

Notes

[1]Naul, Roland. "Elite sport in Germany: The 1990s," *Journal of the International Council for Health, Physical Education and Recreation.* 28 (1992), pp. 17-22.

[2]Auerbach, K., and L. Rausch. "Uberlegungen und Vorstellungen zu einem kuenftigen Sportunterricht in den fuenf neuen Bundeslaendern", *Sportunterricht.* 40 (1991), pp. 20-23; Hummel, A., and W. Knappe. "Thesen zum Schulsport - ein fachspezifischer Beitrag zur grundlegenden Erneuerung des Bildungswesens," *Theorie und Praxis der Koepkultur.* 39 (1991), pp. 131-139; Doering, W. and G. Keil. "Erneuerung des Schulsports. Diskussionsangebot der Arbeitsgruppe Schulsport," *Koerpererziehung.* 40 (1990), pp. 449-452.

[3]Ministerium fuer Bildung, Wissenschaft und Kultur des Landes Sachsen-Anhalt (Ed.). *Vorlaeufige Rahmenrichtlilien: Sekundarstufe, Foerderstufe und Bildungsgang Realschule, Sport.* Magdeburg: Garloff, 1991.

[4]Sieben, B., and W. Vollmar. "Lehrerfortbildung in Brandenburg - ein Praxisbericht," *Lehrhilfen fur den Sportunterricht.* 41 (1992), pp. 53-57.

[5]Porschuetz, W. "Selbstaendigkeit, Leistungsstreben, Ordnung. Diskussion der not wendigen Komponenten im motorischen Lern und Uebungsprozess," *Sportunterricht.* 40 (1991), pp. 77-381.

[6]Schmidt, W.D. "Neue Aufgaben im Sport und fuer den Sportlehrer", *Koerpererziehung.* 41 (1991), pp. 49-53.

[7]Naul, Roland. "German Unification: Curriculum Development and Physical Education at School in East Germany," *The British Journal of Physical Education.* 23: 4 (1992), pp. 14-19.

Chapter 19

Elite Sport in a United Germany: A Study of the German Sports Union November 9, 1989-October 3, 1990

Michael J. Vitelli and Darwin M. Semotiuk

The last three years have seen tremendous change and upheaval in the realm of international sport Several traditional sports powers have undergone radical change or disappeared entirely, while new participants have emerged to fill the void. Perhaps the most significant of these recent changes have been the demise of the once dominant German Democratic Republic from the world sports scene, and the emergence of a united Germany in its place. The purpose of this chapter is to examine the changes that took place in East German sport following the collapse of the Berlin Wall, the impact of these developments on German efforts to merge the sports systems of the two countries, the process of amalgamation, and the nature of the elite sports system put in place in a united Germany. Results show that the East German sports system was largely dismantled in the post-Wall period and that few of its elements were incorporated into the unified German sports structure. Instead, the West Germans simply imposed the existing sports structure, in the Federal Republic, on the athletes and territory of the former GDR. The chapter concludes that these developments were all but inevitable given the desperate financial state of East German sport in the post-Wall period, the lack of public support and enthusiasm for elite sport in the East, and the determination of the West German government and sports establishment to construct a unified sports system based primarily on West German programs, institutions and practices.

If the East German sports machine that emerged in the late 1960s was merged with its West German counterpart, this formidable combination would have swept every Olympics between 1972-1988 except for the boycotted Games of

Moscow and Los Angeles, and the Winter Games at Innsbruck. At the Summer Games in Seoul, for example, athletes from the German Democratic Republic (GDR) won a total of 102 medals, while those from the Federal Republic of Germany (FRG) won 40, for a combined medal total of 142, ten more than the top-placing Soviets.[1] While the above would seem little more than an illustration of the excellence achieved by the elite sports systems of East and West Germany, the events of 1989-1990 brought a whole new significance to this equation. With the decline of Communist rule in the GDR, in the Fall of 1989, and the subsequent reunification of the two German states one year later, the existence of a unified German sports power is now a reality. The emergence of a united Germany is significant in that its athletes have the potential to dominate international sport for the remainder of the decade and into the next century. In addition, German reunification offered the opportunity to construct a new sports system incorporating the best elements of the East and West German approaches to elite sport. Before any of this could occur, however, German sports officials first had to find a way of reconciling two very different and diametrically opposed approaches to elite sport.

This chapter examines the impact of German reunification on the elite sports systems of the German Democratic Republic and the Federal Republic of Germany, focusing on the process through which the two German states combined their respective elite sports systems, the ultimate outcome of this amalgamation, and the consequences and ramifications associated with this development. In addition, an effort is made to explain and interpret the changes that took place in East German sport during the 11-month period beginning with the opening of the Berlin Wall (November 9, 1989) and ending with the emergence of a united Germany (October 3,1990), and to assess how these developments impacted on the effort to combine the two sports systems. The chapter concludes with an overview and analysis of the elite sports system that was ultimately put in place in a united Germany, its specific characteristics, and the consequences of such an outcome for the new German state and for international sport as a whole.

The topic is relevant for a number of reasons. Because an amalgamation of the sports systems of a former East bloc country and a Western nation had never before been undertaken, it is important to understand how the Germans achieved this complex and difficult task, especially given the nature of the relationship that had existed between the two countries. In addition, it would be useful to examine the specific characteristics of the new unified German sports structure, given its potential for achieving success at the international level.

An historical method was utilized in the gathering and analysis of information for this study. This methodology was used to generate both a chronology of events during the period under study, as well as to interpret the significance of those events in the context of wider social, political and economic developments. The primary limitation of this approach was that the researchers were forced to rely on secondary sources of information since they did not travel to the former German Democratic Republic or the Federal Republic of Germany.

East German Sport: A System Under Siege

The period following the opening of the Berlin Wall on November 9 1989, was a time of extraordinary change and upheaval for East German sport. Practices and institutions that had existed for decades disappeared overnight; officials who had played a prominent role in the organization and operation of East German elite sport were dismissed; the extensive state support once provided sport was drastically reduced; coaching and administrative positions were eliminated; sporting priorities and philosophies were challenged; and, a system used to operating in a closed and secretive manner was thrown wide-open to public scrutiny. Long heralded, by the ruling Sozialistische Einheitspartei Deutschlands (SED), as a good example of the superiority of the GDR over the Federal Republic and the other nations of the West, the East German sports system became a prime target for the incredible public rage and frustration expressed following the collapse of the Wall. Resentful of the many privileges enjoyed by top-level athletes and the excesses of sports officials, the East German public demanded sweeping reforms to the country's sports establishment, reforms that ultimately led to the systematic dismantling of the East German sports machine.

Within days of the collapse of the Wall, news reports reached the West of the formation of a violent public backlash in the GDR directed towards current and former elite-level athletes.[2] While many of these reports of violence, abuse, and vandalism ultimately proved to be exaggerated or false, the tremendous public resentment towards the sports community in the GDR was very much real. As Janofsky[3] described it at the time, "in the midst of political change... East German citizens began protesting against the Communist government, its priorities and corruption... the sports system became an easy target." The sports system in the GDR was seen to embody all of the misdirected priorities, excess, privilege, and corruption associated with four decades of Communist rule. Public indignation towards the sports establishment only grew in the post-Wall period, fueled by the new East German 'glasnost' and revelations concerning the privileges of athletes and the corruption of sports officials. For example, it was revealed publicly that East German gold medal winners, in Seoul in 1988, were each awarded bonuses of 35,000 DM by the SED, while silver medal winners received 20,000 DM.[4] In November of 1989, it was disclosed that 300,000 DM had been found stuffed into the desk of Franz Rydz, Vice-President of Finances for the DTSB.[5] Episodes such as these led to a growing public debate over the future of East German elite sport. For the first time in the GDR's forty-year history, people openly questioned why it was necessary to put such a focus on elite sport and to pour such huge resources into its programs. Faced with enormous social and economic problems, and the complex task of making the transition to a more democratic society, many East Germans concluded that the all-consuming pursuit of gold medals and world championship titles could no longer be justified. As Hughes put it, "sport gold medals, the symbols glorified and financed by government to prove its system superior to capitalism in general and West Germany in particular, [had] become irrelevant."[6]

In the months following the collapse of the Wall, pressure from the public and the transitional government of Hans Modrow forced the new leader of the DTSB, Klaus Eichler, to introduce sweeping reforms to East German sport. These included changes to the basic structure of the East German sports system, the adoption of a new fiscal attitude, and a shift in emphasis away from elite sport to sport for the masses. Structural changes became necessary not only because of the introduction of democratic reforms in the GDR, but also due to the drastic reduction in state financing provided to the sports establishment. At an historic two-day, closed-door session held in Kienbaum on November 29-30 1989, the leadership of the DTSB agreed on the need to create a more efficient and streamlined sports bureaucracy. It was decided that the DTSB administration would have to be reduced from over 12,000 people to about 1,500.[7] Moreover, Eichler sought to create a more independent DTSB by ending its long-standing ties to the SED. He announced that his agency "would unshackle itself from the Communist Party... and demand direct access to hard currency earnings."[8] Finally, steps were taken to create a more decentralized sports structure in the GDR. As one East German professor put it at the time, "we have abolished Stalinist, centralist administration... and will create autocracy among individual [associations] and local organizations."[9] This represented the most significant change of the post-Wall period, as the DTSB had relinquished its 35-year-old role as the preeminent organizer of sport in the GDR. These structural changes were accompanied by growing fiscal responsibility on the part of sports leaders. As one official described it, "success at the top will not be ignored, though this time it will be with an eye on the dollars."[10] To generate new sources of income and replace lost government funding, the GDR's sports clubs and associations were encouraged to send athletes abroad to compete for hard currency earnings and to make use of Western-style sponsorship. The DTSB even created a private agency, called SportAgentur, to negotiate sponsorship deals with the West.[11] In spite of these changes, the leaders of the East German sports establishment ultimately found themselves caught up in the midst of a precarious balancing act, trying to keep up with the pace of political reforms in the country on the one hand, while trying to preserve the effectiveness of East Germany's elite sports system on the other.

For East Germany's elite-level and developing athletes, the post-Wall period was a time of great confusion and uncertainty. Athletes at every level of the East German sports system experienced significant disruptions in their training and development programs. Coaches reported that they were "finding it difficult to motivate their athletes, many of whom [were] struggling to come to terms with the dramatic political changes."[12] As sports facilities, once reserved for the exclusive use of elite athletes, were opened to the general public many athletes reported drastic cuts in the quantity and quality of training time. As Olympic swim champion Heike Friedrich described it, "everything is different... Now the pool is closed most of the time, and for many of us, we have no chance to train on a daily basis. We can't get into the swim hall when we need to."[13]

The impact on developing athletes was no less severe. Whereas, in the past, parents of children attending one of the GDR's 25 Kinder und Jugendsportschulen (KJS) had to pay only 35 DM per month for the privilege, there was discussion of increasing the fees to 140-240 DM per month.[14] The prospect of increased costs and the new freedom in East German society led many parents to pull their children from the special sports schools. As East German Athletics head Heinz Kadow put it, "at the moment, children are staying home... It's difficult to calculate, but I'm sure there are thousands of children who have been selected who are now going to be lost."[15]

With the reduction in funding and change in priorities, nearly every facet of the once extensive support system for elite-level athletes in the GDR was dismantled or severely cut back in the post-Wall period. Critical preventative and rehabilitative medical services were lost as the Sports Medicine Service (SMD) was phased out and its doctors reassigned to work with the general population. The world famous Deutsche Hochschule für Korperkultur (DHfK) in Leipzig found its staff reduced, its research curtailed, and its curriculum restructured to focus on leisure sport and physical education programs. Finally, thousands of coaching and sport teacher positions were eliminated, forcing many highly qualified and experienced East German coaches to relocate to sports clubs and organizations in the West or to abandon the profession altogether. These developments, coupled with the loss of state subsidies and special privileges, led to a mass exodus of athletes from the GDR to the West in the Winter of 1989-1990. Over 200 athletes made the move to West Germany alone, seeking lucrative professional contracts, advertising deals, and a more stable training environment.[16] West Germany's sports clubs and associations were more than ready to strip the East German sports system clean of its most promising athletic talent, a development that caused tremendous bitterness and resentment in the East. For those athletes unwilling or unable to move to the West, the post-Wall period brought continued uncertainty and ever-increasing disruptions in training.

By March of 1990, it was clear that the East German sports system was on the verge of collapse. Efforts to create a more efficient, self-sustaining sports system, to develop new sources of revenue, to stem the flow of athletes westward, and to bring order and stability back to East German sport had all largely failed. Episodes such as the resignation en masse of the entire central administration of the DTSB, on December 12, 1989, left the impression that no one was providing direction to the country's sports bodies. As Holchak described the situation, "it's sort of a mirror image of the government... you don't really know who's in control of the government at this point, and you certainly don't know who's in control of the DTSB."[17] The election of Martin Kilian as leader of the DTSB, in March of 1990, and the formation of a new coalition government under the leadership of Lothar de Maiziere, did little to improve the situation. For example, sports leaders insisted that they would require 120 million DM to cover operating costs for the remainder of 1990 plus a further 33.6 million DM for social benefits paid to former workers, but the East German Ministry of Youth and Sport provided only 99.69 million DM.[18] Ultimately, by the Spring of 1990, most sports officials in the GDR had resigned themselves to the fact that it would not be possible to preserve their sports system given the tremendous political and economic changes in their country. As a result, sports leaders began to look to the West, concluding that the only realistic hope for the long-term survival of the programs and institutions of the East German sports system lay in a union with the sports bodies and organizations in the Federal Republic.

The Process of Amalgamation

In essence, the process of bringing about an amalgamation of the elite sports systems of East and West Germany involved not one union, but dozens of different ones. Negotiations took place not only between national level sports bodies like the DSB, DTSB, and the two National Olympic Committees (NOCs), but also between each of the individual sports associations in the two countries. This two-tiered approach to the negotiating process was seen as the most efficient way of bringing about the union of such a vast array of sports bodies, organizations, and institutions.

Informal negotiations between the various sports associations in East and West Germany began soon after the collapse of the Wall. The aim of these discussions was to establish a working relationship for future in-depth negotiations, to build cooperation, and to begin the long process of integrating the athletes and programs of the respective associations. For example, representatives of the West German Athletics Association (DLV) met with their counterparts in the DVfL for the first time in the post-Wall period on December 18, 1989. These initial talks led to more intense negotiations on January 20-21, 1990, in Darmstadt, and to the signing of a formal agreement entitled "Agreement Between the DLV and the DVfL of the GDR."[19] This agreement focused on issues not only in the area of elite sport, but also in youth and mass sport. Under its terms, a series of congresses and seminars were arranged to allow for the exchange of technical knowledge, expertise, and coaching techniques. In addition, a number of joint training camps and competitions for both senior and junior-level athletes were organized, and long-term planning was begun concerning the participation of German athletes in the 1992 Summer Olympics. Finally, questions of structure and leadership were addressed, and a timetable was established for the final unification of the two associations. Most of the other 25 groups of Olympic sports associations held similar discussions and reached similar agreements during the Spring and Summer of 1990. In the end, virtually all of the sports associations completed their final mergers in the three-month period between October 3, 1990, and January 1, 1991.[20]

The larger issues and more complex questions associated with the sports union were negotiated by the leaders of the DSB, DTSB, the two NOCs, and selected government officials. Discussions held in May of 1990, in East Berlin, led to the creation of a special interdisciplinary negotiating commission which was charged with negotiating the specific points of the German sports union. The commission was composed of four technical working committees, each of which focused on one of the following areas: "structures, administration, finances," "mass sports," "competitive sports," and "education, further training, sciences, health."[21] The DTSB/ DSB Special Commission delivered its findings in a report entitled "Competitive Sports," which was adopted by DTSB President Martin Kilian and DSB President Hans Hansen on June 28, 1990, in Offenbach/Main.[22] The agreement outlined principles of integration in such areas as honorary leadership, federal structures, subsidiarity, and neutrality in terms of party politics and ideology.[23] It also provided for a gradual transition to a unified sports structure following reunification. As Rydzy-Gotz described it at the time, "in competitive sports a system of gradual harmonization of the differ-ing sports promotion schemes will be implemented."[24] According to the agree-ment, regional sport organizations were established following the creation of new federal states in the East. These sports bodies then affiliated themselves with the DSB. The DTSB was allowed to continue to function until the sports union was completed, then was phased out according to its own statutes and articles. Finally, the sports associations of the East and West were instructed to proceed with their mergers according to their own timetables and agreements. The leaders of the two German National Olympic Committees created a similar negotiating commission, which resulted in an agreement outlining the terms for the formation of a unified German National Olympic Committee. This agree-ment was approved and adopted at a special Olympic Congress held on November 17, 1990, in Berlin.

Elite Sport in a United Germany

The German Democratic Republic ceased to exist at the stroke of midnight on October 3, 1990, absorbed into the Federal Republic of Germany under Article 23 of that country's Basic Law or constitution. Under the terms of the treaty governing German reunification, the territory of the GDR was divided into five new federal states, or Lander, based on boundaries that existed in 1952. The new Lander were accorded the same rights and recognition given the 11 already existing Lander in western Germany. The most significant aspect concerning the nature of the new German state, and one which had a tremendous impact on the final outcome of the sports union, concerns the dominant position enjoyed by West German structures, ideals, and institutions in the new Germany. As Schweigler described it at the time, "the West Germans... seem to [be]... insist-ing... that the East Germans submit as much as possible, at as little cost as possi-ble, to West German norms and values."[25] The West Germans exhibited little interest in experimenting with the formula that had proven so successful and were very determined that the model of the Federal Republic would serve as the blueprint for a united Germany. This was the central philosophy that guided the creation of the unified state. Ultimately, no segment of the East German popula-tion came to regret this development more than the athletes, coaches, and sports leaders of the East German sports system.

The organization of sport in a united Germany is very decentralized in nature. Authority for planning and coordinating sports activities, including those in the realm of elite sport, is divided among three different groups of sports bodies. At the national level are the Bundesausschusses für Leistungssport (BAL) or Federal Committee for Competitive Sports, Deutscher Sportbund (DSB), and the German National Olympic Committee. At the lower levels of the sports structure are the 16 regional sport organizations (landessportbunde) and the 54 individual sports associations (spitzenverbande). As Figure 1 illustrates, the DSB is situated at the center of the unified sports structure, where it serves as the central umbrella organization in German sport. Virtually all of the sports organizations and institutions in a united Germany are affiliated with and consult with this agency. The BAL, one of eight special committees of the DSB, is a specialized sports body that focuses on organizing and implementing programs solely in the area of elite sport. It is also responsible for distributing funds provided by the Federal Government to the country's sports bodies and organizations. The Bundesministerium des Innern (BMI) or Federal Ministry of the Interior serves as the link between the German sports establishment and the Federal Government in Bonn, while the regional sport organizations represent local sports bodies in dealings with the Governments of the Lander.

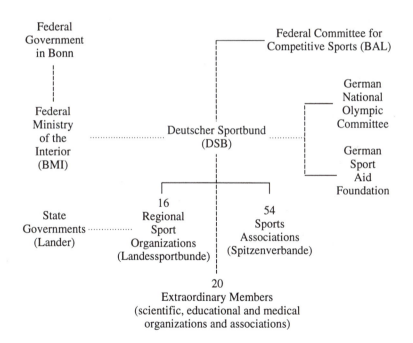

Figure 1—The Organization of Sport in a United Germany (1992); Adapted from Bundesministerium des Innern, 1990, *Siebter Sportbericht der Bundesregierung* [Seventh sport report of the Federal Government], pp. 174-175.

While the effective operation of the unified sports system depends on the inter-action of all these various sports bodies and levels of government, it must be remembered that no single agency has the authority to force another to follow its policies or programs. Instead, the onus is placed on voluntary cooperation between organizations for the development and implementation of programs in elite sport. It is significant to note that the sports officials of the former GDR have been almost completely shut out from holding positions of authority in the new German sports structure. The leadership of all the key bodies, like the BAL, DSB, the German NOC, and the vast majority of the senior administrative positions in the individual sports associations, are all held by former West German officials.

The West German system of organizing athletes into performance groups has been transferred to a united Germany. The four categories are designated the A, B, C, and S-groups. The A group is the top performance category and is reserved for athletes who have attained world-class performances at the interna-tional level. The most exceptional members of this group receive about 1,200-1,300 DM per month in government financial aid, with the remaining athletes receiving 800-900 DM per month.[26] The B group consists of athletes who have not quite achieved world-class performances, while the C group is composed of junior athletes who are members of national teams in their respective age groups. Athletes in the B group receive 500-600 DM per month, while those in the C group receive 250-300 DM per month.[27] The S group is reserved for ath-letes who are temporarily unable to qualify for one of the other performance groups due to injury or some other difficulty. Overall, it is estimated that about 2,400 athletes from the former GDR have been placed in the German perfor-mance groups in addition to the 3,300 athletes already covered in western Germany.[28]

Additional assistance for athletes is provided by the German Sport Aid Foundation. This private organization raises funds through corporate sponsor-ship, public donations, and promotional campaigns. The performance level of the athlete determines the level of monthly funding received. Beginning on January 1, 1991, approximately 2,000 athletes from the East began to receive assistance from Sport Aid.[29] For the period extending from 1991-1992, the Bonn Government has provided Sport Aid with 18.6 million DM in emergency fund-ing to help it meet increased costs associated with providing assistance to east-ern athletes.[30]

Initial planning called for the preservation of the system of special sports schools (KJS) that was in place in the GDR and the creation of similar schools in western Germany. It was envisioned that the KJS could continue to play a key role in the development of athletes, if certain modifications were made. These included raising the minimum age for entrance, dropping political prerequisites for admission, and devoting more time to academic lessons.[31] In January of 1991, however, sports leaders were forced to abandon this plan when members of the Bundestag or Federal Parliament made it clear that they would not provide funding for the preservation or expansion of the KJS.

Funding was provided for the creation of new training centers for elite athletes. Prior to reunification, a total of 15 federal and 27 Olympic training centers were in place in the Federal Republic.[32] With the completion of the sports union, it was determined that six new Olympic training centers would be built in Berlin, Cottbus, Halle, Leipzig, Potsdam, and Rostock to complement the system of training centers in the West.[33]

The number of full-time professional coaches employed in a united Germany will not be significantly greater than the number employed in the Federal Republic prior to reunification. In 1989, West Germany had in place 115 full-time, national level coaches in 50 sports, 220 honorary or volunteer coaches in the Lander, and 200 honorary coaches at work in the training centers.[34] After reunification, only 120 full-time professional coaches from the former GDR were hired to work in the unified sports system.[35] For most East German coaches, the sports union brought an end to their coaching careers. For example, out of a total of 350 East German gymnastics coaches, only seven were offered positions in the new unified sports association.[36] Virtually all of the top coaching positions in the unified sports structure ultimately went to West German coaches, even if there was a more experienced and successful candidate available from the former GDR.

The development and preparation of coaches in a united Germany will be based on the West German model. Volunteer coaches will be trained through a three-tiered certification program while the preparation of full-time professional coaches will be supervised by the Trainerakademie based in Cologne. The training program offered through the DHfK in Leipzig has been abolished. Following directives issued by the State Government of Saxony, the DHfK was refounded as a faculty of physical education associated with Leipzig University on January 1, 1991.

The extensive sports medicine support system (SMD) that was in place in East Germany was dismantled with the completion of the sports union. There had been pressure by the German and International Federation of Sports Doctors to preserve the SMD but with reduced staff levels and greater services for recreational athletes. Due to lack of finances, however, and the fact that there was no mechanism in place in western Germany for the licensing of specialist sports doctors, this plan had to be abandoned. Instead, elite-level athletes will receive medical care from general practitioners and physiotherapists employed by the individual sports associations.

Every elite-level athlete in the united Germany will be subject to random doping checks under the program known as Doping Controls Between Events. Each month, 80 athletes will be selected at random by a computer for testing of performance-enhancing drugs.[37] Increased efforts in doping controls were spurred on by a series of damaging revelations made in March and November of 1990. These reports confirmed that top sport leaders had established an extensive and systematic doping program in the GDR and that vast numbers of athletes, including many Olympic champions, had benefited from the program.[38]

In the last year before reunification, the West German Federal Government spent 269.13 million DM on sports activities of all types.[39] Of this amount, approximately 150 million DM was budgeted for elite sport.[40] Following the completion of the sports union, the Bonn Federal Government announced that it was providing an additional 71.6 million DM for 1991 on top of its regular funding for elite sport to help cover the cost of building new training centers, hiring increased numbers of coaches, and preparing the unified German teams for the 1992 Olympic Games.[41] The Government made it clear to the country's sports leaders, however, that this was a one-time, lump sum payment and that government funding levels for elite sport development would revert to pre-reunification levels following the Barcelona Olympics in 1992.

Conclusions

In the final analysis, the union of the East and West German elite sports systems involved not so much an amalgamation, but an absorption of the East by the West and the imposition of the sports structure of the Federal Republic on the athletes and territory of the former GDR. The much discussed combination of the best elements of each country's approach to elite sport into a unified sports system never took place. Instead, most of the East German sports system was dismantled, and the few surviving elements were absorbed into the existing West German sports structure. As a result, the sports system in a united Germany is a virtual mirror image of the system that was in place in the Federal Republic prior to reunification.

Three conclusions have been drawn concerning the final outcome of the German sports union. First, it was not realistic to expect that much of the sports system in the GDR could have been preserved after the collapse of the Wall and transferred to a united Germany. The financial resources and public will simply did not exist in the East to support even a scaled-down version of the East German sports system. Furthermore, those in the West had made it clear that a united Germany would be built on West German ideals, structures, and institutions, and that there would be little room for East German practices and institutions.

The unified German sports structure may find that it is plagued by many of the same inefficiencies, problems, and shortcomings that affected West German sport prior to reunification. Because the German sports system relies almost exclusively on West German practices, programs, structures, and personnel, it seems likely that many of the problems that existed in the organization and operation of elite sport in the Federal Republic will carry over to the unified German sports system.

Finally, a united Germany will probably not develop into the dominant sports power it was originally forecast to become, and may even experience difficulty in matching the success achieved by the GDR alone prior to the sports union. Over the short term, the influx of athletes from the East, and the temporary increase in government funding provided elite sport, should result in a strong showing by the unified German teams in Albertville and Barcelona in 1992. Germany's success at the international level over the long term, however, may be compromised by its inability to replace the current crop of talented elite-level athletes and by reduced government commitment to elite sport development after 1992.

Notes

[1]Starkman, R . "Can Germans build new dynasty? East, West will have trouble getting together." *The Toronto Star,* June 4, 1990, p. D4.

[2]Hughes, R. "East German sport stars living in fear." *Sunday Times* (London), November 19, 1989, p. A26.

[3]Janofsky, M. "In East Germany, trauma between two eras." *The New York Times,* April 15, 1990, sec. 8, pp. 1, 4.

[4]Fitness and Amateur Sport *German Democratic Republic.* Memorandum issued by the International Relations Directorate, Ottawa, April 1990, p. 1

[5]Janofsky, M. "East German perquisites draw fire." *The New York Times.* December 11, 1989, p. C4

[6]Hughes, p. A26.

[7]Tagliabue, J. "Political pressure dismantles East German sports machine." *The New York Times,* February 12, 1991, p. B10.

[8]"East Germany plans to retune sports machine." *The Calgary Herald,* December 1, 1989, p. D4.

[9]Miller, D. "World sport may lose as map is redrawn." *The Times* (London), March 17, 1990, p. 54.

[10]Coleman, M. "Financial support will extend to all." *Times* (London), November 14, 1989, p. 44.

[11]Janofsky, April 15, 1990, p. 4

[12]Starkman, p. D4

[13]Holchak, V. *The Inside Track: The End of the Miracle Machine.* Radio program broadcast by the Canadian Broadcasting Corporation. Produced by Mel Broitman. 11 minutes. January 12, 1991, transcript, p. 1.

[14]Kassner, F. "Lehrplan ist nicht mehr masgeschneidert " [Training plan is no longer tailor-made]. *Sportecho* (East Berlin), September 4, 1990, p. 3.

[15]Kadow quoted in Woodward, S. "Reunification splits sports community." *USA Today*, August 20, 1990, pp. B 1.

[16]"Lockruf des geldes: West deutsche klubs plundern den amateursport der DDR systematisch aus" [The call of money: West German clubs systematically plunder the amateur sports of the GDR]. *Der Spiegel,* June 4, 1990, p. 183.

[17]Holchak, V. *The Inside Track: Report from the GDR.* Radio program broadcast by the Canadian Broadcasting Corporation. Produced by Nancy Lee. 7 minutes. December 16, 1989, transcript, p. 1.

[18]Schmickler, E.D. "Financial aid criticized: DTSB runs out of patience." *Frankfurter Allemeine Zeitung,* July 28, 1990, p. 2

[19]Deutscher Leichtathletik-Verbands. *Vereinbarung Zwischen dem DLV und dem DVfL, der DDR* [Agreement between the DLV and the DVfL of the GDR]. Press release issued by the DLV on January 26, 1990, West Berlin, pp. 1-6.

[20]Rydzy-Gotz, M. *Fragen zur deutsch/deutschen Einigung der Olympischen Spitzenverbande* [Question of the German/German agreement for the Olympic sports associations]. Report issued on September 20, 1990, by Deutscher Sportbund, Frankfurt, pp. 1-4.

[21]Rydzy-Gotz, M. *The Process of Integration in German Sport.* Report issued on August 10, 1990, by Deutscher Sportbund, Frankfurt, p. 1.

[22]DTSB/DSB Special Commission. *Leistungssport* [Competitive sports]. Agreement signed by the DTSB and DSB in Offenbach/Main, June 25, 1990. Issued by Deutscher Sportbund, Frankfurt, pp. 1-15.

[23]Rydzy-Gotz, August 10, 1990, p. 1.

[24]Rydzy-Gotz, August 10, 1990, p. 2.

[25]Schweigler, G. "German reunification: The social issues." In G.L. Geipel (Ed.), *The Future of Germany.* Indianapolis: Hudson Institute, 1990, p. 8.

[26]Schmickler, E.D. "When the going gets really rough, there's still an S-group: A look at competitive sport in a united Germany." *Frankfurter Allemeine Zeitung,* August 17, 1990, p. 4.

[27]Schmickler, p. 4.

[28]Schmickler, p. 4.

[29]Stiftung Deutsche Sporthilfe. *Stiftung Deutsche Sporthilfe* [German sport aid foundation]. Report issued by the Stiftung Deutsche Sporthilfe, Frankfurt, December 1990, p. 7.

[30]"Medaillen kaufen: Bonner politiker befurchten, das steuergelder von den sportverbanden misbraucht werden" [Buying medals: Bonn politicians worry over the misuse of finances by the sports associations]. *Der Spiegel.* (November 5, 1990), pp. 250-251.

[31]Baker, J.A.W., Baskau, H. and Eden, R. "Reunification of Germany: Pathway to Olympic Domination?" Manuscript submitted for publication, 1991, p. 21.

[32]Bundesministerium des Innern, p. 239.

[33]Baker et al., p. 19-20.

[34]Kruger, A. "Pop the magic dragon (or what will be left of GDR sports?)." *Journal of Comparative Physical Education and Sport,* 12 :2, (1990), p. 5.

[35]Baker et al., p. 20.

[36]"Das gelbe vom ei" [The cat's meow]. *Der Spiegel,* October 1, 1990, pp. 235, 238.

[37]DTSB/DSB Special Commission, p. 10.

[38]Fiedler, T. and Hagele, M. "Doping: Der beweis - Wie die DDR sieger machte" [Doping: The proof - How the GDR creates winners]. *Stern.* November 29, 1990, pp. 202, 203A-G.

[39]Bundesministerium des Innern, p. 299.

[40]Neumann, H. (Sport: The eighth muse (Top performance sport in the Federal Republic). *Scala,* November/December l989, pp. 28-39.

[41]"Medaillen kaufen", p. 250. Also see, Beyme, K. von. "Transition to democracy - or anschluss? The two Germanys and Europe." *Government and Opposition.* 25:2, (1990), pp. 170-190; Coleman, M. "East Germans agree new sports deal." *Times* (London), November 18, 1989, p. 49; "Communist sport machines." *The Economist,* December 22, 1990, pp. 67-68; "Doors opened for East Germans." *The Times* (London), January 19, 1990, p. 39; Fisher, M. "The Berlin Wall has crumbled, a sports power may be next." *The Washington Post,* December 26, 1989, pp. Dl, D6; Gowan, G., J. Bales, B. Thomson, and D. Smith, *A Report on a Visit to the German Democratic Republic and the Federal Republic of Germany to Examine Coaching Structures and Coaching Programs.* Ottawa: Coaching Association of Canada, 1986; Johnson, W.O.,

and A. Verschoth, "Out of the shadows." *Sports Illustrated,* November 27, 1989, pp. 16-21; "Leaders of corrupt East German sports body resign" *Gazette* (Montreal), December 13, 1989, p. F2; Macleod, I. "East Germany's future: What are the prospects for the GDR's showpiece sports, athletics and swimming, as the country's clubs and institutions adjust to the new order?" *Athletics,* July 1990, pp. 12-13; McAdarns, A. J. "From the East German volkskammer election to a new Germany." In G. L. Geipel (Ed.), *The Future of Germany* Indianapolis: Hudson Institut, 1990, pp. 18-36; McElvoy, A. "Wall of privilege comes down." *The Times* (London), November 25, 1989, p. 50; Miller, D. "Unity short-changes East German sportsmen." *Times* (London), February 18, 1991, p. 34; Munnings, F. "Can East German athletes hold their competitive edge?" *Physician and Sportsmedicine,* 18 :4, (1990), pp. 111,114-115; Nationales Olympisches Komitee fur Deutschland. *Bericht* [Report]. Report of the Board of Directors of the German National Olympic Committee to the General Assembly on November 17, 1990, Berlin; Nationales Olympisches Komitee fur Deutschland.. *NOK-Mitliederversammlung in Berlin* [NOC - General meeting in Berlin]. Report issued by the Executive of the German National Olympic Committee on November 20, 1990, Berlin; Nordland, R. "Taking aim on the Games: Is Germany the next Olympic juggernaut?" *Newsweek,* February 26, 1990, p. 29; Schmickler, E. D. "The sports medicine service in the GDR is on the way out." *Frankfurter Allgemeine Zeitung,* August 10, 1990, pp. 8-10; "Sportpolitik: Fest im wurgegriff" [Sport politics: Solid in its stranglehold]. *Der Spiegel,* May 21, 1990, pp. 208-209; "Talentforderung: Groser knall" [Talent promotion: Large cracks]. *Der Spiegel,* January 21, 1991, pp. 159,162-163.

Chapter 20

Sport in Modern Europe: Perestroika in the USSR— Revolution of the East— Integration of the West

Oleg A. Milshtein

Sport in Modern Europe, and a large part of the world, is on the threshold of a radical political, economical, and social renewal. Perestroika in the former Soviet Union, the revolutions in Eastern European countries and the integration of Western Europe has set in motion processes, and caused problems, that were apparently beyond the imaginations of the initiators of these transformations.

All these factors have an impact in the area of sport: the previous high level sport, mass sport, and physical education in the former Soviet Union. The achievements of the European "Socialist" countries" have been replaced by serious social problems connected with the further development of sport and with the implementation of Western European democratic models of sport.

What is the role and the significance of Soviet perestroika in this global village? What are the social changes and social processes in these areas? What will produce new ideas, provoke contemporary routes of sport and physical education development and deepen cooperation between sport scientists in Europe and the rest of the world?

Different scientists give different answers to these questions. For example, the well-known sport-philosopher and sociologist from Poland, Z. Krawczyk, advances the following four criteria:

- economical incapacity,
- conceptual and ideological inadequacy,

• organizational disfunctionality; and
• institutional disfunctionality.

On this basis, he next distinguishes four basic tendencies:

• So far the economic basis of sports has been grounded on
the state ownership of resources and sports facilities (wherein social subjects were partially entrusted.), the central planning, the subsidies and control of various activities. The
income of the sports institutions was minimal and it
occurred only in sensational events. At present, the economic system of sport tends toward self-financing of its activities, socializing or privatizing its resources.

• The new philosophy of sport turns away from socio-political
values, usually associated with institutions of a totalitarian
state. The new philosophy is grounded in categories such as:
society, nation, and man. Thus, the absolute reduction of the
propaganda and political aims of sport in preference to
humanizing and personalizing benefits is executed. In the
place of the "state-run physical culture," universal
Olympism is being introduced together with individualized
health culture and "sports for all."

• The institutional and organizational configuration of sport
will be created from "the bottom up," voluntarily and
autonomously. Hence, its main structures should have a self-
governed and individual character. The state will act as
sponsor, and coordinator of strategic activities. It will keep
its primacy only in the process of physical and health education of youth.

• Either the traditional elite administering sport broke up or
the pace of the "changing of the managing personnel" was
accelerated. The main criteria of choosing new people to the
sport's elite are: connections with other new sports elites,
professionalism, and being a member of the young or middle-aged generation.[1]

G. Foeldesi, a sociologist of sport from Hungary, pays attention to other aspects
of this problem in the sphere of mass sport in Eastern Europe. The Eastern Bloc

countries had very unique conditions to develop "sport for all" compared with Western countries. In Western democracies "sport for all" can be set as a goal but such an aim can hardly be realized. Specifically, in any democratic country it is each citizen's right to decide what to do and what not to do. Sport involvement can be encouraged by providing opportunities, and equality of access can be ensured but sport participation cannot be forced. Conversely, totalitarian states can not only influence but, in many cases, also strictly determine their citizens' social behavior.

Though there were significant differences between Eastern Bloc countries, the historical periods of their existence were totalitarian. Their political power was absolutely centralized. They were based on a one-party system, with planned economy and culture. Moreover, they declared themselves communist, and according to this ideology, respect for privacy was very limited. As a consequence of all this, strange though it may seem, these political structures could have been favorable for the development of their populations' physical activity.[2]

Another internationally recognized sport scholar, American anthropologist and ethno-historian of sport, G. Eisen, following major issues, lists the following topics as examples of the drastic transformation of Eastern European sport:[3]

- The status of the elite athlete: backlash and redemption.
- The decline of the state subsidized sport establishment.
- Privatization of sport.
- New class structure and sport participation.
- Human rights: drugs and anabolic steroids.
- Human rights: the sports for all movement.
- Integration into "world-sport: the new professionals."
- The future of the Olympic Games.

With regard to the situation in the former Soviet Union, I find myself in strong agreement with the position of the Estonian sociologist M. Arvisto with his co-authors:

> Sport was strongly programmed into the model of socialism, and on the level of competitive sport has been put into practice. The model functioned in order to achieve top results — mass sport was largely 'fabricated.' The reported number of sport participants did not reflect the reality, but rather the wishes of top administrators. Sport functioned mostly according to the programmatic-normative model which presupposed

conformity (sports participation). Currently this mechanism has broken down. Coercion and economic stimuli have disappeared. The previous organization of sport has been destroyed, while the new one is not functioning yet, especially at the lower levels (local physical culture group sport club). It is difficult for sport managers and functionaries to overcome a psychological barrier that hinders them in actively pursuing their activities in the context of the new opportunities. They are still waiting for official subsidies, for official orders. But no subsidies or orders can come from above because of typical incompetence in sport of the new leaders. Elite sport is currently very clearly divided in two — professional sport (which attracts the best athletes from the homeland) and amateur sport of much lower quality. The main trouble with sport for all is its commercialization and the lack of support from the state and local authorities. Support is not given to "mass sport" which has compromised itself by militarism and falsifications.[4]

Generalized from the enumerated points of view, opinions of other authors, and on the basis of my own analysis, the social mechanism changing in sport presents itself in the following way. Perestroika in the USSR, which was launched by Mikhail Gorbachev and his companions from the CPSU in April 1985, began as a revolution from the upper structure. The aim of Perestroika was to renovate socialism by means of democracy and openness in internal policy (glasnost), economy, culture, and education. In foreign policy renovation was implemented by the termination of the arms race, de-ideologization of international relations, and recognition of values common to all people.

In the field of physical education and sports, as well as in culture and education in general, innovations were to be implemented by a new policy of financing, freedom of creativeness, and liquidation of the state monopoly. The accomplishments attained during the last six years resulted in:

<u>Changes of internal policy</u>

• imbalance between old and new structures

• fierce ideological and political conflict between liberal, democratic forces and destructive, conservative ones

- significant lag of economic reforms due to political changes

- the polarization of society

- coup d'état

- cessation of the USSR Communist Party monopoly and attenuating of military complex

- transfer of power to democratic forces in central Russia

- freedom and sovereignty of the Baltic Republics

- nationalistic tendencies in Republics and autonomous publics and the independent formation of the Commonwealth

- failure of the socialist idea

- disintegration of the state structures including the system of physical education and sports.

- destructive tendencies in the organization of physical education and sports

- devaluation of values of the socialistic sports

- legalizing of the professional sports

- decrease of donations to sport from trade unions

- privatization and cooperation of small sports organization

- conservatism and potential abilities of the elite sport and Soviet Olympic Movement

- effectiveness and scientific potential of the Soviet school of sports training and system of preparation of personnel

- vitality of the idea "arms race" in sports

• loss of athletes and coaches due to foreign employment

Foreign policy changes

• revolutions in Eastern Europe–countries of the former socialistic bloc

• ruination of the Empire

• reunion of Germany

• democratization processes in countries of Eastern Europe

• similarity of trends and policy in the sports practice of these countries and realization of the new sports policy

• economic instability of the former socialist sports

• economic, political and sociopolitical-cultural integration of Western European countries

• common economic space and new immigration policy

o aggravation of legal aspects of the international sports movement

• consolidation of the Olympic Movement and potential crisis of international sports and Olympic movements

• "race of disarmament" in politics and strengthening of conservative forces

• help from the West—economics and sport

• uniqueness of the European situation of 1990s

• new tasks of the sport science

• necessity of the international project "Europe as an element of culture, way of life and social policy (SPORT-EUROPE)."[5]

At the Second International Conference of Ministers and Leaders of Physical Education and Sport (ICMLPES-II) held in Moscow, during November 1988, several actual initiatives pertaining to the upcoming 100th Jubilee of Modern Olympic Movement were suggested in the report made by the Soviet delegation. It was suggested that the United Nations, together with the International Olympic Committee, should declare 1996 as the "International Year of Sport and Physical Education." UNESCO, together with the IOC, would declare the Jubilee Olympiad (4 years between XXVI Games and XXVII Games, 1996-2000) as the Olympiad of Sport and Peace or World Peace Olympiad.[6] This and other projects are united by the world campaign the "Jubilee Olympiad," initiated in our country for the 1991-2000 period and presented to UNESCO, COI and other organizations.[7] This campaign is a multipurpose one committed to further development and promotion of the Olympic philosophy to strengthening the connection of sport with education, public health, culture, environment protection, improvement of the standards of living in the North, South, West, and East. The main aim is to promote the removal of the imbalance between elite and mass sport ("sport for all" or massovost). The latter point is marked as one of the most important of the Moscow declaration adopted by the Second International Conference of Sports Ministers and had been under permanent discussion during all prior European conferences since the first one held in Vienna in 1973 to the 20th conference in Sofia, the capital of Bulgaria, in 1989. It is this very point (contradictions and disharmony in the development of mass and elite sport in Europe) that has been taken as a basis of the International Research Project "Sport-Europe." This point was included in the program of the World campaign "Jubilee Olympiad."

The following characteristics demonstrate that sport integration in Europe is continuously developing:

- the permanent bilateral and multilateral sports relations of the Northern and Southern, Eastern and Western Europe,

- collapsing socioeconomic structure and political system,

- the far-flung network of sports events and exchange,

- the origin and rapid development of the "sport for all" movement on the continent,

- almost 20 years of positive experience of the European Sports Conferences,

- activities and presence in Europe of the headquarters of UNESCO, IOC, CHIEFS, and most of the international and European sports federations, unions, and associations,

- the First and Second International Conferences of Sports Ministers held in 1976, in Paris, and in 1988 in Moscow,

- activities of the Sports Commission of the European Council; and

- sports science.

However, it must also be pointed out that this ongoing process has its share of problems and contradictions. As an example, some Western countries undertook interesting and topical international investigations of the state in sport, the problem of violence and doping in sport, sports economics, etc. In the framework of fruitful scientific cooperation, the socialist countries have carried out some comparative scientific projects concerning the role of sport in lifestyle, interrelations between sport and culture. National projects on development and prediction in sport were conducted, during the 1980s, in Great Britain, Hungary, GDR, France, Finland, West Germany, and other countries. Most important is the fact that all European countries have accumulated a great deal of social experience in the spheres of sport and the sports policy of states, and governmental, non-governmental and public organizations. A database and a computer center of sport scientific literature have been established and have been working successfully in the Cologne Federal Sports Institute with the active assistance of CHIEFS and its committees, as well as the International Association of Sports Information. In the united Germany, the German Olympic Institute and European Institute of Sport Research have been created. There are other examples.

Everything mentioned above, and also substantial, functional and organizational peculiarities of sport development in every European country and in modern Europe in general, are under the influence of the new positive economic and political changes that have occurred in international relations within the European Community as well as in the World Community. Evidence that work is being done is the lasting practical work of the Committee for the Development of Sport, the Council of Europe, the activities of the Clearing House (Brussels), the work of the European Association of the National Olympic Committees, and other sports organizations. However, more work is needed.

We have, in modern Europe, good sports legislation that covers such topics as:

- the desirability of including a right to sport in the European Convention of Human Rights,

- the desirability of updating the European Sport for All Charter, and possibly preparing a European Sport for All Convention,

- the importance of governmental/non-governmental relationships in the future as stressed in the Paris Summit "Charter for a New Europe,"

- the role of Council of Europe Recommendations and Sports Ministers' Resolutions in providing a common basis for converging technologies,

- the preparation of basic legislation for sport (cadres/ framework laws) necessarily implied the elaboration of implementing instruments (degrees, regulations, etc.) which was often an even more lengthy process; and

- the need for sport to bear in mind not only its "rights," but also its obligations (e.g. environmental, social, etc.).[8]

The traditions of European culture, trends toward the economic integration of the European countries, scientific and cultural relations, international cooperation of nations, successful realization of the Helsinki Agreement, and an improved political climate in modern Europe serve as a foundation for the development and improvement of the European sports integration as a whole and consolidation of research efforts in particular.

The new political realities, the new political thinking, democratization of the political life in East European countries, significant perspectives in the humanitarian sphere laid in Vienna and Paris Agreements, all these trends toward European security and integration, toward cooperation and mutual understanding are the basis for research on the state and perspectives of sport in Europe. Taking these ideas into consideration, the Soviet-Italian scientific group has elaborated an international project and a program of a common European comparative study on the theme, "Europe: Sport as an Element of Culture, Life Style and Social Policy" or briefly, "Sport-Europe." The suggested project is designed for 1991-1995 and involves all European countries on a parity and voluntary basis. A solution of some of the generally scientific, theoretical, applied, and practical tasks is also envisaged. Despite the difficulties (organizational, financial, technical, methodological—there exists no precedent either in sport science or in sport practice for such a study), the investigators believe that the scientific project will be supported by the international participants and will produce an important social impact. Besides the vitally important theoretical and practical results, there will be a precedent for All-European collective scientific collaboration in sport. The precedent for the consolidation of scientific efforts of all-European countries will also be laid down. A basis will also be established for similar investigations in science and sport, in the future, which will reach far beyond the boundaries of Europe. During the Ninth European conference on sports (in Sofia during October 1989), the Ministers of Sport and administrators of the European countries, the members of 26 delegations and the scientists—all the participants of that forum—supported our initiative.[9]

Sports studies, in the relationship of three most important social phenomena, culture, lifestyle and social policy, may really reflect sport's functioning as a social institution, and so unveil disproportion in the development of "sport for all" and elite sport. In turn, they may also reveal the social mechanism of the contradiction between physical activity and consumption of sport as a spectacle.

According to the research plan, the first stage envisages gaining socioeconomic, cultural, sociological, and statistical information of the "desk–research" type concerning the state and development of sport in every European country in the period between 1980 and 1989. A total of 167 such values made up the dynamic process during a decade. The next stage is a mass poll of all national selections by a unique uniformed method aimed at gaining access to the attitudes towards sport of various sociopolitical-demographic groups in European countries, their sports activities, and realization of every person's right for physical activity. A poll of 35 expert groups will be conducted in each country, and five groups on an all European scale after the principal population poll. The experts are the specialists who form public opinion, public disposition, social consciousness, social behavior towards sport and also form and implement sports policy. The third stage, combined with analysis of data gained country-wide, will be to conduct a comparative international analysis and, on the basis of it, to predict the future development of "sport for all" and elite sport, to lay down the process of their harmonization in Europe in general as well as in other countries.

The following is planned:

1. to outline the ways to increase sports activity,

2. to exchange the advanced experience and achievements,

3. to optimize strategy and tactics of sports policy,

4. to strengthen the consolidation of all European sports organizations simultaneously with the development of national features, original form, and traditions; and

5. to expand peace-making trends of further development of support, as a factor of inter-group, international, humanitarian communication of the European nations in terms of building a new common European home.[10, 11]

Notes

[1]Krawczyk, Z. "Sport in the era of structural social changes: The example of Eastern Europe." *Sport: social change and social process seminar ICSS.* Tallinn, (June 1991), pp. 12-13.

[2]Foeldesi, G. "Mass sport as the object of social constraint in Eastern Europe," *Sport: social change and social process seminar ICSS.* Tallinn, (June 1991), p. 25

[3]Eisen, G. "Perestroika and the 'Red Sport Machine'". *Sport and revolution in East–Central Europe.* Unpublished abstract. p. 2.

[4]Azvisto, M., A. Semyonov, and E. Truu, "Social background and typical contradictions of organizational renewal of sport (Estonian case)," *Sport: social change and social process seminar ICSS.* Tallinn, (June 1991), p. 24.

[5]Milshtein, O. "Sport-Europe: Cooperative and cross-cultural international research project." *The Report at the 7th International Conference of the International Society for Comparative Physical Education and Sport.* Bisham Abbey, 1990. p. 17. (unpublished)

[6]Milshtein, O. "On the eve of the golden games." *Olympic Panorama.* 2 (1989), pp. 44-46.

[7]Milshtein, O. "On the threshold of the jubilee." *Olympic Panorama.* 1 (1991), p. 12.

[8]Committee for the development of sport, workshop on sport legislation, Council of Europe. CDD, Strasbourg, 90: 44 (November 1990), p. 3.

[9]Milshtein, O. "Europe: sport as an element of culture, life style and social poli-cy." *The report at the tenth European conference on sports*. Sofia: 1989, pp. 44-46.

[10]Milshtein, O., and M. Abis, "The program of the international scientific project of the European countries," *Europe: Sport as an Element of Culture, Life Style and Social Policy*. Moscow-Rome, 1990, p. 86.

[11]Milshtein, O. and M. Abis,. "Working program of the international scientific project of the European countries," *Europe: Sport as an Element of Culture, Life Style and Social Policy*. Moscow-Rome, 1989, p. 7.

Chapter 21

The Final Game for Soviet and CIS Sport

Soeren Damkjaer

The Olympic games at Barcelona in 1992 saw the beginning and the end of the Unified team. The Unified team represented what was left of the "Big Red Machine," the Soviet structure of elite sport which existed since 1952. The Unified team consisted of the athletes from the 11 members of the Commonwealth of Independent States (CIS), and those athletes from Georgia, which was not a member of the CIS and had followed its own course since the dissolution of the Soviet Union. Following the coup, in August 1991, which led to the rise of Yeltsin and the dissolution of the Soviet Union in December 1991, the Unified team competed in the 1992 Olympics for the first and last time. All of these events led to an unprecedented situation in elite sport. The three Baltic republics gained full independence in October 1991 and, owing to their pre-war status in the IOC, gained full admittance to the Games before the end of the year. The short existence of the Unified team ended 40 years of Soviet elite sport on the international scene, which began in 1952. Contrary to many expectations and forecasts, the Unified team did well, securing a first place in the unofficial medal tally, ahead of both the United States and the reunited team from Germany. In fact, the Unified team did win the number of medals predicted by the Russian experts of the interim bodies that had supplanted Goskomsport. It was a dramatic year for Soviet society, for the international community, and for Soviet sport, which ended in what was a triumph for the remnants of the formidable performance of the CIS team. This was the final event, indeed the final competition for what was left of the elite sport machine of the former Soviet Union. Before the Olympics began, the new independent states had participated in international events as independent nations. The Unified team was a peculiar creation for just two events, the Winter and Summer games of the 1992 Olympiad.

Cultural Change Since 1985

In the span of just a few short years, all the aspects of the sports system of the Soviet Union had changed. Centrifugal forces were at work before 1991, leading to the growing independence of federations from Goskomsport. The massive infrastructure of teaching and research, and development in the world of sport was exposed to the winds of change, the watchwords being commercialism and capitalism. Despite the undeniable success of the CIS Team in 1992, the elite sport system of the 15 independent states had been exposed to the highly uncertain economic and political situation in the former USSR. This situation can only be compared to the revolutionary changes in Germany and the unification of the sports systems of the two Germanys. The smaller but highly successful sports machine of East Germany was dismantled and the remaining parts were integrated into the sports structure of West Germany. The "Big Red Machine" was kept alive for just one year in order to compete successfully in the Olympics. As a result of the aforementioned events, the international sport scene changed dramatically. Political influence in the sports arena disappeared, as did the confrontation between East and West. Will the result be a global village or a global market? Maybe the demise of the Soviet Union and the CIS is yet to be seen? The consequences of this will probably defy simplistic interpretations of the global village or the global market. The historical course of events at any rate defies simplistic forms of analysis. These events were not predicted, their effects were not foreseen, and the final outcome was quite surprising. These major events in recent sport history represent a challenge to historical and sociological analysis.[1]

Centrifugal Forces

The slogans of perestroika, glasnost, and democratization had a peculiar relevance to sport in the Soviet Union in 1985. The boycott by the United States and other western states of the Olympic Games in Moscow, in 1980, diminished the prestige of the games and the Soviet effort. The withdrawal of the Soviet and other socialist teams from the Olympic games in Los Angeles, in 1984, demonstrated the dependency of elite sport on the interest of state policy. Years of preparation were wasted and the order to withdraw was resented by athletes and officials of the sport bureaucracy. Therefore the elite system had its own reasons for severing the tight connections with the party-state. What followed was a centrifugal process that accelerated between 1988 and 1990, with no clear direction, similar to the political, cultural and economic spheres of society at the time. Goskomsport wanted a greater independence from the state and the party. Federations wanted larger independence from Goskomsport. Individual athletes and trainers openly voiced their dissatisfaction with pay, prize money, and authoritarian methods. The Baltic republics established direct links with the IOC and sports organizations in other states to obtain their independence. The first steps to professionalism, based on commercial and capitalist principals, was obtaining contracts with western soccer clubs, which now became a possibility. The reduction of political tutelage and the reduction of the influence of communist ideology led to a vacuum and to new initiatives. In 1990, Olympic Academies and Olympic Societies were formed to fill the vacuum left by the decline of the influence of party ideology. The need for reorientation was felt, and the slogans of commercialism, sponsorships, and total independence were formulated, particularly by the younger generation. During 1990, the economic crisis was growing acute and was accompanied by political disorientation. The deterioration of living conditions led to a decreased participation in mass sport. The prestige of elite sport was lowered. The conservative backlash manifested itself.

1991 was to become the fatal year for the Soviet Union and Soviet elite sport. Athletes from the Baltic republics withdrew from the Soviet teams. The prestige of elite sport was at its lowest. The August coup led to the dissolution of the Soviet Union and to the prohibition of the Communist Party. In December the Commonwealth of Independent States was formed. The Baltic republics had already obtained international recognition of their independence in October. Georgia, under ultra-nationalistic President Sviad Gamsakhurdia, did not join the CIS. The break-up of the Soviet Union was followed by the dissolution of the centralized structure known as the Union Ministries and Committees. Goskomsport suffered the fate of the other Union structures and was dissolved in late November 1991.

Crisis

These events took place during final preparation for the Olympic year. The crucial question in the months to come was, would there be a team for the Olympic games in Albertville and Barcelona? Time was a critical factor. The dissolution of the Union and the bankruptcy of Russia created a huge problem for financing CIS participation at the Olympics. Tense negotiations followed in Lausanne with the President of the IOC. V. Smirnov, President of the NOC of the former Soviet Union, and vice president of the IOC, played an important role in these negotiations. Ukraine demanded to appear with a Ukrainian team and was opposed to a United team. Georgia, which had not joined the CIS, was definitely against a United team. For the IOC, the break-up of the Soviet Union was also crucial for ex-Soviet participation was vital to the prestige of the Games.

The nightmare of the boycotts of 1980, and 1984, was not forgotten. But the participation of 15 new nations in Barcelona would mean a further overcrowding of the already overcrowded Games. What followed was intense negotiations on the conditions of participation at the Summer Games. On March 18, the final solution was reached in Lausanne. The Unified team was formed, comprising athletes from the 11 members of the CIS and Georgia. Ukraine and Georgia had to accept this solution in order to participate at all. All 12 states were accepted (as independent national Olympic committees), as a concession for the future. Details of ceremony were also agreed upon. The Unified team was born, creating a temporary solution that would last one year. In fact, the Unified team was dissolved immediately following the Barcelona Games.

A new period began following agreement, in March, on the conditions for the Unified team's existence. In retrospect, this could have been considered planning for "the final game." The problems ahead were quite formidable. Time was short. The Russian state had ceased to finance elite sport as had the other CIS states. The rapidly expanding inflation rate of 2,000%, per year, made planning difficult. Sponsors supplied foreign currency to finance the costs in Barcelona. Some training centers were inaccessible because of civil war. The organizational structure responsible for both the selection of the athletes and the financial support needed during the games came from the newly formed national Olympic committees of the 12 states. The Olympic committee played the dominant role. Smirnov was undoubtedly the key figure in the eventual construction of the Unified team. Although Goskomsport had been dissolved in November 1991, some of its personnel staffed the new organizational structure. The Russian committee for the support of the Olympic year seems to have had no particular influence. Adidas and Smirnof were the chief corporate sponsors, whereas neither the government of the CIS nor the individual states supported the Unified team. The Unified team was, therefore, the last appearance of a "Soviet team" and the first venture into the future of emerging commercialization of elite sport. The legal foundations were shaky. It was not until June that a new law was passed in an attempt to regulate elite sport in Russia. Although the rest of the economy was in a desperate condition, the last showing of the Soviet system of elite sport demonstrated the effectiveness of the old apparatus and its ability to improvise in a critical situation. In the absence of the former centralized command system, and at a time when the new nations wanted to promote their own athletes, the selection process for the team proved difficult. After the Barcelona Olympics, Smirnov complained of the chaotic and overtly political decisions that had been made.[2] This is hardly surprising considering the exceptional situation in which the Unified team was formed. After all, Ukraine and Georgia had opposed the idea of a Unified team, and had only agreed to participate on the team after being threatened with not being able to compete at all.

The Games in Barcelona

The contingent of the Unified team consisted of 498 athletes from 12 states along with 150 officials including trainers, staff personnel, and administration. Of the athletes, 277 came from Russia, 80 from the Ukraine, 53 from Belrussia, 21 from Kazachistan, 19 from Uzbekistan, 11 from Georgia, 10 from Moldovia, 5 from Azerbaijan, 5 from Armenia, 3 from Kyrgistan, 3 from Tadjikistan, and 1 from Turkmenia. Five athletes from Latvia had to be added to the Unified team. Before the Olympic Games, specialists predicted that 45 gold medals would be won by the Unified Team. The actual harvest of medals was 45 gold, 38 silver, and 29 bronze, making a total of 112. The United States came in second with 37, 34, and 37, and Germany came in third with 33, 21, and 28 respectively. Contrary to many predictions in the West, the Unified team did triumph in the last show. Despite the unsettled situation in the CIS, the uncertain situation for the athletes, and the complicated political maneuvers that led to the formation of the Unified team, this was indeed proof of the ability of the remnants of the "Big Red Machine" to produce extraordinary results. This was an unprecedented situation, and the Unified team responded with a show of strength, despite being a sports system on the verge of dissolution. The Russian sports periodicals responded with both pride and regret. But resignation in the face of the inevitable had been the tenor of the Russian press for years.

There is limited evidence of the attitudes and motivations of the athletes involved in the Barcelona Games. Many, if not all, seemed to deplore the dissolution of the Unified team. They trained together and competed together irrespective of national origin. Most seemed to blame the politicians for the dissolution of Soviet elite sport. Elite sport fell victim to the ambitions of individual republics. After the Olympic Games some athletes would start careers in the West, or continue careers already underway there. But numerous athletes and trainers would return to an uncertain future in the independent states. Smirnov tried to reassure the athletes and trainers that there would be a future and that no one would be fired. The Unified team had proven its ability to survive. Smirnov stated his conviction that the results had shown the necessity of future cooperation within the areas of research, training, and facilities. If not, all states would suffer. With this mixture of triumph, resignation, and plans for the future, the unique event of the Barcelona Games ended.

The Future

Before the Games, the selection process of the athletes for the Unified team had reflected the national interests of the individual states. Smirnov concluded, even before the Olympic Games, that Russia would have to prepare its future sports system on its own premises. There was, however, an interest in not severing the ties to the other states of the former Union. Smirnov repudiated attempts to revive the old structures of the Union or the CIS. There would be no CIS federations. There would only be clear-cut national Russian federations. This was an allusion to the attempts to form, or retain, the all-union federations of the past. Undoubtedly, a struggle was still going on regarding the issues of the organizational principles of the future. In broad outline, the future structure had been decided upon. The sole responsible agent will be a combination of an independent Russian Olympic committee and the federations of the independent states. The principles of operation will be, to a very large extent, commercial. Income for the federations will come from lottos and from foreign and domestic corporate sponsorships. There seem to be no prospects for any substantial support from the Russian state. The decreased prestige of elite sport, and the financial difficulties of the Russian state, seem to dictate such an outcome. While many questions arise from this scenario, they can only be answered within a perspective of the years ahead, because they are intimately connected with the fate of Russian society in general.

The infrastructure of the elite sport system is crumbling. The elite sports schools are closing because unions or other bodies cannot afford to support them. The rising costs of renting stadia and training halls are ruining elite institutions. The famous teaching and research institutes like the Central Institute of Physical Culture and Sport, in Moscow, are organizing such commercial activities as aerobic classes to supplement their budgets. Financing even the most central training centers is left to the initiatives of federations and individuals and their success finding sponsors. The optimism of Smirnov is contradicted by trainers and presidents of federations who predict a catastrophe for Russian elite sport within the next five years. Already, Russia, Ukraine and other states are supplying talented young athletes to the international market. Disciplines like fencing and archery, with little or no commercial potential, already suffer. The ambition of Soviet elite sport was to be the best across all disciplines, in all competitions, at all times. This ambition will have to be sacrificed. Amateur sport is in a dismal situation because of the lack of training halls and equipment. The desperate everyday life of the population is not the kind of situation that predisposes a broad movement toward sport. What was virtually free now commands a price that few can afford to pay. Creating voluntary associations to supplant the centrally organized activities requires a change in cultural values.

Cultural Theory and the Study of Change

Evaluating the monumental changes in all aspects of sport, in the former Soviet Union, is a challenge to the sociology and history of sport. These changes have taken place within a couple of years and the most spectacular changes have occurred within one year. The first phase is to analyze the events on the basis of some theoretical guidelines of importance. Sport, as a social institution of organized games, is just one aspect of a broader movement culture. A particular activity like soccer is embedded in an immediate social and cultural context, implying a specific cultural use of sport. Further, there is the organizational structure typified by the centralized planning system of elite and amateur sport in the former Soviet Union. This whole complex, which can be visualized as Russian dolls, one within the other, has finally established different, distinct relationships outside the political and cultural spheres of society at large. This gives elite and amateur sport a distinctive cultural significance within a given society. One can examine the different aspects of sport in Soviet society utilizing this cultural theory of sport. Such a theory is certainly needed to analyze periods of revolutionary change in society and sport. According to this theory Soviet elite sport has, within a few years, seen changes in all parameters. The immediate context has changed, the organizational structure has changed, and so has the whole complex of distinctive ideological, political, and cultural affinities with other areas of culture. Soviet elite sport was a modern enterprise, promoted for ideological and political reasons. Now it finds itself within a society in a state of unfinished modernization. Elite sport in Soviet society was a state within a state. Amateur sport was uniform, militarized and has not appealed to the populace for years. A number of preconditions for modern movement culture are simply lacking. The breakdown of the system consisting of modern, semi-modern, and pre-modern elements of movement culture has laid bare the working principle of this system. The dissolution of the system gives a unique insight into the mode of functioning of the system. The break-up of a system leads to the very real problem of defining chaos. Social theory is used to describe and explain order, system, and function. The Russian system of sport is presently in a state of partial chaos. The performance of the Unified team conceals the fact that the results in 1992 were due to improvisation by the remaining elements of the centralized structure. The revolutionary change in the former Soviet Union, and its sports system, represents a particular challenge to the theory of cultural change in physical education and sport. The global significance of the changes is an intensification of certain tendencies already present in culture, such as commercialization, promotion, and equality of the main elements in elite systems. But this globalization does not work in a unilinear fashion. Sport, as an institutionalized structure of activities, represents a cultural edifice with many levels of meaning. In Russian society, before and after the revolution of 1991, a coexistence of the old and the new meanings is evident in sport. This was apparent in the Olympic effort to construct a Unified team, to participate in the Olympic games of 1992, and to find a new role for elite sport in Russian society. This is not a uniform process, and the results will only be seen within the perspective of several years. It will take different forms in each of the 15 states that emerged out of the former Soviet empire.

Notes

[1]Riordan, J. *Sport in Soviet society.* Cambridge: Cambridge University Press, 1980.
[2]*Sovietsky Sport,* 1992.

Chapter 22

Sport and Glasnost:
A Case Study of Estonia

Reet Howell

Estonians have developed a strong cultural identity and part of this heritage is their extremely powerful and stubborn national self-consciousness as well as their intense pride in their "isamaa" (fatherland). Throughout their long history, Estonians have experienced many vicissitudes predominantly because of the strategic location of their land on the Baltic Sea. Since 1227, Estonia has been part of the Danish, Swedish, German, and Russian Empires and, despite this colonization and political subjugation, Estonians have steadfastly maintained their unique culture and language. The Estonian national movement, after 1861, was expressed through the Estonian Alexander School Movement (Eesti Aleksandrikool), the Society of Estonian Literati (Eesti Kirjameeste Selts), and all Estonian Song Festivals (Eesti laulupidud).[1] The Song Festivals were of particular significance as they served as a means of expressing nationalism and achieving a sense of unity and togetherness. When the Estonians overtly expressed their desire for independence from the Soviets, in late-1988, they manifested it through 'song' and it was known, in the West, as the "Singing Revolution."

Beginning in the 1860s another major feature of Estonian life was the emergence of local societies and clubs organized for the advancement of music, theater, adult education, and sport. F.R. Kreutzwald compiled the national epic, Kalevipoeg (The Son of Kalev), which affirmed the historical existence of the Estonian nation, and Kalev became the symbolic epic hero of the nation. Organized sporting activities started around 1860 with the formation of gymnastics ("turner") associations, and gymnastics was included in the curriculum of the parish schools. By 1900, sports competitions were conducted in cycling, gymnastics, weightlifting, and wrestling. Traditional folk games and Estonian folklore, such as Kalevipoeg, emphasized athletic prowess and physical strength, so it was natural that the sports of weight lifting and wrestling would gather the most followers, even among women. These sports were also the first to bring international recognition to Estonia. Three of Europe's greatest strongmen at the turn of the century were Georg Hackenschmidt, Georg Lurich and Alexander Aberg. They traveled the world exhibiting their exceptional skill and performing legendary feats.

After the collapse of the Tsarist regime, in February 1917, Estonia fought a successful War of Independence and achieved autonomy for the first time since 1227. For the next 22 years it existed as an independent free nation, and established a democratic egalitarian constitution, modeled principally on the French system. Economically, the country progressed through rapid industrialization and established a prosperous agricultural base. The stability of the country was assured and resulted in a high standard of living comparable to Finland and other Western European countries. The introduction of a comprehensive school system, with compulsory schooling, ensured a literacy level of 98% by 1934, with university standards equivalent to those in Germany.

On a global scale it is difficult for a small nation to make its mark but, for Estonia, such was achieved through sporting successes in the international arena. Even before it became a member of the League of Nations (in 1921), Estonia was admitted into the Olympic movement and participated in the 1920 Olympic Games. The Estonian Olympic Committee was formally accepted into the International Olympic Committee (IOC) and Friedrich Akel and Joakim Puhn were elected as IOC members. An analysis of the all-time "super achievers," based on gold medals per capita, placed Estonia 15th in the 1936 Olympic Games.[2]

In the five Olympic Games that Estonian athletes competed in, a formidable 21 medals were won: six gold, six silver and nine bronze. Of these medals, 11 were in wrestling, seven in weight lifting, two in track and field, and one in sailing. The Olympic Games was only one arena in which sporting success was achieved. In the sport of shooting, Estonian marksmen became World Champions in 1937 and 1939, winning the most coveted shooting trophy in the world, the Argentine Cup. The status of Estonia in the sport of weightlifting was acknowledged by its hosting of the World Championships at Tallinn in 1922. At the various World Championships from 1898 to 1939 a total of 136 medals were won: 71 gold, 32 silver and 33 bronze.

While outstanding athletes were achieving success overseas, the sport and recreation movement was effectively and efficiently organized within the country. Sports clubs were formed in cities, towns and in rural areas, and a plethora of sports were readily accessible to the populace. A style of "voimlemine" (gymnastics), developed by Ernst Idla in the 1920s, captured popular interest, particularly among women, and became an exercise "cult." Idla also inaugurated the "Eesti Mangud" (All Estonian Games) where, as well as sports competitions, there were mass "voimlemine" (gymnastics) demonstrations. Along with the traditional Song Festivals, these Games fostered national pride and nationalism. Sports were an integral component of the nation's cultural life.[3]

By 1939, Estonia was no longer an emerging nation nor an underdeveloped country. Its agriculture was modernized, the economy was industrialized, and the populace was fully literate. Thus, before the nation became a Soviet state, it had developed a strong scientific, economic, educational and sporting base.

With communist Russia to the east, and Nazi Germany to the south-west, Estonia was caught between the ambitions of the super powers and, as a relatively small, insignificant country, it became part of the Western powers' appeasement policy to Germany. In 1939, the signing of the Molotov-Ribbentrop Pact placed Estonia under the Russian sphere of influence, and Soviet occupation. In 1941 the German army occupied the country but, by 1944, the Soviet Army had "reliberated" (or reoccupied) Estonia and forcibly incorporated it into the Soviet Union. As a republic of the Soviet Union, the political, economic, and cultural institutions in Estonia were transformed to conform to the Soviet model. This included collectivization of agriculture, nationalization of all property and industry, suppression of religion, and the installation of Marxist-Leninist ideology. The Sovietization of Estonia was accompanied by intense suppression of nationalist and "bourgeois" elements, by mass deportations of approximately 10% of the population and the genocide of some 96,000. Accurate demographic consequences of this Sovietization have largely been unknown due to the veil of secrecy thrown up by the Soviets. However, between 1940 and 1959, there was a decline in the population by 33.2% or 455,000.[4] Of these, approximately 75,000 were fortunate enough to flee to the West. Among those fleeing were members of the cultural and intellectual elite. Strong emigrant communities were established, and Sweden and Canada became the principal centers of Estonian exile culture, scholarship, and political activity.

With the imposition of Soviet rule, all social, political, and economic organizations underwent radical reorganization. The organization of sports societies under the Central Athletic League was abolished, as was the Physical Culture Foundation of the Cultural Fund, and youth organizations such as the Boy Scouts/Girl Guides and the YMCAs. Among the many sports leaders accused of treason and targeted for persecution were the two IOC members, Puhk and Akel, both sentenced to death by the KGB for their "public" activity. The Estonian Olympic Committee was forced to discontinue its activity (de facto). However, since it was never formally abolished, it has never ceased to exist (de jure).

The organization and administration of Soviet Estonian sport and physical education were forced to conform to the All-Union model and the republic level organ was responsible to the Estonian SSR Council of Ministers as well as to the Soviet Physical Culture and Sports Committee at the USSR Committee Ministers. Many of the leaders in the sports movement had dual appointments. For example, Communist Party member Arnold Green, Deputy Chairman of the Council of Ministers of the Estonian SSR, was also president of the Wrestling Federation. Reginald Kallas, editor of the sports newspaper, *Spordileht,* was also head and secretary of the party section for the daily newspaper, *Ohtuleht,* as well as the propaganda and agitation instructor for the Central Committee of the Estonian Communist Party.[5] It was a Soviet system imposed by Soviets on Estonia. It was a foreign system with complete contempt for past traditions. Acculturation was enforced by the Soviet Army and KGB.

The physical culture movement, like all aspects of life in the Soviet Union, was directed, fostered, and controlled by the Communist Party of the Soviet Union; hence, it reflected the needs and desires of the party. The state-controlled system included the national physical fitness program, Valmis Tooks ja Kaitseks (Be Prepared for Work and Defence), which was integrated into the school system and work place. The All-Union Sports Classification system was a sports ranking pyramid aimed at achieving excellence in specific Olympic sports. These two systems were designed to achieve the two underlying principles of the sports movement, 'massovost' (mass participation) and 'masterstvo' (proficiency and achievement). Integral to the total model were the Pioneer Palaces, where the average child could pursue recreational pursuits, and the Sports Schools, where the elite children and youth honed their skills and talents.

Sport in the Soviet Union maintained a position of rare prominence in not only the national cultural life, but also the political sphere. Victory in the international arena was seen as an indicator of the superiority of the Soviet athlete, the Soviet populace, and the Soviet system. Thus, sports served as a vital cog in the foreign policy of the nation. It brought prestige and international recognition while, internally, the victories enhanced the system and the Party. Consequently, the funding for such a system was unlimited with the Party coffers keeping the sports system well oiled. The payoff was worth the price as the

Soviet team took top medal honors in six Summer and seven Winter Olympics since its debut in 1952.[6]

While the Soviet system exalted these successes, and the western world marveled at their magnificence, the simple fact is that there were athletes from 15 separate republics feeding into the Soviet team, and this was never acknowledged by zealous Marxist advocates. Also, invariably, in the Western press, the team would be referred to as "Russian," which was incorrect, ignorant, insensitive, and insulting. Of course, the Russian Republic provided the most athletes, as would be expected, being the largest and most populous republic (approximately 51% of the total population). The principal training and scientific centers were also situated in the Russian republic.

Estonian athletes competing in CCCP (USSR) uniforms have achieved 12 gold, 11 silver, and 11 bronze medals in summer Olympic Games. Of these, 10 were won by members of the basketball, volleyball, and water polo teams. It must be emphasized that Estonians only constituted 0.56% of the Soviet population. While these results could certainly be considered excellent for a population of only one million, several mitigating factors have kept the numbers down. First, the policy of "Russian first, and other nationalities last," has definitely permeated all levels of the sport system and Russian athletes have received favored treatment in the talent identification system and selection process.[7] Second, a political commitment to the communist regime was mandatory for all athletes, and those considered "politically unreliable" were denied permission to travel "valismaale" (overseas). Hence, Heino Lipp, Soviet champion 12 times, holder of 10 Soviet records and six European records, and ranked number one in the world in the decathlon, never competed in the Olympic Games. However, in Barcelona, with Estonia competing in the Olympics for the first time since 1936, the Estonian team was led into the stadium by Lipp proudly bearing the blue-black-white tricolor flag.

Access to the international arena was also diminished due to the increase in "internal" competition. Estonian athletes had to defeat, or surpass, the elite from 14 other republics before being selected for the "national" team. In sports such as track and field, gymnastics, wrestling, weight lifting, and cross-country skiing, the competitive standard within the Soviet Union was extremely high, and could be compared to trying to make the U.S. team in the 100m sprint race! As a consequence, Estonians have not achieved their pre-war international acclaim in wrestling and weight lifting, winning only one Olympic gold medal in wrestling in 1952 (Johannes Kotkas), and one gold and one silver in weight lifting, in 1968 and 1972 (Jaan Talts). Correspondingly, these sports have declined dramatically in popularity as new sports, with more potential for advancement, emerged.

While sports and sporting achievements were exploited and directed toward politically inspired goals, they nevertheless became one of the best avenues for safely expressing Estonian nationalism. Included in the annual republic "spordi-mangud" (Sports Games) were special sessions devoted to traditional Estonian folk games. In the prescribed All-Union school curriculum, Estonians argued for the right to include traditional Estonian folk dances in the physical education syllabus. Perhaps one of the most obvious displays has been the utilization of the name "Kalev" for the Republic's sports society, and also for teams and clubs. Kalev, the Estonian epic hero, is a strong, powerful man who defeats all opponents. The word, Kalev, is tinged with nationalistic implications and generates emotive feelings among the populace. Also, sports competitions offered spectators an opportunity to express anti-Russian sentiments. When Russian teams appeared in the stadium or on the court, they would be met with jeers and whistles, or a resistance of silence.[8] When overseas teams competed, they would always be supported, particularly if they were from the U.S.A. or other Western countries. Finally, although successful athletes internationally were credited to the Soviet Union, intense pride was developed by the accomplishments of "meie vabariigi" (our republic) athletes.

Estonians seized the opportunity to dramatically display nationalism at the reception given to their Seoul Olympic Games medalists, Erika Salumae (gold in cycling), twins Toomas and Tonu Toniste (silver in 470 sailing), and Tiit Sokk (gold in basketball). Very pointedly, bronze medalist Vladimir Reznitsenka, a Russian-Estonian, was not included in this reception. In early September 1988, over 100,000 people gathered at the Tallinn "lauluvaljak" (Song Festival Amphitheater) and, with the blue-black-white tricolor flag flying, they sang patriotic songs. The "Singing Revolution" had truly begun! One month later, the returning Olympians were received like heroes, "in the spirit of the old tradition."[9] The "free" Estonian flag was everywhere, children were dressed in traditional folk costumes, and the songs of Estonia were sung. At the ceremony, in the old Town Square in Tallinn, the restoration of the Estonian Olympic Committee (EOC) was publicly voiced for the first time. Arnold Green, Chairman of the Estonian Sports Conference and Foreign Minister of the Estonian SSR, and Atko Viru, Professor of Physical Education at Tartu University, became the first two EOC members. Green's selection demonstrated the difficulty that sporting, as well as political organizations, faced in breaking with the past communist bureaucracy.

Fundamentally, Estonia has historically pursued a course where cultural nationalism has appeared to be stronger than political nationalism.[10] Even in 1918, the initial predilection was for autonomy within a democratic Russian federation, and it was only with the complete collapse of Tsarist Russia, and the resulting societal chaos and the imposition of Soviet rule, that political sovereignty for Estonia was demanded. With the crushing of the underground guerrilla movement in 1953, armed resistance to the Soviet rule ended. Reality, and practicality, led to a tacit acceptance where citizens opted "to play the game" and work within the system. As university professor Toivo Jurimaa stated: "We said the slogans and words they wanted to hear, but in our minds, we thought otherwise and in our hearts we remained free."[11] While accepting the inevitability of communist rule, Estonians tenaciously clung to their culture, and rejected, in any and every way, Russification. The massive and deliberate migration of ethnic Russians to Estonia was deeply resented, and resisted; however, by 1970, Russians made up 24.6% of the total population.[12] Most (89.0%) were in compact urban districts, principally in the area around Narva, on the eastern Estonian-Russian border. In other centers, the Russians were segregated into enclaves such as "Mustamaa" in Tallinn, and "Hiinalinn" (Chinatown) in Tartu.

The pragmatic course of the Estonian people continued with the advent of glasnost (openness) and perestroika (restructuring). They were, however, at the forefront in expressing their nationalistic ambitions, being the first to openly take the historic stance in September of 1988. They never opted for the confrontalist approach of the Lithuanians; consequently they also did not suffer from military reprisals! Their diplomatic-pragmatic approach was also realized in the sports domain. In 1990 and 1991, Lithuania refused to take part in any Soviet league competitions and Lithuanians declined membership on Soviet teams. These decisions effectively denied Lithuanian athletes' access to international competitions and, indeed, confined them to competitions within their own borders. Estonian officials placed no restrictions on their athletes or teams, although individual athletes were presented with a choice. With Lithuania not competing in the national basketball championship, Estonia 'Kalev' became the favored team. When the 1990-91 All-Union Basketball Championship was won by Kalev, defeating the Russian team, the resulting euphoria could be compared to the Australian victory over the United States in the America's Cup in 1983, or the American victory over the Soviet hockey team in 1980. For Estonia, it was an historic moment, an opportunity to revel in their national superiority over the Russians in their debut in sport.

In March 1985, the liberalization policies of glasnost and perestroika were launched by Mikhail Gorbachev, when elected as General-Secretary of the

Communist Party of the Soviet Union. As Estonia had the highest living standards in the Soviet Union, he turned to this republic to test his reform plans and ideas. As an agrarian nation, Estonia had always grown much of its own food and it exported meat and dairy products to Leningrad (now St. Petersburg). Price liberalization started in Estonia where, along with Latvia and Lithuania, they became the first Soviet republics to develop democratic parties and hold free elections. The local communist parties were soundly defeated and Estonia then became sovereign in all but name. The red Soviet Estonian flag was replaced by the blue-black-white tricolor; the Russian Cyrillic script disappeared from road and street signs; "unofficial" border patrols guarded the "unofficial" borders; Estonian language lessons were carried on radio; and, in January 1991, even the massive statue of Lenin in Tartu "disappeared" during the night.

On June 1, 1991, Lennard Meri, Foreign Minister of the Estonian SSR, stated: "The Soviet Union sociological experiment, a society based on Marxism-Leninism, a theory hostile to life itself, has run its course and the Soviet Union now stands on the brink of catastrophe."[13] Meri, on that June day, could not have realized how near the total collapse was as he looked down from Toompea, the site of the Estonian Parliament, and viewed the rock barricades erected by Estonian nationalists. In 1917, Lenin and his fellow Bolsheviks needed only ten days to establish Communist dictatorship; but it took 74 years to disintegrate! Following three days of an abortive hardline coup the final death knell to communism sounded. In the midst of the coup, Estonia took advantage of the chaos of the central government and declared independence on August 20, 1991. Cultural independence had brought political independence.

While the tiny country of Iceland was the first to acknowledge Estonia's sovereignty, gradually all Western countries accorded formal recognition, with Canada and Australia following suit on August 25. Finally, on September 6, the Soviet Union accepted the inevitable and acknowledged Estonia's independence. A few days earlier, the USSR Olympic Committee gave formal recognition to the existence of the Estonian Olympic Committee. This was an unprecedented move in a country where sport had been so state controlled, and followed only government commands. One could possibly interpret this move as the rare occasion when sport actually led politics! The final international acceptance came on September 17 when Estonia was accorded United Nations membership, and then the following day, September 18, the International Olympic Committee reactivated the Estonian Olympic Committee. Estonia regained the Olympic status it had been denied for half a century.

Soviet rule has brought the Estonian people nothing but incalculable suffering, deprivation and degradation. Collectivization was a disaster, as there is less land under cultivation now than in the 1930s. In starting their new life of freedom, Estonians have been left with the telltale scars of Soviet reality: drab shops, empty shelves, broken trolley-buses, fume-spewing cars, pot-holed streets, polluting factories, an ecologically damaged environment, and a bureaucracy that was corrupt, inefficient and ineffective. Most damaging of all has been the destruction of the "work ethic." Building a new political, economically viable state can prove to be almost as daunting as the achievement of the dream of freedom. Pride and self-reliance have been the Estonians' weapons of resistance, and now these must serve as the basis for the building of the new nation.

The rebuilding of Estonia is being assisted by the "valis eestlased," or emigrants, who have voluntarily initiated fund raising and appeals. For example, the Australian Estonian Society, with a membership of some 6,000, raised U.S. $25,000 for hospitals and medicine, as well as U.S. $8,000 for the Barcelona Olympic team. Even more substantial aid has come from Canada, Sweden, the U.S.A., and Great Britain, as it was imperative that, despite the economic depression, Estonia should take its rightful place at the world's greatest festival, the Olympic Games.

The 1992 Winter Olympics in Albertville served, for Estonia as well as Latvia and Lithuania, as a perfect stage on which to revel in their nationhood. While the United Nations' sessions are restricted for the public, the Olympic Games are viewed by millions around the globe, and no better forum could have introduced this new nation to the world. Smiles and cheers greeted these athletes, proudly dressed in their new Finnish-donated uniforms and walking behind their blue-black-white flag. In sharp contrast, the poverty-stricken remnant of the once-powerful Soviet sports machine marched behind the Olympic flag, wore a variety of different uniforms, waved little flags from different republics, and called themselves quixotically "UT" (the Unified Team). At Barcelona, the 35-member Estonian team performed above expectations, with nine placing in the top six in their events. Tonu and Toomas Toniste again medalled, taking the bronze in the 470 Class in sailing, while cyclist Erika Salumae repeated her Seoul victory in the sprint. However, this time the blue-black-white tricolor of Estonia was raised. It was an historic moment.

While Olympic participation, under Estonian colors, was no longer a dream, the reality was hampered by finances. The government committed, in February, $46,200, of which $23,100, was a loan to the EOC, while the EOC Olympic Solidarity Fund gave $20,000. These commitments did not even meet the accommodation costs, U.S. $78,000, for the 35-member team in Barcelona. The EOC was promised by the IOC that some additional financial support would be awarded to Estonia. Fortunately, clothing worries were alleviated by the Finnish clothing firm, Terinit, which donated clothing for both the summer and winter Games athletes. Also, the ASA insurance company provided complimentary insurance. Individual athletes have initiated their own sponsorships such as Erika Salumae from the "Estravel" and Juri Tamm with the Tallinn Travel Bureau "Raeturist." Fund raising is now a major concern for the EOC, which formed a separate body called the Estonian Olympic Fund (EOF) on April 26, 1989, to coordinate financial matters for the Olympic movement in Estonia. The mega corporation Coca-Cola, for example, donated U.S. $10,000 to the EOF.

Although finances were the major concern of the EOC, their thorniest problem rested with the citizenship issue. With the restoration of independence, the government has endeavored to establish the right of Estonian citizenship. Estonian citizens were decreed to be those who had citizenship rights in 1938, and their direct descendants. This effectively denied citizenship to approximately 35% of the population, who were principally Russian and had migrated to Estonia after 1945. They were deemed as being "foreigners" and part of the occupying force. Also, the many Russian-Estonians, even those who have lived there for 40 years, that had not bothered to learn the Estonian language, were now barred from government and public service jobs, as Estonian is now the official language. It is also a requirement for citizenship. A detailed debate of the citizenship issue is not within the realm of this chapter; however its implications with relation to the Olympic Games is certainly relevant. The general consensus has been that only Estonian citizens should be part of the Estonian Olympic team. At the beginning of June, the Estonian government "granted" citizenship to two basketball players, two track athletes, and one fencer of Russian descent. Such a move has been severely criticized by the majority of the populace, and the other Olympians. Only one of these achieved a placing in the top six at the Games, and ethnic Estonians were the medal winners and top achievers.

The IOC further complicated this issue when Samaranch announced that athletes from the Baltic states were permitted "to compete in the Unified Team, effectively the former Soviet team, in volleyball, rowing and other sports they are not strong enough to enter a whole team."[14] In Latvia, this issue divided the nation, and particularly a family, as Raimonds Miglinieks elected to play for Latvia while his brother Igors, a member of the 1988 Soviet gold medal team, decided to play for the Unified Team. For Estonian cross-country skier, Urmas Valbe, his nation's independence resulted in a separation from his Siberian-born wife, Jelena, and four year-old son, Franz. With the break-up of the Soviet

Union, Jelena chose to compete for the Unified Team, stating that "she had been brought up as a Soviet."[15]

As national training centers were located throughout the Soviet Union, the breakup of the union and the independence of nations have affected the utilization of these facilities. While for the 1992 Winter Olympics it appeared as if there were no barriers erected, utilization really depended on money available by the national federation. For example, Otepaa in central Estonia was the Soviet cross-country training center and, in June 1991, the Soviet team completed their regular training at the site. The Estonian team trained at Kaariku as they could not afford the costs at Otepaa. After independence, the Russians (or CIS) were still permitted to train at the site as long as they paid. As the economic situation deteriorated in 1992, and as Russia was demanding that Estonia pay in hard currency (dollars) for its oil supplies, Estonia retaliated. Thereafter, the Russians could no longer pay in roubles for using Otepaa, but were required to pay in "valuta" (dollars), which was virtually impossible for them. Further complicating the issue was the insistence by the Russians that "they" (the Soviets) built the facilities, and hence should be reimbursed for associated costs. In reply, the Estonians claim it is their land, and the Russians were illegally in the country! New property laws have nullified all the nationalization of land and property effected by the Soviets and restored pre-war ownership! Meanwhile, the Estonian 1992 Olympic cross-country skiers accepted an invitation to train in Finland.

As sport was a propaganda tool for the Soviet government funding, which has been the bane of amateur sport in Western countries, was never a concern in the USSR. "Money, simply, was not a problem,"[16] stated the General-Secretary of the Estonian Sports Union in 1991. Sport administrators never had to court corporations, woo television sponsors or convince politicians. When the centralized economy and political organization collapsed, and the trade unions, which have for decades helped finance sport, were no longer solvent, sport, like all else in the country, found itself in dire straits. Facilities are now run down and are not being repaired. Equipment is broken and cannot be replaced, and sports schools are closed. There is, simply, no money for such endeavors. The percentage of cutbacks is unknown, principally because exact gross amounts were previously unknown, even to top-level administrators. According to Toomas Tonise, Secretary-General of the newly-formed Estonian Central Sports Union (ECSU), one of the major problems to be faced is making out a budget, as they never had to work out an annual budget which took into account all expenditures. Despite the lack of fundamental business skills in organizing and administering a major organization, the ECSU is endeavoring to reorganize, revitalize, and resurrect sport in Estonia.

One of the major problems facing the Estonian Central Sports Union (ECSU) is "sport for all" (tervise sport), which had been neglected in the old Soviet system. The ECSU is committed to the democratic principles which underpin the new nation. Offering and encouraging sport and physical activity for the total populace is seen as a top priority. However, the current economic crisis will likely restrict any positive and idealistic plans of the ECSU. Also people, after several decades of communism, are accustomed to the State providing everything. They must be re-educated to provide for themselves and pay for programs and facilities. Moreover, with daily survival everyone's concern, most people do not have the time and energy to "recreate."

While the VTK (Valmis Tooks ja Kaitseksor, "Be Prepared for Work and Defense") was one of the linchpins of the Soviet system, and theoretically fostered fitness and exercise among its masses, its functionalist quota system and para-military base literally alienated people. Estonian physical educators and sports administrators flatly stated that VTK was dead. The old quota system had been a farce. The figures for years had been meaningless as there had been so much falsification and fabrication. No one paid any attention to the norms or quotas of the Soviet system except for Western scholars beguiled by the system. In searching for a new battery of physical fitness tests, exercise scientists and physical educators turned to the international standards and tests adopted in 1964 in Tokyo. While evaluating these tests they considered Estonian traditions and the current situation. For example, the lack of hand dynamometers negated the utilization of this test of muscle power. The final decision was to adopt an eight-item battery, utilized in Finland, and then to send teachers/researchers to Finland for training.

The dismantling of the regime has meant that the elite sports establishment has been disinherited. Elite athletes who previously were well-endowed with state support have had to seek sponsorship arrangements to finance their training. Erika Salumae, after her gold medal win in Seoul received, from the government, a large private house (at that time private houses were not available for the average citizen), and all the necessary house furnishings. Now, in 1992, Erika has had to seek private sponsorship. For example, "Estravel" is fundraising her overseas competitions. Shot putter Juri Tamm signed contracts with Tallinn Travel Bureau 'Raeturist' and 'Tallinna Keskkonaamet' to finance his preparations for Barcelona. Some, however, have turned to overseas companies, such as the cross-country skiers, financed by Fischer, Atomic, and Karhu. The Estonian Football Union has signed a two-year contract with the Italian company 'Lotto.' Lotto is giving the national team all the gear they need from boots to bags in return for playing in Lotto colors and using the Lotto ball.[17]

As funding for sport has shifted from a state to a private and commercial basis, the privileged state amateurs are starting to decline. Those in low-profile sports, such as fencing, speed-skating, rowing, archery, and even yachting, are finding considerable hardship in maintaining a full-time athletic career. Others, in more commercial sports such as cycling, football, basketball, and hockey are becoming professional athletes, openly accepting money, principally from the West, for their athletic prowess. Now that state-imposed travel restrictions have been removed, the "brain and body" drain to the West will have a devastating effect on local development potential. The most talented athletes are "fleeing" to the West where facilities, equipment, and general living standards are far superior. Estonian cyclists and basketball players have been the first to profit from glasnost. Such professional traffic is not all one-way, as the national 'Kalev' basketball team has acquired the services of a black American player, George Jackson.

For the past several decades, the Soviet sport system has been admired and envied by the West. Its success in the Olympics and other competitions seemingly verified, and dramatically demonstrated, the superiority of the communist system. Furthermore, it was argued that while capitalist sport was dehumanizing and exploitative, communist sport was founded on the noble aims of Olympism. The laudatory comments on the Soviet system were perpetuated by academics, particularly sport sociologists, through the 1970s and 1980s. Glasnost and perestroika have swept aside, forever, the idealized picture of the Soviet sport system and, as communism collapsed, so did the dependent sport system. Hypocrisy, corruption, and cheating permeated the system for decades. This has now been readily admitted by Estonian sports administrators and athletes. Newspapers openly carry articles on previously forbidden topics such as drugs and, virtually every day, new exposures are brought to world attention. There is no question that performance-enhancing drugs were part of the system, as drug-taking was financially supported, approved, and administered by the state. Records and figures were falsified; nothing was sacred. Although "massovost" or "sport for all' was an avowed aim of the system, it was too costly and of no benefit to the Party for it brought neither prestige nor glory. Sports for the handicapped were totally ignored as, theoretically, "handicapped" people did not exist in a society where only perfect health was possible. The system has been exposed and the challenge is to rebuild from the ashes.

In summary Estonia, prior to Soviet occupation, was a developed Western country with a sound economic, social, and educational base. Its sports system had developed parallel in form and structure to that in Western Europe. During the independence years, its system was superior to that in Soviet Russia. The Soviet system that was imposed on Estonia after 1945 was an alien one, with no regard for Estonian traditions or heritage. It was all-encompassing and all-embracing, and it was all part of the Russification process.

Estonia has now freed itself from the shackles of Russian imperialism although, in June 1992, nine months after international acceptance of its independence, 25,000 Russian troops still remained there. Sport, like all social institutions, is endeavoring to move away from the previous dominance of a centralized command system characterized by bureaucracy, and has rejected previous hypocrisies and 'shamateurism.' While the current economic situation is grim, the future for sport is seen to be in the evolution of a system that is reflective of and, responsive to, the needs and desires of Estonians, as well as integral to the Estonian culture.

Notes

[1]Raun, 1987, pp. 57-80

[2]"Scorecard", *Sports Illustrated.* (September 14, 1988), p. 110.

[3]Nurmberg, R. A. "Sport and Physical Education in Estonia." Unpublished Ph.D. dissertation, University of California, Berkeley, 1972

[4]Parming, T. "Population changes and processes," In, T. Parming and E. Jarvesoo (eds.). *A Case Study of a Soviet Republic: The Estonian SSR.* Boulder, CO: Westview Press 1978, pp. 21-74

[5]Nurmberg, 1972, p. 228

[6]Wallechinsky, D. *The Complete Book of the Olympics.* London: Autumn Press, 1992, pp. xiv-xvii

[7]Personal interviews, May 1991

[8]Personal interviews, May 1992

[9]Estonian Olympic Committee, 1991

[10]Pennar, J. "Soviet nationality policy and the Estonian communist elite," In, Parming, T., and E. Jarvesoo (eds.) *A Case Study of a Soviet Republic: The Estonian SSR.* Boulder, CO: Westview Press, 1978

[11]Jurimaa, 1991

[12]Parming, p. xiv.

[13]"Free Estonia key to Soviet recovery," *Weekend Australian,* (June 2, 1991), p. 17.

[14]"Larger team gets Olympic blessing," *Baltic Independent.* (April 10-16, 1992), p. 7. 1992

[15]"Eesti sport", *Vaba Eestlane,* (March 26, 1992), p. 6.

[16]General Secretary of the Estonian Sports Union, 1991

[17]Estonian football," *Baltic Independent.* (April 24-30, 1992), p. 10; Also see, "Baltic states ready for Albertville," *Baltic Independent.* (January 24-30, 1992), p. 6; "Eesti opilaste kehalised voimed on rehuldavad," *Eesti Spordileht.* (January 27, 1992), p.2; Howell, M. L., and R. Howell, "The 1952 Olympic Games: Another Turning Point?" In, P. J. Graham and H. Ueberhorst (eds). *The Modern Olympics.* West Point: Leisure Press, 1976, pp. 187-198; Nurmberg-Howell, R. "Physical education and sports," In, T. Parming and E. Jarvesoo (eds.). *A Case Study of a Soviet Republic: The Estonian SSR.* Boulder, CO: Westview Press, 1978, pp. 223-244; and, Raun, T. H. *Estonia and the Estonians.* Stanford, CA: Hoover Institution Press, 1987.

Chapter 23

The Influence of the Political Changes on the High Performance Sport Organization in Czechoslovakia

**Jaromir Sedlacek, Rotislav Matousek,
Roman Holcek, and Roman Moravec**

The sports movement in Bohemia and Slovakia has rich traditions that can be compared with advanced countries. Evidence for this can be found in the spontaneous development of the club physical education movement in the second half of the nineteenth century, the early foundation of the Czech Olympic Committee (in 1899), and regular and abundant participation in the Olympic Games in the first half of the twentieth century. Further quantitative and qualitative growth of the sport movement came after World War II. This has been manifested through improved achievements in succeeding Olympic Games. The most points ever scored were in Tokyo and Mexico where, in the unofficial evaluation of nations, Czechoslovakia occupied 10th and 11th place with 101 and 103 points respectively.

| | | | MEDALS | | |
	POINTS	PLACE	Gold	Silver	Bronze
Tokyo	101.0	10th	6	6	3
Mexico	103.5	11th	7	2	4

Figure 1—The Best Olympic Games Results of CSFR

In 1968, when the democratic social evolution ended, officials representing the new communist political order were interested in demonstrating their economic prosperity by excelling in sport.[1] As a result of the communist party central committee this interest grew in the early 1970s into the so-called "Czechoslovak System of High Performance Sport" accord. This new system was designed to identify a number of gifted athletes and provide them the best possible conditions for training. This included the development of new institutional structures, the preparation of scientific and methodological direction of the sport training process and, of course, the selection and preparation of gifted athletes.

The purpose of this chapter is to review the existing system of high performance sport in Czechoslovakia, evaluate the influence of the new social, political and economic conditions on changes in the organization of the high performance sport movement, and to outline the fundamental differences between the Czech and Slovak Republics and other countries of the former East European bloc.

The Czechoslovakian system of high performance sport is composed of two related parts:

- The selection and preparation of gifted athletes; and
- The development of high performance centers.

The selection and preparation of gifted young athletes takes place according to the following process:

1. Testing and selection of elementary school pupils (age 7). In 1988 approximately 55% of the Slovak population had been tested. Those children determined to be "gifted" (approximately 20% of the school population) were allowed to enter special small games and participate in more physical education classes.

2. Testing and the selection of pupils ages 9-10. Selected pupils (approximately 10% of the school population) enter "sport classes" or "school sport centers."

3. Testing and the selection of pupils who are 14 years old. These selected pupils enter "training centers of youth," "sport schools," or "centers of high performance sport for youth." In 1990 there had been approximately 6,200 young athletes in this and related institutions representing approximately 2% of the population of the Slovak Republic.

Testing (age in yrs)	Location	% of Population
17-18	Training Centers of Youth Sport Schools High Performance Centers	2% of Slovak republic (6200 sportsmen in 1990)
14	Sport classes Sport school centers	10% of school population
9-10	Special small games Extra P.E. lessons	20% of school population
7		55% of elementary population

Figure 2—Selection and Preparation of Sport Gifted Youth.

Young athletes finish a first level by the time they are 17-18 years old at which time they pass on to a different level. Successful completion of the lower level allows athletes to enter the second level including centers of high performance sport (see Figure 3). The main purpose of these institutions is to prepare the athlete to represent Czechoslovakia in international competition. These centers of sport performance were affiliated with the Ministries of Education, Defense, Interior, Czechoslovak Union of Physical Education and/or the Union of Cooperation with the Army. In the last 20 years these institutions prepared from 70-100 % of the Czechoslovakian representation in most sports.

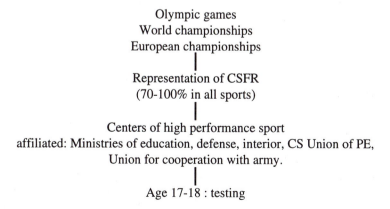

Olympic games
World championships
European championships
|
Representation of CSFR
(70-100% in all sports)
|
Centers of high performance sport
affiliated: Ministries of education, defense, interior, CS Union of PE,
Union for cooperation with army.
|
Age 17-18 : testing

Figure 3—High Performance Sport Centers.

Twenty years of building and developing this system has produced both positive and negative outcomes. Some positive factors include:

- Preparation of high quality conditions for athletes.

- Provision of a rational administrative structure.

- Introduction of scientific and methodological influences in training.

- Reasonable selection and preparation of "gifted" athletes.

- Successful integration of sport training with education or work.[2]

Negative outcomes to be considered include:

- Overly strict centralism and imperative direction.

- Alienation of the talented athletes from other average athletes and from the wide voluntary physical education movement.

- Minimal commitment from most subjects (coaches, teachers, sportsmen/women, managing staff, etc.).

- Unjustified glorification and politicization of high performance sport.

- High pressure (political and economic) in high performance sport with regard to reaching international success.

- Blood doping in high performance sport.[3]

The comparison of fundamental practices between the Czechoslovak system of high performance sport and some other former East European countries leads to the conclusion that the Czechoslovak system has not been as centralized and intensive as in East Germany, Bulgaria, and the U.S.S.R.

The second basic difference between Czechoslovakia and other East European countries, after World War II, in physical education is the existence of voluntary associations in Czechoslovakia. In most eastern countries 'physical education and sport' committees controlled by the government were created and given relatively great power. Because of the voluntary associations in

Czechoslovakia the state influence on high performance sport had not been as strong and centralized as it had been in other countries. Many complications were witnessed between the Czechoslovak Union of Physical Education and Ministries of Education Health and Defense as dual participants in the high performance sport organization.

Today a new social, political and economic situation in Czechoslovakia is creating fundamental change even in the sphere of high performance sport. Many negative features of the former system have disappeared with changes in the social system. Further positive changes will most likely come with additional structural changes. New physical education associations are developing including the Czechoslovak-Slovak Automotorclub, Union of Technical Sports and Activities, Czechoslovak Eagle, Czechoslovak Sokol just to name a few. There is change in the structure of the Czechoslovak Physical Education Organization which still has mass appeal at 1.3 million members, along with the Czechoslovak Olympic Committee whose once tarnished respect has been renewed. Today the entire physical education and sport movement in Czechoslovakia is directed at the local, district, national and federal levels.

The relative independence, at the national level, brings different opinions on how to solve the problem of high performance sport. The Bohemian government is making an effort to abolish, or to transfer all of the institutions for the selection and preparation of gifted athletic youth, including the administration of centers of high performance, sport to non-governmental agencies (sport clubs) Opinion in the Slovak republic is that the entire system of high performance sport that has been built for the last 20 years, and has absorbed enormous sums of money, should be preserved and coordinated with today's social needs. The system ought to be created on a national basis establishing regular testing of the school population and with voluntary participation following in a variety of institutions (see Figure 4.).

Under the current constitution the Ministries of Education and Health, as well as Physical Education and Sport, are not under significant influence from the federal government. The degree of state involvement, with regard to sport gifted youth, high performance sport and sport representation of the Slovak Republic, should continue in the national training centers. Research, medicine and information centers should be developed on a national basis as well.

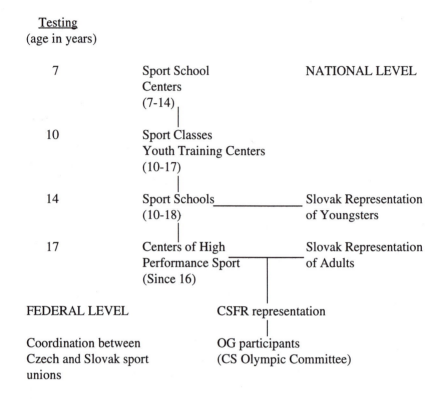

Testing
(age in years)

7   Sport School   NATIONAL LEVEL
          Centers
          (7-14)

10   Sport Classes
          Youth Training Centers
          (10-17)

14   Sport Schools_____   Slovak Representation
          (10-18)   of Youngsters

17   Centers of High   Slovak Representation
          Performance Sport   of Adults
          (Since 16)

FEDERAL LEVEL   CSFR representation

Coordination between   OG participants
Czech and Slovak sport   (CS Olympic Committee)
unions

Figure 4—New High Performance Sport Organizing Structure Proposal
          (Slovak Republic)

Financial support should be guaranteed by the Slovak Union of Physical
Culture, Ministry of Education, Youth and Sport, Ministry of the Interior,
Ministry of Defense, and the Olympic Association of Slovak Republics and
sport clubs. Financial needs are estimated per year at 150 million crowns
(approximately 5 million United States dollars). This amount represents approximately 10% of the money spent in sport in Slovakia each year.

Conclusions

1. The most positive feature in the "Czechoslovak system of
high performance sport" has been the formation of a huge
network of institutions that are linked and supplement each
other. The system enables the identification and preparation
of sport gifted athletes. Today it is completely under the

guidance of highly qualified teachers and coaches. This system proves that it is possible to combine education and high performance.

2. Further development of the system will follow the political changes in Czechoslovakia. It may be necessary to blend the two national systems, Czech and Slovak. There will need to be federal cooperation on both sides from federal sport unions.

3. Except for national differences, even positions between the Slovak Union of Physical Culture and the Ministries of Education, Interior and Defense have been cleared up. This is especially true from the point of view of the Slovak government and other supporters of high performance sport.

4. The system described lasted until 1992 Olympic Games in Barcelona. Ironically it corresponded with the latest elections and political development in Czechoslovakia.

Notes

---

[1]Riordan, J. "Soviet sport and perestroika," *Journal of Comparative Physical Education and Sport* .XI: 2 (1989), pp. 6-18; Semotiuk, D. "East block athletics in the glasnost era," *Journal of Comparative Physical Education and Sport.* XII: 1 (1990), pp. 26-29; and, Havlicek, I. The methodological approach and the system of the selection of sport gifted youth in Czechoslovakia, Conference europeenne sur1' EPS. January 1992.

[2]Broom, E. F. "Lifestyles of aspiring high performance athletes: A comparison of National models," *Journal of Comparative Physical Education and Sport.* XIII: 2 (1991), pp. 24-55, 1991.

[3]Semotiuk; and, Sedlacek, J. *Efektivita vyberu talentovanej mladeze v behoch na kratke vzdialenosti.* KDP, Bratislava, FTVS UK, 1992, p. 124.

Part 6: International Sport

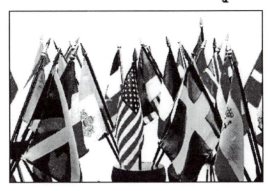

Part 6: International Sport

Part Six contains three different examinations of international sport, all of which look in some way at the need for, or consequences of, success at the highest level of sport. Clumpner evaluates the various factors that are likely to lead to success in elite international sport. Ironically, Semotiuk's subject—how the Canadian government responded to the shame of Ben Johnson's drug-assisted "victory" in the 1988 Olympic 100 meters—centers on how values can, and often do, get distorted when the pressure for success in elite international sport becomes too great. McGehee gives a historical perspective of four different series of regional games in which nations of the Americas participate.

Clumpner focuses on the Olympic Games in his assessment of factors necessary for success in international competition. Adequate financing is almost always a sine qua non, at least in the more "technical" activities, because money can provide training centers, qualified and knowledgeable coaches, good medical support, and time for athletes to train. Sometimes it provides for so much time, ironically, that athletes—particularly younger ones—suffer from overuse injuries. The second factor for success is a well-connected support system that enmeshes athletes in an unbroken system from initial selection, to high level competition, to retirement and helping the next generation. It is quite clear that totalitarian regimes can achieve this more readily than the hit-and-miss of private enterprise that lacks government backing. One of the ironies of the former Soviet Union was the excellence of sport communication in a society not otherwise noted for good telecommunications. The third factor for success is having a large and physically diverse population from which to select, and having this in place for very young potential athletes. Casting the net as widely as possible is also helpful. Sometimes, economics can restrict access to sport but religion and gender bias, and cultural bias can be restrictions, too.

For many in Canada, Ben Johnson came to represent all that was worst about elite international sport. In the subsequent Dubin inquiry (named after its chairman) ethics and morality were as frequently considered as one suspects they are usually assiduously ignored. The inquiry was convened four months after Johnson's disqualification from the Olympic Games for having tested positive for a banned substance. It is significant because it represents one of the very few serious government attempts to review and recommend change in a country's approach to sport from largely an ethical point of view. Unfortunately, implementation has proved much less easy to either do or fund. The inquiry was noteworthy because it struggled with two problems that often confront scholars in our field: first, are mass and elite sport friends, enemies, or in symbiosis; and second, is it appropriate for governments to "use" elite sport for political ends? The recommendations were generally well received; however no one seems to know how they can be implemented without money, and no money appears to be forthcoming. Cynics also doubt there is the will to implement them among the general population. However, in the sense that the Canadian government recognized the power and influence of sport in society, were forced into disclaiming the status quo, and are (still!) thinking about reform, they are surely to be commended.

McGehee gives a historical view of the Central American and Caribbean, Pan American, Central American and Caribbean University, and Central American Games. This is a useful compilation, especially for the non-Spanish speaker, because three of these Games are not very well known, and what information does exist is mostly in Spanish. At least two attempts at holding regional games were made in the early 1920's but were not continued. Then in 1926, 14 nations attended the first Central American (later Central American and Caribbean) Games, in Mexico. Since then, a four-year cycle has been maintained with only minor variations. Cuba and Mexico have won the most medals. The Pan American Games were scheduled for 1942 and 1946 but had to be canceled owing to the war. 1951 was thus the date of the first Pan American Games, and they have continued every four years. The United States and Cuba have garnered the most Pan Am medals. Recently, and perhaps surprisingly, winter games have been added—in 1989 they were canceled due to lack of snow in Argentina, but were held in 1990. The Central American and Caribbean University Games were first held in 1972 and they have been dominated by Cuba. The Central American Games (without any other areas added to this designation, so excluding, for example, the domination of the United States, and Cuba, and Mexico) began in 1973, and were held also in 1977, 1986, and 1990. Guatemala has won the most medals in these games. The success of scheduling these various games, and each country's individual success rates, have varied enormously and serve to highlight the vast discrepancies in availability of the factors needed for success as outlined by Clumpner, and they thus illustrate his point.

Shirley H.M. Reekie

Chapter 24

21st Century Success in International Competition

Roy A. Clumpner

This chapter prescribes several factors necessary for international Olympic success. It is based on an examination of descriptive research on various elite sport systems. Vertinsky notes that:

> The utility of such research lies in providing an intuitive basis for identifying common elements among disparate systems. Such a portfolio may be a mechanism for the transfer of "know-how" and technologies. The reader from one culture makes his/her own sense of the pattern in another culture and selects those features which appear relevant to her/his own culture and problems. "Thick descriptions" of systems also provide a basis for theorizing about the globalization of processes and about what distinguishes one system from another. It is a necessary step in developing a general multinational paradigm for research and a normative basis for a globalized profession.[1]

This chapter suggests that there are ingredients which ensure success in the world of Olympic sport. Indeed, from this perspective, the author would agree with Krueger's[2] assertion that the amount of difference between countries is constantly decreasing, and as a result sport systems are rapidly moving closer together. This author contends that successful countries in international elite sport incorporate more of the factors pointed out in this study than the unsuccessful countries. Awareness of these factors by sport administrators and their implementation can make a difference in a country's success in the international Olympic arena providing the country in question has control over these forces. Many countries do not. By analyzing these factors with respect to the forces which can be controlled in their respective countries, greater chances for success can be ensured and more realistic, obtainable goals can be set by countries interested in better performance in the international arena.

Broom[3] inadvertently outlined a prescription for international success when he suggested that the essential ingredients for success in international competition involved linking talent and education and providing training with competent coaching. For several years in undergraduate classes, this author has used this as a model for assessing a country's potential for international success. However, linking talent and education, and providing training with competent coaching, while valid, have been found to be too limiting as a prescription for success. In all fairness, Broom did not set forth to pick out specific ingredients for success but rather was describing various systems in place at the time. Broom's latest work[4] seems to address this topic even less. The need for a more definitive measurement to assess a country's potential for international success has resulted in the following prescription using Broom's work as a foundation. It suggests that three major factors are responsible for international success: (1) financial support, (2) an ongoing integrated Olympic Sport system, and (3) talent. While on the surface these three headings do not differ greatly from what Broom originally outlined, the subfactors within each of these ingredients expand greatly Broom's ingredients and shed greater light on forces responsible for success.

I. Financial Support

It has been said that money is the root of all evil. In international sport, sad to say, money is the chief ingredient for success. However, the acquisition of money does not alone ensure success, rather it is what is done with that money that ensures success. Financial support for any program should support two primary areas: Training Centers and Personnel.

A. Financial Support for Training Centers

Accessible training centers with adequate supplies and equipment are essential for international success. This would include not only athletic supplies but medical supplies as well. Once adequate equipment and supplies are provided they must be used in such a way as to maximize participation and practice time in an efficient manner. Ideally, training centers should be located near the athlete's home, especially if the athlete is school-aged. While the trend, in recent years, in several countries has been to establish sports boarding schools, it is questionable whether the results warrant such a practice. Moreover, the entire practice of having youngsters 12 years old, and even younger, leave the home environment at such an early age should be increasingly questioned from an ethical standpoint as the quest for international success intensifies.

B. Financial Support for Personnel

Financial support for personnel includes providing athletic talent with the time necessary to train, with well-qualified coaching and with scientific and sports medicine backup.

(i). Providing Athletic Talent with the Time Necessary to Train

No country can achieve international success in sport without athletic talent. However, having talent alone does not ensure success. Having the time to train is essential. How much time should be made available to train? This is a double-edged sword. On the one hand, if excellence is to be achieved, then the more training (within reason and based on science) the better. On the other hand, too much training can be detrimental. In sports such as swimming and gymnastics the norm is often 30+ hours a week for talented 11- and 12-year-old youngsters, not counting the hours spent in travel. To begin with, a question of ethics arises. Child labor laws in most civilized countries outlaw work outside the home for this age group, yet this practice is continually overlooked, even in the most progressive countries.

From a practical point of view excessive training can be quite injurious to the athlete both psychologically and physically. For instance, spending long hours in training can often turn sport from a play experience for a child to a work experience. Rather than the sport experience being joyful it turns into drudgery. The result is burnout and dropout. There are examples of this occurring in both the United States and Canada in sports such as hockey, baseball, football, and basketball. In addition, it is not at all unusual for a youngster to be asked to make a choice at an early age as to the sport he/she will specialize in and train year round. Here again dropouts are inevitable as interest wanes and boredom sets in.

A successful sport system should be able to maintain the interest of its young athletes as they develop up through the system. Similarly, such a system should have provisions for those athletes who wish to enter sport at a later stage in life (late bloomers) or for those who have dropped out and wish to return (a return loop).

Interestingly, concern for the training load of American athletes has resulted in limitations in the number of hours athletes can spend in training each week. This action, however, was not taken to protect young athletes but was implemented by the governing body of major collegiate sport, the National Collegiate Athletic Association. The limitation which restricted the time in which coaches may hold practice to 20 hours a week during the season and 8 hours a week in the off-season (other workouts must be voluntary and unsupervised) was imposed primarily to force men's basketball and football to have their athletes spend more time studying. This move backfired when Janet Evans and Summer Sanders, two top swimmers on the U.S. team, relinquished their remaining collegiate eligibility at Stanford University because the restrictions made it impossible for them to train while in college. Such a scenario demonstrates just how difficult it is to develop international training guidelines so that there is a "level playing field."

Another frequently overlooked aspect of intensive training for youth has been the long-term effects of such sports as gymnastics (low back and joint problems in later life), soccer (vertebrae problems from heading), and American football (degenerative disk problems in the neck).

Making time available for athletes to train for most sport systems usually includes dovetailing the training system with the education of youngsters.[5] Such concepts as specialist classes in which athletes combine sport and education, and extending education, have been deemed to be essential to the success of an elite sport system. As was noted earlier, however, the needs of athletes training for elite sport can clash with policies set up by educational sport bodies (e.g., number of hours allowed to train). It is entirely possible for school-age athletes to succeed in international sport without attending school. In point of fact, young athletes who face a full-time, intense training program not only cannot be expected to succeed in a normal school situation but realistically should not be expected to carry much, if any, of an educational load if the current training practices of extensive hours continues to rise. This tug-of-war between schooling and training will only get worse in the coming years as training and the importance of athletic achievement increases, especially if the athlete competes within the school's competitive setting. The need for international agreements in this area, particularly in the maximum training time allowable for school-age children, is inevitable while differences between what school leagues dictate and the needs of elite performers pose a more difficult hurdle.

(ii). Providing for Well-Trained, Full-Time Coaches with a Low Athlete/Coach Ratio

Ideally a sport system would have all coaches well-trained. The former Soviet Union provided the ultimate model for coaching effectiveness in that specific degrees in coaching were required of all coaches and ongoing training of coaches was the norm. The reality in North America, and numerous other countries, is just the opposite as the study of sport coaching is virtually nonexistent. Those wishing to pursue high level coaching often are forced to obtain higher level degrees in noncoaching disciplines such as education or counseling in order to be employed in universities of higher learning, even though their jobs do not entail teaching in the area in which they receive their degrees. Such a system, tied to education, forces future coaches to divert their interests away from coaching in order to be employable and does not allow for in-depth study of a sport. International experience as players and coaches is also an essential ingredient if optimal coaching practices are to be employed. Several countries require experience at the international level in order to coach internationally, under the belief that you cannot understand it or teach it if you have not been there!

In addition to well-trained coaches, there is evidence that high performance sport requires a low coach/athlete ratio, in some sports as low as 1 coach to 3 athletes (gymnastics). It would seem that as the importance of international success increases, the use of personal trainers will increase thereby bringing the ratio of coach to athlete even lower. It is also important that qualified coaching be available at all levels not just at the elite level and/or for only older athletes. This, of course, again takes money. An ongoing worldwide problem is the dilemma of educating, training and upgrading volunteer youth coaches through certification programs. Unless there are incentives and/or the training is free, volunteer coaches tend to withdraw their services and/or refuse to participate in such programs.

3. Providing Scientific and Sports Medicine Backup

Today, high performance sport demands state-of-the-art techniques in sports medicine especially when it come to surgery, repair and reconstruction. This, of course, limits developing countries drastically. How can a country justify such expense if it cannot meet the bare minimum health requirements necessary for its people? On the other hand, Western medicine is so far removed from natural medicine that countries practicing only Western medicine are at a distinct disadvantage. Centuries-old medicines and treatments are often equal to, if not better than, modern medicine. A combination of the two medical practices would be ideal; however, it is impossible in today's high-tech sports medicine world to survive without modern, highly trained sports medicine personnel to back up the athlete.

II. Ongoing Integrated Olympic Support System

A. An Unbroken Line Up Through the System

A successful system that allows the athlete to continue in a straight line up through the system rather than force the athlete to switch back and forth between various sporting bodies and/or organizations is one that will succeed in the 21st Century. The idea of using the school as the center for the training of elite athletes through interscholastic sport as found in the United States is increasingly becoming obsolete. Broom[6] noted the limitations to this system in that it makes no allowance for the intellectually deficient athlete who cannot get accepted into higher education, and it has no provision for those who graduate (a new system must be found).

Of more significance, however, is the built-in contradiction that exists between sport and education. Ideally, interscholastic sport has as its primary purpose the development of an educational experience for the athlete, not to win or develop the elite athlete. These educational goals can be in direct conflict with the goals of developing an elite sport system for high international performance sport. Often the educational value of sport is compromised at the expense of developing elite athletes. The idea of a sport season ceases and year-round practice becomes the norm. Exposure to a variety of sporting experiences no longer matters, and becoming socially adjusted in a school setting ceases to be an objective. As was noted earlier, American educational sport-governing bodies at the collegiate level have recognized the impact of long training hours on the athlete and have responded with training restrictions of their own, thereby limiting the use of the educational model as an ideal sport model. This has not as yet occurred at the interscholastic level but conflicts have occurred, and it is inevitable that this problem will surface and have to be dealt with since the goals of each program are so different. It would seem that, in the future, elite international athletes in an educational setting would not compete in the educational setting but would use the educational setting with its educational and sport training facilities to advance and develop. The three-in-one training system currently in France attempts to combine the more favorable aspects of a school-based sports model without the inherent problems that come with it. Under this concept permanent training bases for national teams are developed at national institutes for sport. Such institutes train not only high-caliber athletes but also teachers, coaches, and sports organizers, and combine sports training with academic studies as well as scientific research in a boarding setting.[7] Tied to this unbroken system would be a method of identifying just where an athlete lies through some sort of ranking or carding system, a practice which is common in most competitive countries.

B. Communication Network which Maintains the System

One can have a well-designed sequential sport system, but it all goes for naught if there is no communication network to maintain the system. This communication network could be in the form of regular training seminars to update coaches in all parts of the country, the mail system, or an advanced system of computer networks such as SIRC to inform sport administrators and coaches. For developing countries high-tech communication systems are out of the question; however, a simplified system can be implemented which does not require such a high-tech price tag. For example, the former Soviet Union managed to maintain an excellent communication network for sport even though it had one of the most antiquated telecommunication systems of any modern society. Such a network ensures an ongoing integrated, unified sport system countrywide, with all coaches and administrators working from the same plan rather than a system that is piecemeal and splintered throughout the country.

C. International Olympic Sport Exposure

Exposure by athletes to Olympic sports is another factor which increases the chance for international sporting excellence. The fact that, for the most part, Olympic sports were the only sports available and/or seen by the populace in the Soviet Union and GDR during their supremacy ensured that few athletes were drained into non-Olympic sports. This problem of non-Olympic sports draining athletes from potential Olympic sports is most evident in the United States with respect to American football. Originally, concern was centered on professional sport and its effect on Olympic sport. Today, however, the competition for athletes comes not so much from professional or non-Olympic sport (American football, baseball, golf, etc.) so much as it comes from the emphasis by the media and the public on high profile Olympic sports (often moneymakers or high profile television sports) such as soccer, downhill skiing, and basketball. This comes at the expense of other lesser known Olympic sports such as luge, team handball, cross-country skiing, badminton, and field hockey. For example, American coverage of the 1992 Summer Olympics, by NBC, excluded coverage of badminton, field hockey, and team handball. As a result young, potential athletes in America were exposed to and will probably gravitate to the high profile, more lucrative sports as opposed to the lesser known. If the Americans ever hope to be successful in sports such as badminton and field hockey, more access and exposure to these sports is a must. This problem exists in all countries throughout the world and will increase as more high profile sport appears on international television. From an international Olympic sport perspective the result will be a stacking of athletes in a few high profile sports such as basket-

ball, track, tennis, and soccer at the expense of the lesser known sports. For a
system to be truly successful in the 21st Century it will be necessary to make
sure that sport exposure is broad rather than narrow.

D. Ongoing International Competition

To be truly successful in international sport an athlete must be exposed not only
to challenging competition but also to the environment in which international
competition takes place. Most countries do not have the luxury of a large stable
of elite athletes in each sport to challenge each other toward superior performance. Similarly, it is impossible to replicate the atmosphere of international
competition on the home front with its mixture of alien advantage if their teams
have limited international competition.[8] Countries isolated from the sporting
mainstream, such as Australia and New Zealand, and developing countries have
inherent built-in problems in this area. Increased expenditures for travel can
alleviate the problem, but this is usually impossible for developing countries.
Some countries like Kenya have developed large groups of highly talented athletes in one sport (such as distance running) and these athletes feed off themselves in intra-country competition; however, the successful examples are few.

III. Athletic Talent

A. Large Diverse Population

Of all the factors necessary for success in international competition the availability of athletic talent looms as the major ingredient for success. Having a
large healthy population pool to draw from is obviously an advantage, and such
countries as China, Germany, and the United States have a built-in advantage
here. However, population size and health do not ensure success in sports which
require specific physical attributes such as basketball (height), and/or a conducive body type. Countries such as Japan, with a diminutive body type, have
little chance of becoming a dominating power in basketball but have a distinct
advantage in such sports as gymnastics, which requires a smaller physique. It
may be that, in the future, countries which have considerable cultural diversity
in their population will have greater chances for success in international sport
because they will be able to draw on diverse body type.

B. Access for All

The successful sport system in the 21st Century would make use of all its available talent and not just reserve sport to a certain part of society. The mere cost

of a sport can restrict its accessibility. Gymnastics and ice-skating facilities, for example, are seldom found in impoverished countries or in the poverty-stricken area of the inner city, thus overlooking a vast source of talent.

Overcoming sexism and/or religious and cultural bias can increase a country's potential for success in the international sporting theater. This belief in the idea of equal opportunity to compete was primarily responsible for the Eastern Bloc's success in international sport. At least half of the medals won by the Eastern Bloc countries were won by females. Today, women in numerous countries are denied access to sport due to sexist practices. Many countries use religious laws to prevent women from partaking in sport. For example, several Islamic countries deny women access to sport citing the Koran, despite the fact that there are also parts of the Koran which accept female participation in physical activity.[9] One need only look at the absence of women in the Opening Ceremonies at the Barcelona Olympics to see which countries continue to deny women access to sport.

Cultural bias can also affect sport success in various ways. For example, Deford[10] noted a Chinese inferiority complex when competing against Caucasian or black athletes. Similarly, cultures which forbid public touching would have a more difficult time enticing male athletes to wrestle than those cultures with no such stigma.

Stereotyping genders into specific "appropriate" sports is another ongoing problem. Males are often encouraged not to engage in such "feminine" sports as figure skating while females are to avoid masculine sports such as field events in track and field. Such barriers need to be destroyed if equal access is to be achieved.

If a country has a large, healthy population with a sport system accessible to everyone, only two more ingredients are needed to complete the puzzle, and they are an early spotting system of athletic talent, and dedicated and motivated athletes.

C. Early Spotting

Early spotting of athletic talent is essential for success but, as pointed out earlier, there are pitfalls which have to be avoided so that burnout and dropout do not occur.

D. Dedicated and Motivated Athletes

Finally, keeping the athletes (and coaches, I might add) dedicated and motivated is another factor which is specific to each culture. For example, in observing what made the GDR's "miracle machine" work, Krueger[11] noted:

> The more facts are known, the more it becomes obvious that half of the success was due to the social conditions. Athletes and coaches were privileged to such an extent that it was most attractive for any person to become part of this system. You had to wait ten years for a car (often twenty) for a new apartment as are [sic] ordinary citizen, but as an athlete you were rewarded for your services by the same item instantaneously.

This system, which Krueger called a system of "deprivation for most," still exists in several countries but would not apply, say, in Canada or the United States. In these countries the incentives take the form of cash subsidies either through a national card ranking system or direct deferred payments for appearances. Not all incentives, however, need to be monetary in nature. During the Cold War, for example, the honor of competing and representing a country often was more of an incentive than capital rewards. Often, just the prestige of competing in an international event can bring honor to the athlete and drive him/her to work harder.

Conclusions

The purpose of this chapter was to expand on Broom's earlier work[12] and describe, more clearly, the ingredients necessary for a country's success in international Olympic sport. Success in international sport today depends upon three key ingredients: financial support, an ongoing, integrated sport system, and athletic talent. By analyzing these three ingredients, and the various subfactors within each, a country's sport-governing body should be able to determine factors over which they have control and make an educated decision about their country's potential in international sport and from there plan a realistic program for success as measured by their own potential.

Notes

[1]Vertinsky, P. "Methodologies of cross-national behavioral research in sport and physical education: Problems and solutions," *Journal of comparative physical education and sport.* XII: 2 (1990).

[2]Krueger, A. "The sportification of the world: Are there any differences left?, *Journal of comparative physical education and sport.*" II: 2 (1989).

[3]Broom, E. "An international perspective of support systems for highly talented young athletes," *Journal of comparative physical education and sport.* VII (1985).

[4]Broom, E. "Lifestyles of aspiring high performance athletes: A comparison of national models," *Journal of comparative physical education and sport.* XII: 2, (1991).

[5]Broom (1985).

[6]Broom (1985).

[7]Xiong, D. "A comparative study on competitive sports training systems in different countries," *Journal of comparative physical education and sport.* X: 2 (1988).

[8]Waiters, T. "Sports report on early edition: Canada's Olympic soccer coach on qualifying for the Olympics," (Radio Show), April, 1992.

[9]Sfeir, L. "The status of Muslim women in sports: Conflict between cultural tradition and modernization," *International review for sociology of sport.* 20: 4 (1985).

[10]Deford, F. "An old dragon limbers up," *Sports Illustrated.* (August, 1988).

[11]Krueger, A. "Pop the magic dragon (Or what will be left of GDR sports?)," *Journal of comparative physical education and sport.* XII: 2 (1990).

[12]Broom (1985).

Chapter 25

Restructuring Canada's National Sports System: The Legacy of the Dubin Inquiry

Darwin M. Semotiuk

The men's 100-meter race, featuring a classical confrontation between Canada's Ben Johnson and Carl Lewis from the United States, was the premier event of the 1988 Seoul Summer Olympic Games. Ben Johnson won the sprint in a world record time of 9.79 seconds and the celebration began in Canada. Canada's elation turned to bitter disappointment in less than 24 hours when it was revealed that Ben Johnson had tested positive for a banned performance-enhancing substance. Who would have predicted that the events surrounding this 10-second experience would lead to a four-year trial of Canada's national sport system?

This study examines the events, developments, and discussions that concern themselves with redefining Canadian sport in response to the Johnson substance abuse scandal. The appointment of The Honorable Charles L. Dubin to oversee a *Commission of Inquiry into the Use of Drugs and Banned Practices Intended to Increase Athletic Performance* served as the catalyst to stimulate an introspective analysis of the structure, function, and future of amateur sport in Canada. Government commissioned studies, and sport community initiatives, gave rise to a spirited debate on the following important questions: What role should government play in promoting sport? Can mass sport and elite sport coexist? Do ethics and morality have a role to play in sport? What does the future hold for sport? These fundamental questions are examined within the context of the changing political and economic reality facing Canada. This study commences with an analysis of the *Commission of Inquiry into the Use of Drugs and Banned Practices Intended to Increase Athletic Performance*,[1] and concludes with a review of the *Minister's Task Force on Federal Sport Policy—Sport: The Way Ahead*.[2] Activities, reports, and conferences taking place between June 1990 and May 1992 are analyzed (see Appendix I). The chapter concludes by offering further comment and observations on what the future holds for Canadian sport.

The Dubin Inquiry: The Catalyst for Change

The political sensitivity and accountability of the Johnson incident forced the federal government to reassess its priorities in the area of sport. The Government of Canada reacted swiftly in announcing, on October 5, 1988 (11 days after Ben Johnson's 100 meter race), that it would be conducting an inquiry into this incident. The inquiry began on January 11, 1989, and concluded on October 3, 1989, after sitting 91 days, hearing 119 witnesses, taking 14,817 pages of testimony, admitting 295 exhibits and costing the Canadian taxpayers $3.6 million. The 638-page report on drug use in Canadian amateur sport was released in June 1990 and offered 70 recommendations to clean up what Justice Dubin referred to as "a moral crisis" in sport.

Dubin openly questioned and challenged the federal government's overemphasis on high performance sport suggesting that federal sports policy, since 1970, emphasized the primacy of high performance sport and the pursuit of excellence at the international level.[3] Dubin criticized the "medals, flags and national anthem" approach to sport by posing the following question: "Have we, as Canadians, lost track of what athletic competition is all about? Is there too much emphasis by the public and by the media on the winning of a gold medal in Olympic competition as the only achievement worthy of recognition?"[4] A dual vision for sport was advocated through Dubin's insistence that "success in national and international sport should be viewed as a consequence and not as a goal of domestic participation in sport."[5] The Dubin Inquiry condemned the athletes, the coaches, and the system within which they exist and held both groups accountable for these indiscretions. By stating that they should not be held solely responsible, he castigated the federal government's prejudicial use of high performance sport.

The Dubin Report strongly suggested that the federal government has a responsibility to provide sport opportunities for all its citizens and recommended:

- a broad participation in sport, not solely for a focus on elite sport.

- access to sport programs for all Canadians.

• encouragement of women in sport by ensuring equal access to sport programs and facilities.

• encouragement of greater participation in sport by disadvantaged groups.

• support for the disabled in sport; and

• amelioration of regional disparities in access to sport programs and facilities.[6]

Structurally, the Dubin Report recommended that government maintain an arm's length relationship with the sports community and that the measure of success of government funding be linked not to medal count, but to the degree to which it has met broader, social, educational and national goals. Social accountability was introduced as an important issue.

The Dubin Report raised questions that provided the stimulus for a re-evaluation of the national sport system. The federal government's responsibility for the provision of sport was not challenged: its focus, emphasis, and leadership were. Following the Report's release, the Minister of State for Fitness and Amateur Sport established a special secretariat to review its contents and prepare a federal response. The Government announced its Phase I response to the Dubin Report on August 9, 1990, in which it addressed 26 of the 70 Dubin recommendations. The Government had accepted and acted upon those recommendations relating to penalties for individuals named in the Report as having been involved in doping activities. The Government also concurred with the recommendation that an athlete's eligibility to compete should be decided by the athlete's sport governing body, and not by the federal government. The Government's Phase II response, released in January 1991, was based on wide consultations and was more comprehensive in scope. A significantly enhanced Canadian anti-doping campaign to include a combination of deterrence, prevention and control measures was suggested. A strategic element of this campaign was the establishment of the Canadian Anti-Doping Organization, CADO (now called the Canadian Centre for Drug Free Sport). The Phase II response addressed an additional 36 of Mr. Justice Dubin's recommendations, with the eight remaining recommendations dealing with broader sport issues, being considered as part of a final response (Phase III review). *The Minister's Task Force on Federal Sport Policy* was released on May 7, 1992.

Structural and Philosophical Reports on the National Sport System

In responding to the Dubin Report, the Government commissioned two separate reports on the structural and philosophical questions facing the national sport system. *Amateur Sport: Future Challenges*, co-authored by Porter and Cole,[7] primarily dealt with the organizational restructuring of the national sport system, while *Values and Ethics in Amateur Sport—Morality. Leadership and Education*[8] investigated the values and ethics of the major stakeholders in amateur sport in Canada.

The Porter and Cole Report focused on the structural changes required to strengthen sport at the national level. By revitalizing the recommendations of *Towards 2000: Building Canada's Sport System*, the Report outlined the specifics of the national sport structure; the importance and rights of high performance athletes; the role of the corporate community in the financial sponsorship of sport; and the role that the federal government has in the provision of high performance sport independently, and in partnership with, the sport community. Highlights of the Report include:

- advocating an athlete-centered system in which athletes' rights and needs are protected.

- a clarification of the term success, wherein Canadian standards be based on national standards.

- a reaffirmation of the jurisdictional responsibility for sport with the federal government responsible for high performance sport and the other levels of government responsible for domestic sport.

- a greater responsibility and role for the educational system in the development of athletes.

- support for the Government's anti-doping campaign.

- support for broader sport participation and better access to sports programs by women, disadvantaged groups and the disabled.

- strongly encourages financial participation by the commercial and business sectors with a goal of achieving a 50:50 balance of government and non- government funding.

- recommended that the federal government take a less active role in daily sports operations and that NSOs be given the autonomy to manage the public resources allocated to them; and

- that the Canadian Sports Council be created with the authority and the autonomy for providing and coordinating future leadership and direction for amateur sport.[9]

The primary focus of the *Values and Ethics in Amateur Sport: Morality. Leadership and Education* study was to investigate the realm of "high performance sport within the broader context of amateur sport as a whole."[10]

The Report studied the contemporary values of sport and described the views of key players in amateur sport. It concluded that a morality vacuum existed within the high performance system and that there is no longer a concern for sport ethics and winning has become "the end that justifies the means."[11] The need for a policy based on values and ethics, and a system which would enforce that policy was strongly advocated. This position supported Justice Dubin's claim of an overemphasis on high performance sport within the system. Highlights of the *Values and Ethics in Amateur Sport* report include:

- there is a moral crisis in Canadian amateur sport due to the absence of values and ethics.

- the rights of high performance athletes are important.

- leadership, or the lack of ethical leadership, compounds the moral crisis in sport.

- education is seen to have the greatest potential to address the moral crisis in amateur sport and is identified as the highest priority focus.

- re-establish the importance of domestic sport in Canadian society and secure a better balance between it and high performance sport.

- acrimonious relations existed between the values and objectives of the national sports organizations and Sport Canada; and,

> • the development of a collaborative education strategy for the moral development of amateur sport in Canada is strongly recommended.[12]

Two additional studies, *For Excellence: A Symposium on Canadian High Performance Sport*[13] and the *Status of the Athlete* study were also undertaken as part of the organizational evaluation. The initial study focused on the structural, technical, and athlete requirements of the national sport system. It advocated an athlete-centered and technically driven national sport system. To date, the *Status of the Athlete* study has not been released to the public. It is generally accepted that the report will outline restructuring recommendations based on the needs of the athletes. If this is the case, these recommendations will be consistent with other reports supporting the need for an athlete-centered model.

The Sport Community Response

While the federal government continued to pursue its introspective analysis, the sport community undertook some independent initiatives in response to the government's ongoing activities. In convening Sport Forum I and II, the sport community moved to meet the challenge by issuing a collective reply outlining a vision for the future direction of Canadian amateur sport. The sport community seized upon this time of uncertainty and change to voice its concerns, needs, and wants to the federal government.

Four issues have become the cornerstone of the self-analysis undertaken by the sport community. They are:

> • the sport community should become proactive and not reactive.
>
> • the sport community should establish a collective voice.
>
> • the sport community should establish a National Sports Council; and
>
> • the sport community should give more importance to the athletes and their needs and rights.

The sport community's evaluation focused on their role in the Canadian sport system and their relationship with the federal government in the provision of sport for Canadians. The philosophical analysis recognized the importance of an athlete-centered national sport system and a balanced Canadian sport system.

These discussions provided the initial impetus towards redistributing the power within the Canadian sport system. A change in the alliance with the federal government, which would permit shared leadership and a more equitable partnership, is of fundamental importance to amateur sport. The sport community is seeking more autonomy and greater involvement in setting financial and policy objectives.

Sport Forum II, held in October 1991, brought together 200 participants to consider a "new global vision for sport."[14] Sport Forum II developed a vision statement and nine directions detailing the course of action necessary to realize this vision. The sport community advocated a future in which:

> ... all Canadians, regardless of ability, race, gender, class, culture or language have access to Sport... it is community based and encompasses the values of equality, fairness and safety... the dual vision of sport is sustained by strengthening sport's intrinsic benefits while maintaining the importance of excellence.

This vision forms the framework by which the sport community proposes to establish its opinions on the following nine directives:

• towards National Goals for Sport.

• towards Removing Roadblocks.

• towards a New Relationship with Government.

• towards Changes in Sport Governing Bodies.

• towards a New Relationship with Education.

• towards Better Communication.

• towards Better Relations with Athletes.

• towards International Leadership.

• towards Collective Action and Leadership.[15]

All directives center around two main foci: the achievement of greater autonomy, and the movement towards collective action. The movement is towards a more equal partnership, characterized by increased consultation and collaboration. To achieve greater autonomy, a "credible overall leadership structure" is required "to chart the direction of Canadian sport in line with our vision... this collective structure must include all the partners in the Canadian Sport System."[16]

Work continues toward putting some substance on the subject of collective mechanism—the mandate of Sport Forum I as directed by delegates of Sport Forum II. In response to the release of the *Minister's Task Force on Federal Sport Policy*, the Sports Federation of Canada has indicated that it would be prepared to coordinate a sport community response to the report.[17]

The sport community's activity and response continues to be characterized by an element of mistrust and a lack of team spirit amongst its members. Many do not have confidence in the Sport Federation of Canada to represent the views of Canadian amateur sport. National level coaches, national level high performance athletes, sport science representatives, the Canadian Olympic Association, and several national sports governing bodies have declined to participate in the Sport Forum conferences. The greatest amount of anxiety appears to surround the decision regarding the mechanism of collective leadership. Individuals in Canada's sport community seem to be unprepared to sacrifice their autonomy and territory for the collective benefit of the national sport system.

Sport: The Way Ahead—Minister's Task Force on Federal Sport Policy

After numerous delays, the long-awaited Minister's Task Force on Federal Sport Policy was released on May 7, 1992. The three-member task force (Cal Best, Marjorie Blackhurst, and Lyle Makosky) was given a sweeping mandate to address:

- the purpose and place of sport in Canadian society.

- the values and ethics that should shape its future conduct.

- the roles and responsibilities of national sport governing bodies; and

- the federal government's future role in sport policy and programs.[18]

The *Minister's Task Force on Federal Sport Policy* made 117 recommendations in its 311-page report. The main ones are:

- governments and sports bodies should develop an integrated sports plan for Canada, based on "a shared vision, essential values and national goals."

- develop strategies to raise the profile of amateur sports in Canada to offset the dominance of professional sports—mostly American and mostly on television. This would include having top Canadian athletes perform more often at home and holding more top-level international competitions.

- develop an approach to sports focused on athletes rather than sport organizations and government agencies. Establish a Canadian Association of Athletes and increase financial support for high performance athletes.

- develop a new sports financing system that would give money to a set of core Canadian sports and reduce the list of financed international sports.

- phase out direct control of how sports organizations spend taxpayers' money.

- develop a system of professional coaching that would certify coaches and give them financial support.

- support the participation of women, natives, the disabled and other disadvantaged groups in sport. For example, the report recommends creation of an independent indigenous people's sport secretariat.

- harmonize financing policies and sports development programs among provinces and the federal government. Promote links between schools and sports clubs.[19]

Reaction to the Task Force Report has been mixed. Generally speaking, Canadian amateur sports officials were impressed with the Report's recommendations, but had one big question: Just where is the government going to get the money to do all this?[20] When asked this question, Sports Minister Pierre Cadieux provided little assurance when he replied, "I don't know." Another observer cynically offered the following views:

> Imagine happy, united Canadians participating in sports, loving fairplay, hosting international competitions and disclaiming professional games on T.V. to watch well trained amateur athletes. A kind of athletic nationalism. Seem a little idealistic? Naive? Yup.[21]

Amateur sports groups have generally welcomed the new focus on cooperative planning in the Task Force Report. However some recommendations, particularly to limit funding to a core of "Canadian" sports instead of the current array of 116 sanctioned games, raised questions.

The Task Force Report will form the basis for a new federal sports policy. Sports Minister Pierre Cadieux is expected to announce this policy in the Fall of 1992 after consulting sports organizations, provincial governments, athletes, coaches and the public.

Notes

---

[1]Dubin, Charles L. *Commission of inquiry into the use of drugs and banned practices intended to increase athletic performance.* Ottawa, Ontario: Minister of Supply and Services, 1990.

[2]Best, J. C., Marjorie Blackhurst, and Lyle Makosky, *Minister's task force on federal sport policy. Sport: The way ahead,* Ottawa, Ontario: Ministry of State, Fitness and Amateur Sport, 1992.

[3]Dubin, p. 52.

[4]Dubin, p. 513.

[5]Dubin, p. 526.

[6]Dubin, p. 527.

[7]Porter, Bob, and John Cole, *Amateur sport: Future challenges. Second report of the standing committee on health and welfare, social affairs, seniors and the status of women.* Ottawa, Ontario: Ministry of State, Fitness and Amateur Sport, 1990.

[8]Blackhurst, Marjorie, Angela Schneider, and Dorothy Strachan, *Values and ethics in amateur sport: morality, leadership, education*. Ottawa, Ontario: Ministry of State, Fitness and Amateur Sport, 1991

[9]Porter & Cole.

[10]Blackhurst, Schneider & Strachan.

[11]Blackhurst, Schneider & Strachan, p. 3

[12]Blackhurst, Schneider & Strachan.

[13]*For excellence: A symposium on Canadian high performance sport proceedings*. Ottawa, Ontario: Ministry of State, Fitness and Amateur Sport, 1990; and, Status of the Athlete Study.

[14]*Towards a new vision for sport in Canada*, Ottawa, Ontario: Sports Federation of Canada, Report of the proceedings of Sport Forum II, November 5, 1991, p. 4.

[15]*Towards a new vision for sport in Canada*, p. 7

[16]*Towards a new sport vision,* Ottawa, Ontario: Sports Federation of Canada, a consultation paper for national organizations, July 30, 1991, p. 7

[17]Sports Federation Communication, April 29,1992

[18]*Fitness and Amateur Sport - Annual Report. 1990-1991*, Ottawa, Ontario: Ministry of State, Fitness and Amateur Sport, 1992, p. 24

[19]Best, Blackhurst, & Makosky.

[20]Starkman, Randy. "Who has money for big list?" *The Toronto Star.* (May 8, 1992), p. D1.

[21]Cox, Bob. "A dose of athletic nationalism," *The London Free Press.* (May 8, 1992), p. A1-2.

Chapter 26

Los Juegos de las Américas: Four Inter-American Multisport Competitions

Richard V. McGehee

International multisport competition among countries of the Western Hemisphere has existed for over 70 years. Four of the principal festivals are the Central American and Caribbean, Pan American, Central American and Caribbean University, and Central American Games. Figure 1 summarizes the years and sites where these events have been held.

First Central American Games—Guatemala, 1921

As part of the centennial celebration of independence of the Central American region in 1921, four countries participated in a sport festival in Guatemala City which was billed as "The First Central American Games."[1] Athletes from El Salvador, Costa Rica, Honduras, and Guatemala competed in 18 track and field events, tug-of-war, baseball, football, tennis, and swimming. It was intended that the competition continue on a regular basis, the second games to be held in El Salvador two years later. However, the 1923 Games were not held and the series failed to develop.

South American Games—Brazil, 1922

In 1922 Brazil held its independence centennial celebration which included athletic games. Brazil, Argentina, Uruguay, and Chile participated, and the events included track and field, and soccer.[2] The attendance was small at these first South American Games, and even less was anticipated for the proposed second Games.[3] Physical education and sport were not highly developed in many of the South American countries. Furthermore, distances were great and travel was difficult between the major cities. Thus, this series did not become established either.

Central American Games	Central Amer & Caribbean Games	Pan American Games	Central American and Caribbean University Games
1) 21 Guatemala City (23 proposed for El Salvador; not held)	1) 26 Mexico City, MEX		
	2) 30 Havana, CUB		
	3) 35 San Salvador, ES		
	4) 38 Panama, PAN (name changed to CA&C Games)		
	{Planned for 42; not held because of war}	{Planned for 42 (BA); not held because of war}	
	5) 46 Barranquilla, COL	{Planned for 46; not held}	
	6) 50 Guatemala City	1) 51 Buenos Aires, ARG	
	7) 54 Mexico City {planned for Panama}	2) 55 Mexico City, MEX	
	8) 59 Caracas, VEN	3) 59 Chicago {planned for Cleveland}	
	9) 62 Kingston, JAM	4) 63 Sao Paulo, BRA	
	10) 66 San Juan, PR	5) 67 Winnipeg, CAN	
	11) 70 Panama, PAN	6) 71 Cali, COL	1) 72 San Juan, PR
1) 73 Guatemala City	12) 74 Santo Domingo, DR	7) 75 Mexico, MEX	2) 75 Mexico City
2) 77 El Salvador {81 proposed for Nicaragua; not held}	13) 78 Medellin, COL	8) 79 San Juan, PR	3) 77 Santo Domingo, DR
	14) 82 Cuba	9) 83 Caracas, VEN	4) 82 Barquisimeto, VEN
3) 86 Guatemala	15) 86 Dominican Republic	10) 87 Indianapolis, USA	5) 86 Havana, CUB
4) 90 Tegucigalpa	16) 90 Mexico {planned for Guatemala}	11) 91 Havana, CUB	6) 90 Guatemala City
5) 93 El Salvador {Originally ceded to Nicaragua}	17) 93 Puerto Rico	12) 95 Mar de Plata, ARG	

Pan American Winter Games
1) 90 Las Leñas, ARG

Figure 1—Four Inter-American Multisport Events with Initial Years and Sites

Central American and Caribbean Games

A key person in the development of inter-American Olympic-type competition was present at the Brazilian Independence Games in Rio de Janeiro. This was Count Henry Baillet-Latour, vice president of the International Olympic Committee at the time, and later IOC president, from 1925 to 1942. He represented the IOC in Rio de Janeiro to promote the formation of national Olympic committees and the holding of regional games.[4] In January of 1923, Baillet-Latour traveled to Mexico where he proposed and encouraged (1) the formation of a Mexican National Olympic Committee, (2) the alliance of Mexican sport federations with the international federations, (3) the participation of Mexican athletes in the 1924 Olympic Games in Paris, and (4) the hosting, by Mexico, of a regional sport festival, to be called the Central American Games, in 1926.[5]

Mexico made its first appearance in the Olympics with a small team that went to Paris in 1924. At that time, representatives of the Middle America region met for the purpose of discussing the initiation of Central American Games in Mexico in 1926, and the regulations for these Games ("*La Carta Fundamental*") were approved.[6] The 14 nations invited to participate in 1926 included Mexico, Guatemala, El Salvador, Honduras, Nicaragua, Costa Rica,

Panama, Colombia, Venezuela, Cuba, Haiti, the Dominican Republic, Jamaica, and Puerto Rico. Only Mexico, Cuba, and Guatemala competed in these first regional games in the Western Hemisphere recognized by the IOC. Exclusively male teams participated in shooting, fencing, basketball, baseball, tennis, swimming, and track and field. In addition to the official sports, President Machado of Cuba sponsored a rifle shooting competition between Mexican and Cuban soldiers. At the conclusion of the Games, there was another exhibition event featuring Tarahumara Indians, who ran 100 kilometers from the town of Pachuca to Mexico City.[7]

The 1926 Games were followed, in 1930, at Havana with more countries in attendance, more sports, and the first participation of women, although that was only tennis competition among several Cuban women.[8] Representatives of Cuba visited all the Central America countries (except Nicaragua) in order to encourage their attendance at the Games. Two Cuban warships were utilized to transport the athletes of the five Central American nations, and Jamaica, to Havana. Puerto Rico made its first appearance at the Games, arriving on a commercial airplane, which was not common in 1930. Soccer and volleyball, sports which had been originally scheduled for Mexico in 1926, were added to the program.

The third Games were held in El Salvador, in 1935, after a one-year postponement due to an earthquake. It had been thought that Guatemala, as one of the original participants in the series, would host the third Games, but they were not able to do so. Beginning with the fourth games in Panama, the name of the event was changed from Central American, to Central American and Caribbean Games. Venezuela and Colombia participated in the festival for the first time in these Games of 1938. Also, for the first time, there were exhibitions and competitions in the fine arts, using sport motifs, and other activities outside the usual athletic events.[9]

Over the years there has been a general increase in the number of participating countries and athletes, and the number of sports in the program.[10] The Games have been held in sites distributed geographically throughout the region, although rarely within the five Central American republics proper, represented only by El Salvador in 1935 and Guatemala in 1950. Until 1950 there had been little construction of new sport facilities for the festival. However, in preparation for the VIth Games, Guatemala built a large stadium, gymnasium, swimming and shooting facilities, velodrome, tennis courts, baseball park, and an administrative center, *El Palacio de los Deportes*.

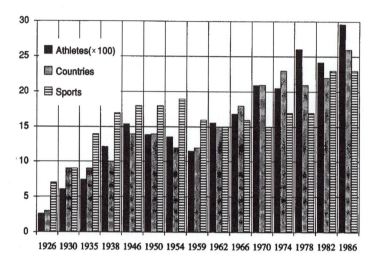

Figure 2—Numbers of Athletes, Countries, and Sports by Year in the Central American and Caribbean Games

Twenty-nine countries, most of them bordering the Caribbean Sea, are now eligible for the Central American and Caribbean Games, which were held for the 16th time in Mexico City in 1990. The latest edition of the Games utilized the magnificent facilities already in existence in Mexico City and other sites within Mexico. The leading Central American and Caribbean Games medal winners are shown in Figure 3. Given the relative geographic areas, populations, and resources of the participating nations, it is interesting to note that Cuba is in first place in medals won and, perhaps even more striking, that Puerto Rico is in third place. Cuba and Mexico have been the principal medal winners since the beginning of the series.[11]

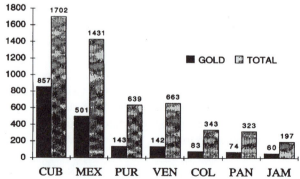

Figure 3—Numbers of Medals of Top Medal Winners in C.A. and C. Games

Pan American Games

The grandest sport festival of the Americas, and the only one that brings together all countries of the hemisphere, is the Pan American Games. At the 1932 Olympics, in Los Angeles, informal meetings were held by the representatives of several Western Hemisphere countries, and Mexico proposed the formation of a Sport Confederation for all the countries of the Americas.[12] Representatives of American nations met again at the 1936 Berlin Olympics and approved the holding of Pan American Games. Avery Brundage, the president of the U.S. Olympic Committee became very interested in this idea, and in 1937 he and George Marshall organized an Inter-American competition in Dallas, Texas. The participants included the United States, Canada, Cuba, Argentina, Brazil, Colombia, Chile, Paraguay, and Peru. This was the first attempt to unite all of the athletes of the Americas in a multi-sport festival. When the XIIth Olympic Games, scheduled for 1940, were canceled because of the war in Europe, the Argentinian Olympic Committee urged a meeting of Western Hemisphere countries. Sixteen countries took part in a congress and set up the Pan American Sporting Committee with Avery Brundage elected as its first president. The first Games were to be held in Buenos Aires in 1942, but they were postponed because of the war. They were planned then for 1946 but again had to be canceled.

At the 1948 Olympics in London, representatives of the Americas held their second Pan American Congress and approved the year 1951 for the initiation of the Pan American Games. In 1959 the Pan American Sports Organization was created. The permanent location of PASO is in Mexico City and its president, since 1975, has been Mario Vásquez Raña, a Mexican newspaper owner and sports enthusiast. From its beginnings, with 22 countries participating in 18 events at Buenos Aires in 1951, the Pan American Games has grown to an immense spectacle last staged in Cuba in 1991. The United States, Cuba, Argentina, Canada, Brazil, and Mexico have won the most gold and total medals (see Figure 5).[13]

Only a few U.S. athletes (including a seven-member basketball team and a single gymnast) made the long, costly trip to the initial Pan American Games, and host Argentina won the most gold and total medals. This was the last time, until the 1991 Games, that the U.S. did not win the greatest number of Pan American gold medals. Baseball was included in the 1951 program and was won by Cuba, as it has been on all but three occasions since the initial Pan American Games.[14] Mexico hosted the 1955 Games and new events included synchronized swimming, volleyball, and women's basketball. The Mexican women won volleyball and the U.S. women won their first of many titles in basketball. The 1959 Pan American Games were originally planned for Cleveland but, in an effort to cut taxes, the U.S. Congress withdrew $5 million of federal funds that had been ear-marked for the Games. Cleveland could not find sufficient financial backing elsewhere, Guatemala City and Rio de Janeiro, the first and second alternates, both withdrew and on August 3, 1957, Chicago was chosen over Sao Paulo, Brazil. Yachting was added to the program and 15 nations competed in the sport. The visitors borrowed U.S. boats for this event, which was held on Lake Michigan. Oscar Robertson led the U.S. basketball team to victory and Althea Gibson came out of retirement to win the tennis singles gold.

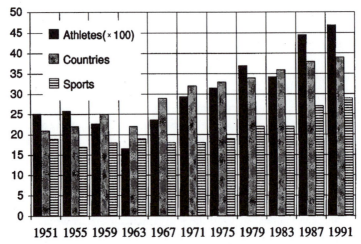

Figure 4—Numbers of Countries, Athletes, and Sports in the Pan American Games

At the fourth Games in Sao Paulo, the sport of judo was added, and the Mexican mixed doubles tennis team won the gold medal for the fourth straight time. For the 1967 Games, in Winnipeg, 29 of the 33 eligible nations sent teams but the U.S. was the only country with a complete contingent. Schollander and Spitz of the United States starred in swimming and Arthur Ashe, in men's tennis. The 1975 Games were originally awarded to Santiago de Chile and then transferred to Sao Paulo, Brazil, but both withdrew, and Mexico City stepped in with only 10 months left for preparation. Thirty-three nations participated, Greco-Roman wrestling was added to the program, and CBS-TV covered the first of three Games. New facilities worth $60 million were constructed for the 1979 Games in San Juan, Puerto Rico. New sports in the program included men's and women's archery, roller-skating, and softball. The detection of widespread drug use

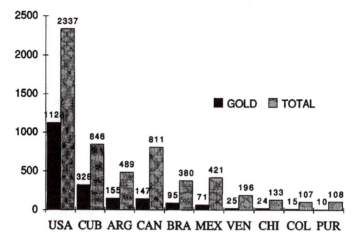

Figure 5—Medals Won by Country in Pan American Games

was the big news from the 1983 Pan American Games in Caracas, and political conflict between the United States and Cuba and Nicaragua was part of the story of the Xth Games in Indianapolis. Carl Lewis bettered the long jump record by a foot and a half in 1987. Cuba's Javier Sotomayor set a new high jump record, and Ana Fidelia Quirot set new records in both the 400 and 800 meters.

Cuba hosted the Pan American Games most recently, in 1991, and new records were set in the number of countries and athletes participating. The United States' economic embargo and travel restrictions made financing the Games difficult for the host. ABC-TV (American Broadcasting Company) had agreed on a figure of $9 million to pay for television rights but, initially, the U.S. Treasury Department would not allow any payment to be made to Cuba. After going through the courts, and further negotiations with Cuba, ABC and Turner Network Television were allowed to send crews and equipment, but ABC was restricted by the Treasury Department to a crew of 300 and a spending limit of around $1.2 million while in Cuba.[15] The events were held in newly constructed facilities, such as the Pan American Stadium, velodrome, and tennis and swimming complexes, as well as in many of the excellent sport facilities already existing in Havana and Santiago de Cuba.

Winter Pan American Games

The first Winter Pan American Games, planned for 1989 in Las Leñas, Argentina,[16] were canceled because of poor snow conditions. However, they were held in September, 1990, and included alpine, Nordic, and freestyle skiing as well as the biathlon.[17]

Central American and Caribbean University Games

The Central American and Caribbean University Games were first held in Puerto Rico in 1972, and the event has expanded from an original program of eight nations, competing in four sports in 1972, to 16 countries in seven sports in 1990. Cuba has dominated this competition.[18]

Central American Games

In the early 1970s, sport leaders in Guatemala received IOC approval for a new series of games which would include only the geographic region of Central America. They wanted to provide more opportunities for competition for the athletes of the countries of the region, without the dominating influence of sport powers such as Cuba, Mexico, and the United States. The central figure in negotiations with Avery Brundage and other IOC officials was the executive secretary of the Guatemalan National Olympic Committee, a woman named Ingrid Keller. Señora Keller began her crusade for Central American sport at the meetings of the Central American and Caribbean sport organization in Panama in 1970. There she was elected to membership in the organization and had an opportunity to speak with General José Clark Flores of Mexico, the vice president of the IOC. General Clark died before she could cultivate any strong support from him, but she continued to travel extensively, mostly at her own expense, to seek the support of Latin American sport leaders and IOC officials. She eventually received approval for the Central American Games from Avery Brundage, just as he was leaving the IOC presidency and then from Lord Killanin, who became president in Munich in 1972.[19]

The Central American Sport Organization was formed, and the first of these Central American Games were held in 1973 at the fine sport facilities that Guatemala had constructed for the VIth Central American and Caribbean Games of 1950. The second Games were held in El Salvador in 1977, and Nicaragua was awarded the third Games. However, the Sandinista revolution in Nicaragua, and subsequent military and economic attacks on their new government, made it impossible for them to host the Games. After a lapse of nine years, Guatemala again took the lead and hosted the event in 1986. Honduras was awarded the fourth Games, which were held in Tegucigalpa in 1990 and set new records in the number of athletes, participating nations, and sports. For the fourth Central American Games, Honduras built extensive new sport facilities

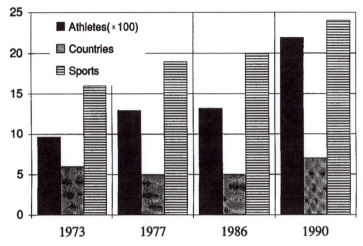

Figure 6—Numbers of Athletes, Countries, and Sports by Year in the Central American Games

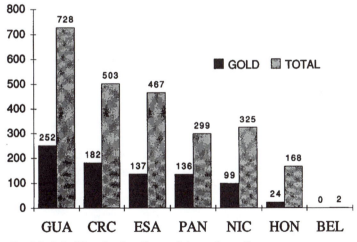

Figure 7—Medals Won in the Central American Games

including baseball and track and field stadia, three gymnasia, tennis courts, and a swimming pool.

Guatemala has won most Central American Games medals. Panama might have had that distinction but did not participate in 1986 and was able to send only two athletes for the 1990 Games, which were held in January, shortly after the U.S. invasion of Panama. Belize, the former British Honduras until obtaining its independence in 1981, has participated in the Central American and Caribbean Games since 1970. However, it was not included in the Central American Games until 1990. Belize was admitted to the Central American Sport Organization just two months before the 1990 Games.

Conclusion

The international athletic games of the Americas have grown and prospered since their beginnings in Guatemala in 1921. The great diversity of resources, national policies and international relations within the Western Hemisphere have been factors in the differing participation rates and athletic successes among the included countries. However, by bringing together individuals from such diverse backgrounds, the Games offer not only opportunities for high level sport competition but, more importantly, possibilities for promoting brotherhood and peace.

Notes

[1]McGehee, Richard V. "The rise of modern sport in Guatemala and the first Central American Games," *International Journal of the History of Sport.* 9 (1992), pp. 132-140.

[2]*"El corredor chileno Plaza ganó la carrera marathon,"* El Demócrata. (September 18, 1922), p. 4; "El evento más popular del programa de los juegos Olímpicos sudamericanos," *El Demócrata.* (September 18, 1922), p. 4;"La comisión olímpica acordó hoy," *El Demócrata.* (September 21, 1922), p. 4.

[3]Aguilar Reyes, A. *México en los IV Juegos Deportivos Centroamericanos y del Caribe.* Mexico, D. F.: La Afición, 1938.

[4]*Memoria del Congreso Técnico de los VIII Juegos Deportivos Centroamericanos y del Caribe.* Mexico, D. F., 1953, p. 35.

[5]*"Mexico es invitado a la Olimpiada del año de 1924,"* El Universal. (February 13, 1923), p. 5.

[6]Montesinos, E., and S. Barros. *Centroamericanos y del Caribe: los más antiguos juegos deportivos regionales del mundo.* Havana, Cuba: Editorial Científico-Técnica, 1983.

[7]*"Los rifleros cubanos derrotaron ayer a los mexicanos,"* Excélsior. (October 30, 1926), p. 3; *"La sensacional carrera de los cien kilómetros,"* Excélsior. (November 7, 1926), p. 1.

[8]Montesinos & Barros.

[9]Montesinos & Barros.

[10]Ferreiro, Toledano, A. *Centroamérica y el Caribe a través de sus juegos.* Mexico, D.F.: Artes Gráficas Rivera, 1986.

[11]Ferreiro.

[12]*Memoria de los VIII Juegos Panamericanos.* San Juan, Puerto Rico, 1979, pp. 23-28; Emery, C. R. *The story of the Pan American Games.* Kansas City: Ray-Gay, 1972.

[13]*Compendium of the results of the Pan American Games from Buenos Aires 1951 to Indianapolis 1987* (4th ed.). Mexico City: Pan American Sports Organization, 1989; Pitts, J. "Cuba concludes Games with gold rush," *USA Today.* (August 19, 1991), p. 1C.

[14]Emery; Plant, G., & B. Gresham (Eds.). *The USA in the Olympic movement.* Colorado Springs, CO.: U.S. Olympic Committee, 1988, pp. 46-50.

[15]Brown, R. "ABC navigating choppy waters to Cuba," *Broadcasting.* 121: 55 (1991).

[16]Miller, P.M. *"Buscando oro (plata y bronce) en la nieve," Américas.* 41:2 (1989), pp. 42-45.

[17]USOC personal communication, June 8, 1992.

[18]*Los VI Juegos Deportivos Universitarios.* Guatemala City; publicity brochure. No date.

[19]*Guatemala Os Saluda.* Guatemala City; publicity bulletin. No date or author.

Part 7: Sport in the Global Village: Comparative Perspectives

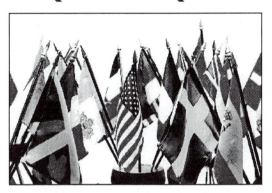

Part 7: Sport in the Global Village: Comparative Perspectives

Part Seven includes nine studies which actually compare various factors regarding sport and/or physical education. One is a comparison of regions within one country, six compare two countries' systems, one is a six-nation study, and one focuses on multiculturalism itself. As such, these are examples of the problem approach to comparative studies and offer good insight into what is effective and less effective in situation-specific examples.

Chapter 31, the inherently cross-cultural study, examines the situations created by what might loosely be called "sport exchanges." Often, individuals assume that an exchange must be successful just because it happens, but the author gives information on how to maximize the opportunities for success in such exchange situations. The conclusions indicate that individual attitudes are vital with respectful, nonjudgmental, people-oriented, flexible individuals being the most successful. This chapter would be useful reading for anyone planning to compete or coach abroad, or take a team overseas, or for someone hosting people from abroad. Further conclusions that include the warning against thinking that "different" is "wrong" or "inferior" should be written on every comparativist's heart.

Chapter 27 compares two regions within one country—the P.R.C.—from the perspective of physical culture educational institutions, where one is state (i.e., national government) funded and one is province funded. Factors compared include administration, staff, programs, financing, and facilities. State funding was found to convey a range of advantages.

In the six two-nation comparison studies, the places represented are the United States, P.R.C., England, Kenya, Hong Kong, Macau, Germany and Czechoslovakia (some countries appearing more than once). The topics compare aspects as diverse as intercollegiate athletics, politics in sport/physical education, women's involvement, sporting excellence, selection and development of talent, and motor performance.

The comparison of intercollegiate athletics was conducted between the United States and P.R.C. and is of particular interest because it is written by a Chinese, and also because it shows how two very different political systems can seek to make use of similar programs, albeit for different reasons and with different philosophies. It is noteworthy that China's interest in intercollegiate sport is in order to promote world class athletic performance, at a time when many suggest that linking athletic success to educational institutions may be detrimental to that success. The author comments on the different interpretations of "amateur" in the two countries, and also on the widely different philosophies that result. For example, in the United States, intercollegiate athletics serve the needs of a variety of people—athletes, cheerleaders, the student body, boosters, administrators, etc.—whereas in China the need is only to develop elite athletes for international competition.

Although juxtaposive rather than fully comparative, politics—concluded to be so important in the Chinese/United States study—form the central topic in the examination of England and Kenya. Selected points of political and sporting interaction are reviewed historically for England, and then for Kenya, with the conclusion that politics and sport/physical education are deeply intertwined in each country.

The mark of colonialism so clear in Kenya's sporting history is also covered in the Hong Kong and Macau comparison of women in sport. Colonized by Great Britain and Portugal respectively, there is a large difference in per capita GDP which may account for some of the variation in sports provision, but in both places opportunities for participation by females are greatest within educational institutions.

Historical comparison is the methodology used to examine sporting excellence in England and Germany. A major difference was that the focus of sport was traditionally on schools in England and more on clubs in Germany, although the underlying philosophies were quite similar. In both countries, however, a growing need to identify and nurture excellence (and perhaps even sometimes at the expense of sport for the many) began to assert itself in the 1970's. This change in attitudes has led to new programs, designed for the elite, being implemented.

The question of how a country develops sports talent is also investigated by Jones in his comparison of provincial swimming in Sichuan, China, and Leicestershire, England. In the former, young swimmers with potential are actively supported by the province as an outcome of the entire sports system in China, and in the latter individuals are very much on their own to do their best in the rather nebulous system of English county sport.

The authors of the final two chapters in this section used quantitative rather than qualitative or descriptive methods of research. The comparison of daily physical activity and motor performance among German and Czechoslovakian children revealed that the Germans spent more time in physical activity but that this by itself did not necessarily lead to an improvement in motor performance. The various cross-cultural differences and their impact on testing were also revealed.

The other study that employed empirical research methods looked into attitudes and youth participation patterns in sport, and included data from six countries. Results are reported by country, by gender, and by whether respondents were players or nonplayers. The instrument was a Likert-type scale of responses to 19 statements about interscholastic sport. There was high correlation between students and across countries to indicate that such sport was valued and a source of pride.

In a time of such rapid change in the world, such studies as these represent honest attempts to evaluate how well a system is delivering what it is supposed to, and suggest where change may be necessary for future success—whatever that success is deemed to be. In every case, however, prevailing cultural traditions and mores are always the greatest determinant of outcome.

Shirley H.M. Reekie

Chapter 27

A Comparison of the National and Provincial Institutes of Physical Culture in the People's Republic of China

Frank H. Fu

Long before the founding of the People's Republic of China (PRC) in 1949, physical culture was very important to the Chinese people. Mao indicated that "physical culture is the complement of virtue and wisdom... Attention should be first given to a child's physical needs, there will be time later to cultivate his morality and wisdom."[1] As in other communist states, the development and promotion of sport continued to be important in China as a vehicle for nation-building, integrating a multinational population, improving defense capability, improving health and hygienic conditions, and gaining international recognition and prestige.[2] This trend was confirmed with the establishment of the Institutes of Physical Culture and Sports Schools in the 1950s. The cultural revolution put a halt to most development in the 1960s and 1970s, but the open-door policy in the 1980s again revived the drive towards modernization and international exchange.

Recent changes in Europe have shifted the focus of international competitions between the USA and the former USSR, to competition between the USA and the PRC. While the centralized approach on talent selection and training has proven to be effective in the former Soviet empire and Eastern bloc countries, its benefits were realized by the PRC only in recent years. There were 17 state-funded institutes of physical culture in China, dispersed in different parts of the country, and many others that were funded by the provincial governments. The importance of the provincial governments as an alternate source of funding in the development of sports talent was realized by the success of the national games held at Guangzhou in 1987. It was also obvious that the success of many of the national teams was dependent on the supply of talented coaches and athletes from the provinces.

This chapter discusses the similarities and differences of the state-funded and province-funded institutes of physical culture. Since they are both breeding grounds for future teachers, athletes, coaches, and researchers, knowledge in this area will contribute to a better understanding of the future development of physical education and sport in the PRC.

General Background of the PRC in the 1990s

The unequal progress made in economical and political reforms during the modernization movement of the 1980s led to the tragic events of June 4, 1989. Some have suggested that this precipitated the changes in Russia and Eastern bloc countries. After a cooling period of two years, Deng Xiao-peng reiterated the need to pursue the modernization program with better control and supervision. This was highlighted by Deng's visit to the Guangdong province and special economic zone in the spring of 1992.

Political influence is strongest in the Hubei province, home of China's capital, Beijing, but the southern coastal provinces are better exposed to outside investors, and this resulted in the formation of various economic zones. The preferential treatment given to the state-funded institutes was slowly matched, if not surpassed, by their province-funded counterparts. Among the 17 state-funded institutes, the Beijing Institute of Physical Education was on the top of the priority list. The Guangzhou Institute of Physical Culture was one of the best representatives of those in the affluent coastal provinces in the south. This chapter will focus on comparing the two institutes in terms of administrative structure, staff resources, programs offered, financial resources, and sports facilities.

Administrative Structure

The comparison of the administrative structure of the Guangzhou Institute or Physical Culture (GI) and Beijing Institute of Physical Education (BI) is presented in Table 1. While the two institutes are of similar size in terms of staff and students, GI has a larger administrative staff. The Communist Party is represented at GI by the President and the Party Secretary. At BI, daily affairs are handled by the President, while the role of the Communist Party is represented by a Vice-President. The state-controlled All China Sports Federation is the highest authority at BI and at GI it is the Provincial Higher Education Authority. The ratio of employees to administrative staff at BI is 5 to 1 and at GI, 2 to 1.

Table 1—Comparison of Administrative Structure.

	Guangzhou Institute	**Beijing Institute**
Highest Authority	Provincial Higher Education Authority	All China Sports Federation
Frequency of Meeting	Six Times Per Year	Four Times Per Year
Highest Authority within Institute	Institute Communist Party Committee	Administrative Affairs (I) Committee and Staff Assembly (II)
Frequency of Meeting	24 Times Per Year	26 Times Per Year (I) and Two Times Per Year (II)
Administrative Staff	President -1 Vice-Presidents-2 Party Secretary-1 Unit Heads-14 Others-244 Total-262	President-1 Vice-Presidents-3 Unit Heads-15 Administrative Asst.-47 Others-63 Total-129

Staff Resources

The student to teacher ratio shows the major difference between the institutes (Table 2). By most standards, the student to teacher ratio of 8.8 to 1 is very good as in the case of GI. At BI, there is a 4 to 1 student to teacher ratio. One would expect the quality of teaching and coaching at both institutes to be excellent.

Table 2—Comparison of Staff Resources.

	Guangzhou Institute	**Beijing Institute**
Number of Administrative Staff	262	129
Number of Teaching Staff	242	488
Number of Students	2136	1928
Student to Teacher Ratio	8.8 to 1	4 to 1
Distribution of Teaching Faculty		
Professor	15	25
Associate Professor	39	162
Assistant Professor	88	187
Instructor	17	114
Other	83	0

The distribution of academic rank in the institutes shows that the state-funded BI outnumbered the province-funded GI. There are 10 more professors, 121 more associate professors, 99 more assistant professors, and 97 more instructors at BI. One of the reasons for the enormous difference is the emphasis on research and graduate programs at BI. The administration/teaching staff to student ratio for BI is 3.1 to 1, and 4.2 to 1 at GI. This is outstanding considering the accepted standard of 10 to 1.

Academic Programs

The academic programs offered at GI were mainly for the preparation of physical education teachers and coaches. There are Master's programs in Teaching Methods with 18 students (Table 3). At BI, teacher and coach preparation programs are offered, but nearly one third of the students major in other areas, such as Wu Shu, Sports Science, Sports Management, and Adult Education. BI also offers a Doctoral program.

Table 3—Academic Programs Offered.

	Guangzhou Institute	Beijing Institute
Undergraduate	2118 Students	1864 Students
Graduate	18	64
Undergraduate Major		
Teaching	1718 Students	789 Students
Coaching	400	590
Other	0	585
Graduate Degrees		
Master's	offered	offered
Ph.D.	not offered	offered
Departments		
Physical Education	offered	offered
Sports Training	offered	offered
Wu Shu	not offered	offered
Sports Science	not offered	offered
Sports Management	not offered	offered
Adult Education	not offered	offered

The emphasis on research at BI might account for the larger graduate program and the employment of more senior faculty members than at GI. As BI is state-funded, this might reflect the government's awareness of the need to train more qualified people in these areas. BI also offers a variety of short-term, nondegree programs for in-service training and the retooling of athletes. It might take some time before this trend will be followed by province-funded institutes.

Financial Resources

While the budget for BI is three times that of GI, the actual difference is probably higher because the cost of living is higher in Guangzhou than in Beijing. The cost per student at GI is about 2,669 yuan per year and, at BI, 7,780 yuan per year.

One might argue that the severe winter in Beijing accounted for a huge maintenance budget, but our findings indicate that maintenance only accounted for about 10% of the budget.

Table 4—Comparison of Financial Resources.

	Guangzhou Institute	**Beijing Institute**
Source		
State (Central Government)	0	88%
Province	100%	0
Other	0	12%
Budget	5.7 million yuan/year	17 million yuan/year
Staff Salaries		
President	380 yuan/year	320 yuan/year
Vice-President	315	310
Unit Head	290	290
Professor	370	305
Associate Professor	310	225
Assistant Professor	270	211
Cost per Student	2669 yuan/year	7780 yuan/year

The salary structure of the senior staff at both institutes reflects the differences in the economic zones of the Hubei and Guangzhou Provinces. While salaries for established posts are standardized in China, special allowances are awarded due to the differences in the cost of living in various parts of mainland China. Since Guangzhou has a higher cost of living than Beijing, the staff salaries are adjusted accordingly. This adjustment is inadequate because official figures on cost of living in more affluent economic zones such as Guangzhou are very conservative and outdated. The only advantage for GI is that it is closer to Hong Kong, and is able to generate income from educational programs offered to Hong Kong residents. Opportunities for academic exchange and commercial sponsorship are also more readily available.

Teaching and Sports Facilities

The mild climate at GI, during the winter months, enables most sports activities to be conducted outdoors year round. Thus, there are more outdoor sports facilities than indoor facilities. At BI, all sports activities have to be conducted indoors during the winter months, but ample outdoor facilities are available (Table 5).

Table 5—Comparison of Facilities.

	Guangzhou Institute	Beijing Institute
Teaching Facilities		
Laboratories	4	41
Special research Labs	0	4
Classrooms	26	38
Libraries	1	1
Outdoor Sports Facilities		
Basketball Courts	10	20
Volleyball Courts	7	8
Softball Fields	1	0
Soccer Fields	2	5
Tracks	2	3
Swimming Pools	2	0
Tennis Courts	3	1
Indoor Sports Facilities		
Swimming Pools	1	1
Badminton Gyms	1	2
Table Tennis Gyms	1	2
Wu Shu Gyms	1	1
Weight Rooms	1	1
Multi-Purpose Gyms	1	1
Sports Hall	1	1
Tracks	0	1

The data obtained indicates that BI has more sports facilities, both indoor and outdoor. Furthermore, on-site visits show that the quality of both teaching and sports training facilities are superior at BI, indicating that funding for constructing new facilities is more readily available from the central government than from provincial governments. It should be noted that maintenance work is performed better at BI.

Compared to similar institutes around the world, BI and GI are of similar size, but BI may be academically superior.

Summary

The state-funded institutes of physical education are much more stable financially than the province-funded institutes, which are more financially stable than teacher training colleges and physical education departments within universities. The increase in funding is reflected in the quality of teaching and sports facilities available at the state-funded institutes, as well as in the number of senior positions established in the administration and teaching faculty. The extra financial resources also allow state-funded institutes to offer a more diversified curriculum with emphasis on graduate programs and research. It is obvious that the number and quality of programs offered at the state-funded institutes will be used to forecast trends for the province-funded institutes, which will always have limited resources.

The role of the Communist Party is represented in the province-funded institutes with established posts, while at the state-funded institutes, they are disguised in the form of appointments of senior posts and by control of the All China Sports Federation. The allocation of resources for nondegree programs at the state-funded institutes will contribute to the development and success of the national teams by offering in-service training and retooling programs for coaches and athletes, and better communication and cooperation between the researchers and practitioners. This is further reinforced by better exchange opportunities with overseas institutes through staff development and consultation. Given the limited resources and restrictions in offering innovative programs, the province-funded institutes can improve their programs if they focus on streamlining their administrative structure, improving on the management of their existing facilities and exploring opportunities of commercial sponsorships in their regions.

Notes

[1]Mao, ZeDong. *Une étude de L'éducation physique*. Paris: Maison des sciences de I'homme, 1962.

[2]Riordan, James. *Sport, politics and communism*. Manchester: Manchester University Press. Also see Brownell, Susan E. "The changing relationship between sport and the state in the People's Republic of China," *The third millennium*. Canada: Les Presses De L'université Laval, 1991; Fu, Frank H. "Delivery of physical education and sport programs in the People's Republic of China and Hong Kong: Comparative analysis," *ICHPER journal*. 26:2(1990); Fu, Frank H. "The effects of urbanization on the delivery of physical education

and sports program in the People's Republic of China," Paper presented at the 24th World congress on HPER meeting, Manila, 1981; Fu, Frank H. "The price of being elite," *Proceedings the sports medicine conference*, Hong Kong, 1987; Hu, C. M. (Ed). *China's encyclopedia of physical education*, Beijing, 1982; Krotee, M. L. and Jaeger, D. M. (Eds). *Comparative physical education and sport*. 3, Illinois: Human Kinetics Publishers, 1986; Lin, S. and Zhu, D. "Bashyiyiming yundongyuande chengcai zhilu," *Xin tiyu*, 10 (1981), pp. 2-4; Ma, QiWei. "The physical education programme and spare time training in primary and high schools in China," *Proceedings of the 1987 sports conference*, Hong Kong, April, 1987; Selection of research papers, National research institute of sports science, Beijing, 1985; Pendleton, Brian B. "China returns: A preliminary prospectus for a study of potential Chinese sporting success and the 1984 Olympic Games in Los Angeles," *Comparative physical education and sport*. Illinois: Human Kinetics Publishers. 3, 1986, pp. 217-226; Rodichenko, Vladimir. "Sport and the state: the case of the USSR" *The third millennium*. Canada: Les Presses De L'université Laval, 1991; Shao, Wenliang. *Sports in ancient China*. Beijing: People's Sport Publishing House, 1986; and Zhou, Yuan. (Ed). *China's contemporary sports*. Hong Kong: Enterprise International Publishing Company, 1986.

Chapter 28

A Comparative Study of Intercollegiate Athletics in China and the United States

Ming Li

It is commonly acknowledged that in order to become one of the advanced nations in sports, China would have to solve several major problems one of which is how to establish a sound intercollegiate athletic system. The purpose of this chapter is to compare the current practices of amateur sports in Chinese higher education with the model of American intercollegiate athletics. It is hoped that, by using a qualitative method of cross-cultural study, some of the existing problems in the Chinese intercollegiate athletic system could be identified. Comparisons were conducted in three areas: philosophy of intercollegiate athletics; social values and attitudes to sports; and administrative issues of the amateur sports programs in higher education. The findings of the study indicate that tremendous differences exist between Chinese and American intercollegiate athletic systems. The results of the study also suggest that in order to develop an effective intercollegiate athletic system, it is critical for China to (1) establish a sound philosophy which properly positions intercollegiate athletics; (2) promote intercollegiate athletics in Chinese society by altering people's attitudes to sports competition; and (3) design and institute a proper administrative structure for intercollegiate athletics.

Introduction

To become one of the world's advanced countries in sports by the year 2000 is the optimistic goal of Chinese sports. This goal was established by the State Commission of Sports in the early 1980s in its strategic plan for sports development.[1] An analysis of China's international success in sports in the past two decades indicates that the country has been making some progress towards this goal. However, as acknowledged by Chinese sports planners, while China is gradually nearing that glorious end signaled by its recent success in the XXVth Olympic Games, there are still some major issues which need to be addressed. Two of these issues are whether the development of its sports programs could be accelerated and the strategic goal could be eventually attained. Another issue is how to reform the current national training structure for world-class athletes in order to establish a new paradigm that is multi-prototypic, multi-strategic, and multi-stratified.

Intercollegiate athletics in the United States, Canada, and the former Soviet Union have long been perceived and used as the breeding grounds for world-class performers. Because of this, Chinese sports planners argued that, in the same manner, its higher education system could be responsible for the strategic development of Chinese sports also.[2] Collegiate athletics in China could be operated as a prototypical athletic farm system for world-class athletes. In 1986 the State Commission of Education[3] granted permission to 53 colleges and universities to establish intercollegiate athletic programs. The Commission hoped that problems in the administrative aspects of intercollegiate athletics could be identified and a productive collegiate athletic farm system could be developed.[4] The five-year implementation did uncover several associated problems with the new system. The lack of a philosophically conceptualized model of intercollegiate athletics was a major problem. The Commission then suggested that it would be worthwhile to establish a theoretical framework of intercollegiate athletics which would match the reality of Chinese society before any further actions would be taken.

Intercollegiate athletics, in the United States, are widely recognized as one of the great collegiate ventures in the world, even though the system has been heavily criticized by the American public since its inception. From its humble student-controlled beginnings more than one hundred years ago, American intercollegiate athletics have grown into a central place in higher education[5] and become a major producer of world-class performers, significantly contributing to America's success in international sports competition. Because of this, it is worthwhile to analyze what American intercollegiate athletics have experienced throughout their entire process of evolution so that China can benefit from America's experiences by imitating its good points and avoiding its mistakes.

The purpose of this chapter is to compare the current practices of amateur sports in Chinese higher education with the model of American intercollegiate athletics. It is hoped that some of the problems existing in the Chinese intercollegiate athletic system could be identified. In addition, it is hoped that some suggestions which may be beneficial to establishing a workable intercollegiate athletic system could be presented. The discussion will center on three primary issues: philosophy of intercollegiate athletics; social values and attitudes to collegiate sports; and administrative issues of amateur sports in higher education.

Philosophy of Intercollegiate Athletics

Philosophy is concerned with the process of pursing the beliefs, values, and truths in ourselves. The philosophy of intercollegiate athletics, then, is the way in which we perceive and believe in the value of intercollegiate athletics. It will provide us the understanding of what intercollegiate athletics are and what social responsibilities intercollegiate athletics owe to society.

It is assumed that intercollegiate athletics are characterized by amateurism in both China and the United States. Nevertheless, the meaning of amateurism is quite different in these two nations particularly with regard to their perceptions of the relationship between higher education and intercollegiate athletics. In other words, how intercollegiate athletics are perceived in higher education and the main goal of the system differ tremendously between the two countries.

Intercollegiate athletics in the United States have long been recognized as an integral part of American higher education. It is generally believed that American higher education has an obligation to provide a large number of curricula and various extracurricular activities to meet the needs of students. A comprehensive intercollegiate athletic program is then offered as evidence of administrative commitment to this responsibility. The intercollegiate athletic program is perceived as an important element in enriching and enhancing the quality of campus life by providing athletic entertainment to students, faculty, and staff. It is also utilized as a critical element in enhancing the prestige and reputation of the institution, indirectly attracting students and financial endowments.

The value of intercollegiate athletics, as defined in China, is quite narrow and one dimensional. It is merely perceived as part of the state's plan for sports development. The ultimate goal of intercollegiate athletics, therefore, is to train and develop more elite athletes for international competition. The development and administration of intercollegiate athletics are invariably associated with the enhancement of the country's political status in the world.

Since the higher education system in China is centralized and controlled by the state government, enrollment and financial stability usually are not a major concern of individual institutions. Accordingly, many people, including school administrators on various campuses, regard intercollegiate athletics as an extension of the university curriculum, not an integral part of it, and in complete consonance with the entire institutional process.[6] The philosophy, which is generally endorsed by Americans, that intercollegiate athletics should be included as a part of the general development of individual student athletes has not yet taken root on many Chinese campuses. This difference in the philosophy of intercollegiate athletics may be attributed to the differences existing in the social values and ideologies embraced by Americans and Chinese, which will be discussed later. American individualism and competitiveness, as well as democratic principles, provide a societal foundation for the formation of such a philosophy of intercollegiate athletics: athletics are an essential part of America's democratic way of life; both are interdependent. "Without democracy, our system of athletics could not flourish, and without athletics, our democracy could lose a vital, invigorating force."[7] To the contrary, communist ideology primarily determines the nature of intercollegiate athletics in China. Intercollegiate sports, like other social transactions, must be responsible for contributing to the national development of sports by devoting itself as if a pawn in a national chess game. A recent document co-issued by the State Commission of Education and the State Commission of Sports, entitled "A Blueprint for Enhancing Interscholastic and Intercollegiate Athletics,"[8] exemplifies this philosophical orientation. "It is imperative to establish intercollegiate athletic programs in higher education and it is the responsibility that the contemporary history endows to the Chinese higher education."[9]

Evidently, the philosophical orientations possessed by the people in these two countries are polarized. The Americans emphasize the achievement of intercollegiate athletics and relate it with the accomplishment of the goals of the individual institutions; whereas the Chinese stress the responsibility of individual institutions and their intercollegiate athletic programs to Chinese international success in sports. Philosophically speaking, the two orientations are not contradictory and exclusive. Instead, they may even be compatible.[10] First of all, intercollegiate athletics could be used as a means of integration for the institutional mission and as a reinforcement of the sense of honor for all segments of the institution. This is the bottom line and main goal of intercollegiate athletics. Without this goal, intercollegiate athletics would not survive because of a lack of needed spiritual "nourishment." Secondly, as supported by evidence, a well-integrated intercollegiate athletic program could be gradually strengthened and sustained both emotionally and financially by the school administration and other involved groups. As expected, a sound nurturing environment for world-class athletes may eventually be created to contribute to the national development in sports. The current practice of Chinese intercollegiate athletics discloses a philosophical dilemma for amateur sports in Chinese higher education, national anxiety for sports accomplishment versus institutional locus for integration.

Social Values and Attitudes to Sports

The public's perception of intercollegiate athletics in the United States is quite unique. Sports and athletic competition are regarded as part of American society. Social Darwinism is the underlying principle explicitly expressed by American sports.[11] Americans are proud of their prestige and culture by claiming that they are born with sports. "Most Americans believe it to be the one quality that has made America great because it motivates individuals and groups to be discontented with the status quo, public perception and with being second best."[12] Competition and success are two major values that are intertwined with American sports and have been internalized by the American people. Participation in sports and athletic competition provide individuals with the opportunity for pursuing excellence and success.

Because of such a value orientation, which highly regards sports and competition, intercollegiate athletics have become a unique emotional outlet for the American people through which their value system can be cherished and nurtured. "Sports and education are inexorably intertwined in American society; colleges without interscholastic sports are so rare that as exceptions they prove the rule."[13] It is commonly recognized that American students, faculty, and alumni often identify themselves distinctly with the athletic programs of their institutions, and the institutional communities enthusiastically nourish a strong emotional bond with their sports programs.

The scenario observed in China is vastly different. Three important principles exemplify these differences regarding the social values and attitudes of the Chinese people to intercollegiate athletics. First, the Confucian view that states, "Those who work with their brains rule and those who work with their brawn are ruled,"[14] has been deeply rooted in the Chinese culture. Accordingly, intellectual development is highly valued in Chinese society, which has also been considerably influenced by feudal culture and ideology for thousands of years.[15] Considerable public attention has always been given to the activities and careers that require intellectual skills, and only the person who possesses these skills is respected by the society as a talent. Moreover, many Chinese people sincerely believe that "those who have brawny extremities are simple-minded." This is another misleading notion that exemplifies the profound impact, of the Confucianism on the attitudes of the masses in China, to sports and athletic competition in general and to collegiate sports in particular.

Contrasting sharply with the attitudes of American educators to intercollegiate athletics, a great number of Chinese educators insist that the academic reputation and prestige of an institution is the major attraction of student enrollment, and the success and reputation of its athletic programs are not of substantial significance.[16] This is another example of why intercollegiate athletics have not been properly installed in Chinese higher education.

The third philosophy that exemplifies the Chinese attitudes to intercollegiate athletics is aptly expressed by Calhoun in the phrase "Chinese non-competitiveness."[17] It is acknowledged that the Chinese people usually show a lack of enthusiasm for competition and winning. "A bird which stands above the rest would be shot first" is a doctrine or norm that takes root in Chinese society prohibiting competition and individuality. Competitions are seen as a threat to society's unity.[18] Thus, it is not surprising that sports competition or intercollegiate athletics per se are not as widely encouraged and welcomed as other social endeavors.

In fact, the winning-losing feature of sports necessitates a better understanding of competition and the development of intercollegiate athletics requires a truthful appreciation of the physical activity and competition. The end result, then, is that for an intercollegiate athletic system to be constructed properly in Chinese higher education, the attitudes of the Chinese people have to be altered.

Administrative Issues of Amateur Sports in Higher Education

Intercollegiate athletic programs in many "big-time" sports institutions in the United States are supposedly the best scenarios if scrutinized by classic organizational principles. Extensively, they are managed independently by separate departments. The athletic department and the physical education department are directed under diverse missions. The daily operations of the athletic programs are supervised by a person (athletic director) who, in most cases, reports directly to the top senior administrator of the institution. The conflict resulting from the dual roles as an athletic director and a faculty member may be minimally reduced.

As one looks back through the evolution of intercollegiate athletics in America, the current, commonly adapted administrative pattern of college sports in the "big-time" sports institutions is the product of continuous modifications. In its infancy, collegiate athletics was part of the administrative structure of the physical education department. Because substantial differences existed between intercollegiate athletics and physical education in terms of their purposes and philosophies, conflicts between these two units were intensified on many school campuses in the 1950s regarding finance, administration, and utilization of facilities. Separation seemed to be necessary. Consequently, independent athletic departments in many big-time football and basketball institutions were established to deal specifically with intercollegiate athletics. In most of those institutions, the athletic directors, the chief executive officers who are responsible for supervising their athletic programs, directly report to the top administrators of their institutions.

All of the institutions in China that have established intercollegiate athletic programs operate in quite the opposite way. The athletic programs are housed in the physical education departments. The entire coaching staff comes solely from the physical education department. That means that the faculty members usually have both teaching and coaching duties. Besides, two programs with different goals and patterns of pursuit are arbitrarily united and managed by the same group of people.

A few drawbacks have consequently been noticed because of this type of administrative structure[19] and lacking reasonable policies and procedures. Conflicts often occur among the programs about authority, responsibility, provision of facilities, and budget allocation. In addition, due to the fact that a consensus has not been reached in terms of what should be used to evaluate the performance of the faculty members who have dual responsibilities, the structure has created problems in determining merit increases and promotions.

It has been assumed that, from the perspective of systematic theory, the performance of the collegiate athletic programs may be maximized if they could be separated from the physical education department.[20] A special administrative structure similar to the athletic departments in American higher education institutions, therefore, is recommended by the nature of intercollegiate athletics in China[21] which is illustrated by Figure 1 shown as follows:

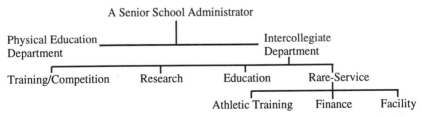

Figure 1—A proposed administrative structure for Chinese intercollegiate athletic programs.

Conclusions and Recommendations

Through analyzing and comparing the practices of intercollegiate athletics in China and the United States, this study concluded that:

1. Tremendous differences existed between the Chinese and American intercollegiate athletic systems in many areas. Due to the differences existing in the social systems of the two countries, it was impossible for Chinese higher education to directly adopt the American model of intercollegiate athletics without any modifications. However, it is the philosophy of intercollegiate athletics and attitudes to sports that the Chinese have to learn from their American counterparts.

2. In order to develop an effective and fruitful intercollegiate athletic system, it is critical for China to resolve the following issues:

   (a) A sound philosophy of intercollegiate athletics has to be established. The philosophy should insist that intercollegiate athletics be bi-dimensional, serving the integrative function of the institution first, and then contributing to the national development in sports.

   (b) Societal attitudes to sports and intercollegiate athletics have to be changed and shaped. The masses should be educated to be able to appreciate the value of sports competition and the functions of intercollegiate sports; and

   (c) Intercollegiate athletic programs should be managed under a specific departmental structure.

Notes

_____

[1] In China, the State Commission of Education is the government agent responsible for all affairs in the educational arena, including sports and physical fitness.

2Wang, C. S. "An administrative model of intercollegiate athletics in higher education." *Collegiate sports in Beijing,* 3 (1988), pp. 21-24.

3State Commission of Education and State Commission of Sports. *A blueprint for enhancing interscholastic and intercollegiate athletics.* 86 #015. Beijing; The State Commission of Education, People's Republic of China, 1986.

4Chen, L. D. "An analysis of collegiate athletic programs and several related issues." *Journal of Wuhan Institute of physical culture.* 2 (1986), pp. 81-82.

5Cady, E. H. *The big game; college sports and American life.* Knoxville, The University of Tennessee Press, 1986.

6Zhang, J. H. and T. L. Yang, "College sports in America and China," *Journal of Shanghai Institute of Physical Culture.* 3 (1989), pp. 17-20; Li, et al, 1989.

7Zahniser, R. R. "Athletics as a motivating force." *Scholastic Coach.* (February 1950), pp. 24-28.

8Chinese State Commission of Education, 1986.

9Bai, J.X. et al. "An analysis of the tryout of intercollegiate athletic programs in Beijing's higher education institutions." *Intercollegiate sports in Beijing,* 3 (1986), pp. 3-15.

10Lui, W. J. "The rationale for collegiate athletic programs." *Forum of sports and physical education.* 4 (1986), pp. 35-37.

11Eitzen, D. S. & G. H. Sage. *Sociology of North American sports.* 3rd ed. Dubuque, Wm. C. Brown Publishers, 1986.

12Eitzen et al, 1986.

13Eitzen et al, 1989.

14Li, Z. S. "Controversy of intercollegiate athletics." *Gengshu scientific research of sports and physical education.* 2 (1989), pp. 68-71.

15Fung, Y. L. *A short history of Chinese philosophy.* New York, The Free Press, 1948.

16Lui, 1989.

17Calhoun, D. W. *Sport, culture and personality.* 2nd ed, Champaign, Human Kinetics Publishers, Inc., 1987.

18Calhoun, 1987.

19Wang, 1988.

20Wang, 1988.

21Jang, S. R. "Discussion of several critical issues of intercollegiate athletics." *Intercollegiate sports in Beijing.* 3 (1988), pp. 25-28.

Chapter 29

Politics in Physical Education and Sport in England and Kenya

Ken Hardman and Jacob S. Nteere

Politics, physical education and sport are terms which have "global" presence; their meanings, however, bound in culture, may have "village" interpretation. The various extraneous constraints imposed upon this chapter render it impossible to dwell on the respective semantics of these terms. Hence, generic definitions of each are employed in order to facilitate examination of a range of physical education/sport political relationships and to provide the necessary common basis for comparison.

Since they are acknowledged for their worldwide application, definitions for "physical education" and "sport" are drawn from Bennett et al.,[1] respectively, they embrace physical activities or systems that are part of the formal programs of educational institutions and institutionalized physical activity in which the rules are fixed externally. Less widely known perhaps amongst physical and sport educators are meanings encompassed within the term "politics." The view that the use of power at varying societal levels as the defining characteristic of politics is the one adopted here, for such power influences decisions taken by governmental agencies and organizations such as schools and other institutional bodies such as sports clubs and associations. Thus, politics is a ubiquitous phenomenon: it cannot be seen as a separate entity; it is "at the heart of all collective social activity, formal and informal, public and private, in all human groups, institutions and societies"[2]: it is all-pervasive. Physical education and sport are then, inextricably intertwined and the cliché that 'sport and politics should not mix' naively ignores the pervasiveness of politics and is at best a pious hope. Even Baron de Coubertin believed in the political expediency of the Olympics in fostering unity and cooperation between nations. It is intended here to highlight only those aspects which serve to illustrate some principal features of the pervasiveness, especially at national and government levels.

In England, Edward IV's ban on football in 1314 to promote archery (for military purposes), and Cromwell's suppression of Sunday sport in the 17th century (as it was seen as a token of opposition to the ruling Parliamentary and Puritan cause), are early illustrations of political intervention in sport. In early, post-industrial society of the 19th century, some industrial capitalists and philanthropic reformers viewed hedonistic pleasures as threats to a work-disciplined labor force and social order, and which also unsettled the internal disciplines of the middle class world; hence, they could not be allowed to develop freely. Once patronized and now abhorred, 'popular' activities were no longer tolerated by the rich; suppression came through legislation and public pressure: bull-running and cock fighting were outlawed (whilst animal sports of the noble and wealthy were protected by Game laws),[3] street football was attacked, nude bathing was banned in London out of a desire for public decency; and children in voluntary societies' established elementary schools were to receive the benefits of physical exercises in the playground in order to "extend the moral influence of the teacher."[4] Alternative forms of 'rational' and 'respectable' activities with an emphasis on order and control were to be provided for exposure to the 'superior example.' The working classes were to be subjected to a process of resocialization.

Individual enthusiasts from the 'leisured' classes pioneered the development of certain organized sports, codified rules and set conventions. Consequently, single sport clubs and associations for individual sports separate from one another were established; voluntary, independent organizations based on a particular social group with a particular social outlook evolved. From this firmly entrenched social base emerged hostility to government interference and control. In the development of a liberal society, the prevailing ideology was that of "'individual' decision-making and 'free' contracting between 'equal' social atoms."[5] Sport was regarded as a concern of the individual. The industrial bourgeoisie shaped sport as a means of molding character and conditioning behavior, acquiring skill, and social accomplishments. Nowhere was it more evident than in the private boarding schools and their later derivatives. The Clarendon Commission, reporting in 1864, considered physical education in the form of organized games as a valuable and essential feature for character building rather than for their physical effects; the associated traits were ensconced in an unwritten code of sporting ethics, and "were intended to prepare (the middle classes) for their future careers principally in laissez faire capitalism or as agents of colonial development."[6]

The requirements of monopolistic capitalism, and Empire, for fit obedient, orderly workers and soldiers assisted in the diffusion of organized sport and physical training to the working classes, prior to which development, social distinction and exclusiveness were widespread as epitomized in "Gentlemen" (amateurs) versus "Players" (professionals) cricket matches and the Amateur Rowing Association's exclusion of watermen, mechanics, artisans, laborers, menial task employees, and a member of a club or a boat containing anyone liable to disqualification from membership. Sporting activity came to be seen as 'rational.' Its democratization provided outlets for energies less degrading and less damaging to society than hooliganism, alcohol and sexual permissiveness. It was beneficial to health and working efficiency, as well as essential to the realization of a physically fit nation of potential soldiers to defend the Empire.

Following the Forster Education Act (1870), which heralded a system of state elementary education, the Government's instrumentary policy orientation was seen in the revised code of regulations permitting drill to be counted as school attendance for grant purposes. The strong military flavor of subsequent Codes of Regulations was related to the Prussian Wars of 1866, and 1870-1, and the rejection of high numbers of potential armed forces recruits on health and medical grounds. This drill (military in form) was the only officially approved form of physical education until 1890; it was introduced to "teach boys habits of sharp obedience, smartness and cleanliness,"[7] and reflected an attitude evidently that education would raise them above their station and business in life. The drill was also 'cheap,'[8] an important consideration given the remit of the Newcastle Commission (1858-61) to recommend "...Measures... required for the extension of sound and cheap elementary instruction to all classes of people."[9] Doubtless, the desire for "obedience" had its roots in the memories of the Peterloo 'massacre' (1819)[10] and Chartism. The uniform regimented rows of children performing exercises in unison were employed to meet national military and industrial efficiency needs. They inculcated "ideas of order, regularity and discipline without which it was difficult to obtain fully qualified soldiers and sailors."[11] In the political arena, it was a struggle between ideals, of a developing social conscience, of militarism, and of a ruling class which determined a specific type of (physical) education of its lower classes.

In the 1930s, the military connection forced physical activity back on to the political agenda, "the... growth of German armaments... petrified nation after nation."[12] Within a month of Chamberlain's (Chancellor) October speech delivered at the Conservative Party Conference on "Defence of Our Country and Our Health,"[13] a Parliamentary Address indicated that his Ministers would submit proposals designed to "improve the physical condition of the nation." Other powerful forces were also central to development in policies based on political expediency. Concerns for social and economic welfare inspired by years of

'Depression' brought debate in Parliament on availability of playgrounds and fields during out-of-school hours and in holidays for 'something to do,'[14] and eventually resulted in physical education having a part to play in "raising the standard of wellbeing—equally important for the social welfare of young people... not least those who are out of employment."[15] The means to achieve this goal were to be local government and voluntary organizations' collaborative action. Their contribution would be "...of inestimable value in the development of a healthy, happy and vigorous community."[16] The rationale was "...Any imitation of the centralized methods in use in some continental countries would be altogether inappropriate."[17] Government was lending a supporting hand. The bottom line, however, was minimum cost to the government purse. A 'White Paper'[18] on "Physical Training and Recreation" preempted the "Physical Recreation and Training Act" (1937), which ushered in a short-lived National Advisory Council (1937-39), commonly known as the National Fitness Council.

Self-proclaimed government support of sport has gradually given way to interventionism since 1960, when the Central Council for Physical Recreation's (C.C.P.R.) sponsored Wolfenden Committee published its Report on "Sport and the Community" and it has gathered momentum ever since.[19] The immediate aftermath of the Wolfenden Report was political party debate in Parliament which resulted in the setting up of a Sports Advisory Council (1965) and a Sports Council by Royal Charter (on January 1, 1972). Significantly, when the C.C.P.R. General Secretary, Walter Winterbottom, was appointed Director of the Sports Advisory Council, and the C.C.P.R. took on the task of servicing the new Council, the government determined its political will to be the final arbiter in conflict of policy in matters of Sports Council terms of reference. Another overt indication of the weakening of the notion of government support and a shift in stance, was seen in the Department of the Environment's 'White Paper' entitled "Sport and Recreation" (1975) when, in acknowledging the importance of physical activity to physical and mental well-being, it indicated that "...the role of government is to *coordinate* [my emphasis] community" and other agencies were to operate "within the framework laid down by the Government."[20] The White Paper also referred to government's right to intervention by citing the Sports Council's Royal Charter requirement to "have regard to any general statements of policy issued by the Secretary of State,"[21] and emphasized its changing position by signaling its intention to strengthen regional level coordination by replacing Recreation with broader consultative and advisory powers.[22] The trend to overt intervention occurred in the choice of a successor to Walter Winterbottom, when the Sports Council's nominee was twice refused by the Minister for Sport (Dennis Howell) in the period 1977-78. Thereafter, interventionist politics have continued unabated. The mythical notion of 'non-political sport' in England was overtly laid to rest with the Government's campaign to boycott the Moscow Olympics, for it constituted a major departure in the relationship between state and sport. The pressure applied to all vested interest public and private sector agencies formed an unequivocal direct attempt to employ sport as an instrument of foreign policy. The Sports Council's opposition to the boycott, as was the decision by 17 national governing bodies to participate, comprised an embarrassment to the government. A cynical interpretation might well be ascribed to the ensuing reduction in the autonomy of the Sports Council in the 'Thatcher' years by appointments of individuals who eschewed the party philosophy.

As the level of its financial support of sport has grown, so government has firmly established sport as an area of policy activity, for many issues impinge on problems of policy communities. The adoption of the 'sport for all' policy has been a policy area of reactive measures and has been dogged by financial stringency. The economic crisis of the 1970s, for instance, deepened and social dislocation manifested itself in delinquency, vandalism, and riots, causing the Sports Council to change tack to target specific social groups, defined as constituting 'social problems.'[23] The chief concern though was with young working class males and 'blacks,' and the programs and measures advocated aimed to integrate them.[24]

The greatest stimulus to change in the last decade has arisen from party policy embedded in political philosophy. The shift of emphasis from public to private funding for sport and increased privatization of services represents a policy reflecting the prevailing government ideology calling for greater efficiency from contracting services. Education has not been immune from such intervention. In 1976, for example, the Education Act illegalised selective entry to secondary level schools (except for music and dance) and so effectively prevented the establishment of sports secondary schools within state sector provision. Physical education and school sport have been at the epicenter of a political battleground. Now teacher contracts specify how extracurricular hours can be used; innovative 'partnership' schemes are evolving, such as the National Coaching Foundation's pilot projects (funded with £700,000 of government money), which raise questions of teacher involvement/non-involvement, as the case may be, and the perceived threat of coaches replacing them, a danger given "added poignancy with the introduction of Local Management of Schools, whereby "employment of part-time coaches (makes)... sound financial if not educational sense,"[25] the debate on a National Curriculum for Physical Education, the introduction of which will, for the first time, make the subject compulsory for all pupils in the age range 5-16; the demise of the local advisory service (itself a reflection of the changes implemented in relation to local government) affecting the support and advice offered in the delivery of the subject in schools; and, finally, the policy initiative announced by the Secretary of State for Education to remove the process of teacher education into the schools themselves, which will have a radical impact on those institutions involved in this area of work.

In Kenya, the historical antecedents of modern physical education and sport lie in the traditional activities employed as instruments for survival and defense against tribal forms of militarism .[26] Pre-colonial, interethnic group warfare was endemic and physical and sporting activities were taught and encouraged for the expressed purpose of development of strength, endurance, and courage, qualities necessary to survive the rigors of life and the hostilities of enemies. Each ethnic group pursued its own rituals of a physical or sporting nature. Competitive activities in running, throwing, and climbing were common among herdboys,[27] traditional wrestling had its champions; the Kalenjin developed strength and endurance while 'farming' cattle at high altitude and so began a tradition of distance running bringing medal-winning performances in modern world championships; the Luo organized boat races on Lake Victoria to test the efficacy of new craft,[28] the Maasi moran (warrior) initiation involved killing a lion with the use of a spear; and young boys among the Maru and Kikuyu engaged in sports activities preparatory to adulthood with the best performers being 'marked' for future leadership.[29]

Within the parameters of an informal education, based in and around the home, where cohesiveness and communal responsibility were fostered and preserved, the instrumental values of physical activity were an integral component of Kenyan tribal society. Typically they were fundamental to social, vocational and, hence, cultural life, embracing recreative play and skills development. With the advent of missionaries and colonial administrators, many were repressed, displaced and eventually replaced, thus characterizing progress towards civilization and imposed westernization. Formal education began with the infusion of European denominational missionary societies, but it was the reality of political control which brought acceptance of British patterns of education, organization of schools' curriculum content and examinations procedures.[30] The imposed system, however, was a poor replica of the British system, being under resourced and subject to poor quality teaching. Physical education was included to achieve the goals of a healthy sound body which would bring a sound character—the ideal colonial citizen. The most striking element was the lack of relevance for the indigenous population as the skills, knowledge and values imparted were based on colonialists' aspirations, whose policies aimed to 'Christianize' Africa, control tribes by a process of isolation, and pursue capitalism through cheap labor and goods.[31] Colonial infusion was accompanied by a colonial passion for sport as well as a concern for the health of the indigenous population. One of the inherent values of sporting activity was its ability to generate social and cultural cohesion: it became part of the fabric of life, facilitating links "between the educated and the uneducated, different ethnic groups, a common language and mode of communication."[32]

The colonial administrators, settlers, and missionaries instituted a framework of sports clubs and brought order to sport (as in the 'mother country') by establishing first, national governing bodies, and then, to meet the demands of international sport, 'umbrella' organizations such as the Kenya Amateur Athletic Association (briefly holding a coordinating role in amateur sport), followed by the Commonwealth Games Association (1952) and Kenya Olympic Association (1954), which merged in 1955. Concomitant with these developments, a hierarchical form of organization of sports competition emerged, ranging from sublocations (intervillage) to national levels, serviced by a network of officials under the ultimate direction of a Colonial Sports Officer. Prestige attached to success was a prime motivation for chiefs who took their responsibilities in sport seriously. At local levels, administrators were empowered to raise revenues, generated from taxation and rates for area services. This system suffered from inequalities between areas and, after Independence in 1963, the central government wrested financial powers from the local authorities and, thereby, 'flagged' the modification of its supportive, to one of a controlling agency, role.[33] During the Mau Mau rebellion (in the early 1950s), which foreshadowed events leading to Kenya's Independence, the Colonial Sports Officer (operating in the Department of Community Development and Welfare) posted trained Community Officers to the Central Province (stronghold of rebellion), to promote sport as a counter-measure to the anomie created by the government-imposed curfew.[34]

Outside the school system, participation in sport by 'Africans' was restricted to opportunities provided by a few missionary boarding schools, the security forces, and a few state-endowed clubs (reminiscent of nineteenth-century developments in England) for 'whites' only. Likewise, Asian immigrants, 'imported' to build the Kenya-Uganda railway, brought their own sport culture and, once settled, introduced their own clubs often restricted in membership by caste or religious affiliation.[35] Such a none too discreet form of 'apartheid' was counter to the participative interest of 'African' Kenyans.

In the immediate post-Independence period, pressing social and economic problems outranked physical education and sport, the former particularly suffering from low status and esteem; but the government soon looked to sport in its route to reconstruction along the lines of Africanization and restoration of pride and cultural heritage. Politicians viewed sport as a vehicle to foster unity amongst disparate ethnic groups, and it became an accepted indispensable component of the diminution of parochialism and process of integration. Politicians were quick to further their ambitions by identifying with successes in sport which, through their ready visibility, also served to enhance national and international profiles. The bronze medal gained by Kiprugut at Tokyo in 1964 was timely for it lifted the morale of the nation and created a sense of national consciousness. President Kenyatta shrewdly welcomed home, from Mexico City (1968), the successful Kenyan athletes, only four years after the Government Minister with responsibility for sport greeted the Olympic team returning from Tokyo with gratitude "...for having shown the rest of the world that there was a country called Kenya..."[36] Subsequent sporting successes achieved by Kip Keino have been accompanied by increased foreign investment. The international sphere has also been utilized to make political points, as witnessed in the Kenyan boycotts of the Olympic Games in Montreal (1976), Moscow (1980), and the Commonwealth Games in Edinburgh (1986).

The growing state influence on sport was reflected in the Societies Act, which created the Kenya National Sports Council (KNSC) in January, 1966. It was a government arm with a mandate to administer, develop, and organize sport, and disburse grant aid to the sports associations whose interests it also represented. In short, a recipe for conflict! It was soon identified with a degree of politicization when Sport Minister Ngala announced approval for team visits into and out of the country would be considered by the KNSC and subject to government approval:[37] government control was being assumed through the KNSC with an implicit deterioration in the position of the voluntary sports associations.

The obligations of the KNSC have brought the development of a network of provincial and district offices which have helped to stimulate participation in sport through 'Harambee' (pulling together) projects in rural areas, partly assisted by government grants. The principle of 'Harambee' has been extended to national sports organizations, which received state monies as subsidy towards sports-related projects. To a large degree, the work of the KNSC has been duplicated by the Department of Sports within the Ministry of Culture and Social Services, set up with an associated National Sports Institute in 1987. The new Department, created to "...implement a coherent and coordinated policy for sports,"[38] functions in an advisory capacity, articulates government policies, has control of sports funds, including approval and auditing of national sports associations' expenditures, and is required to collaborate with the Ministry of

Education to promote sport in the school curriculum. This latest government initiative has to be seen in the context of power politics and policies in furthering the cause of central control.

Such centralized control has pervaded the school curriculum, especially in primary schools where the Institute for Education (K.I.E.), answerable to the Ministry of Education, exercises tight control. It was not until 1979, that a physical education specialist was appointed to advise on curriculum matters in secondary schools (between 1963 and 1979, the subject had been under a music specialist). One year later, President Kenyatta made physical education a compulsory subject, since when it has gained in prestige and now is regarded as worthy of study at postgraduate level. As a subject, it has moved part way to gaining the "respect and support of the government, the education profession... and the community at large" which, according to Habte,[39] it had not previously enjoyed. The 'Africanization' of a foreign founded and based system has been, and is being, reformed to better meet the educational and development needs of the country and the people. The role of physical education in this process is envisaged as a 'model' to build unity and a sense of national cohesiveness, as well as contributing to a "healthier life-style, building interpersonal relations and increasing intergroup respect."[40] Physical education, like sport, is intertwined with politics!

Concluding Comments

This overview of physical education, sport, and politics in England and Kenya demonstrates they have not, and do not, function independently. Clearly, politicization of physical education and sport is a reality with interwoven relationships within and between these entities at all institutional levels. Power is at the very core and such power has substantially influenced decision-making and taking in the two countries; it is a phenomenon which, if anything, seems to be on the increase everywhere as the "village" becomes "globalized."

The historical antecedents and developments of the two delivery systems reveal the all-pervasive nature of politics. Instrumentary policies, in nineteenth-century England and colonial Kenya, respectively show suppression of 'popular' pastimes with gradual replacement by 'rational' and 'respectable' forms of physical activity engagement and ethnic groups obliged (sometimes forcibly so) to abandon traditional pursuits integral to their world. Likewise, the concern for health and fitness and disciplined, obedient working classes, fed a diet of military drill and later physical training based on therapeutic gymnastics is paralleled in Kenya, with colonialist attempts to transplant a formalized education which comprised a physical education curriculum designed to produce a healthy, responsible and content workforce. A feature somewhat reminiscent of the 'civilizing mission' of nineteenth-century 'rational recreationists' of the 'mother' country.

The ubiquitous incursion of politics in physical education and sport has been sustained throughout the second half of the twentieth century with evidence of acceleration in both countries since the 1960 C.C.P.R. inspired Wolfenden Committee's Report, and Kenya's attainment of Independence in 1963. Programmed intervention is manifested in the introduction of a compulsory National Curriculum in Physical Education in England, and central government control of the curriculum in Kenya, in British central and local government and other agencies' sports-related policies, which impinge upon provision, participation, law and order, social welfare, drugs, development of excellence etc., and extension of political control through the sports administrative organization within Kenyan government ministerial departments and agencies. Physical education, sport, and politics do mix!

Notes

[1]Bennett, B. L. et al. *Comparative Physical Education and Sport*. Philadelphia: Lea & Febiger, 1975, p.3

[2]Leftwich, A. *What is Politics?* Blackwell, Oxford, 1984, p. 63.

[3]Interestingly plebeian sportsmen were nearly always prosecuted by the R.S.P.C.A.

[4]Committee of Council, *Annual Report.* (1839), p.19

[5]Riordan, J. "The Political Role of Sport in Britain and the U.S.S.R." Centre for Leisure Studies, University of Salford, Salford, 1986, p.2.

[6]Riordan, p.3; and, Clarendon Commission *Royal Commission on Public Schools.* (1864).

[7]Committee of Council, *Annual Report.*(1870), p. cxxxvi.

[8]The Codes of Regulation stipulated that instruction was to be given by non-commissioned officers, employment of whom did not require considerable outlay of monies.

[9]Newcastle Commission (1858-61).

[10]The "Peterloo massacre" occurred when 60,000 people assembled in St. Peter's Fields in Manchester to hear the radical orator Hunt. Some 400 people were wounded and 11 killed when mounted yeomanry, sent by magistrates to arrest Hunt, charged the crowd.

[11]*Parliamentary Debate* House of Commons, London. Vol. 223, (1875), Col. 1203-1204.

[12]*The Times* Editorial. June 1, 1935.

[13]Chamberlain, N. "Defence of Our Country and Our Health" (1936).

[14]*Parliamentary Debate* House of Commons, London. Vol. 234, (1930), p. 2122.

[15]Board of Education *Physical Education.* Circular 1445. London: H.M.S.O., January 13, 1936, p. 2.

[16]Board of Education, 1936, p. 8.

[17]Board of Education, 1936, p. 4.

[18]A "White Paper" is a government policy statement.

[19]Wolfenden, J. *Sport and Recreation in the Community.* Report. London: C.C.P.R., 1960.

[20]Department of the Environment *Sport and Recreation.* London: H.M.S.O., 1975, p. 4.

[21]*Sport and Recreation,* 1975, p. 6.

[22]*Sport and Recreation,* 1975, p. 10

[23]The Sports Council *Sport and the Community.* London: Sports Council, 1982.

[24]Hargreaves, J. *Sport, Power and Culture. A Social and Historical Analysis of Popular Sports in Britain.* Cambridge: Polity Press, 1986, p. 256.

[25]Fisher, R. J. "The Changing Face of Sport and Physical Education in the United Kingdom," Paper presented at the 2nd Conference of the British Society for Comparative Physical Education & Sport, St. Mary's College, February 29, 1992, p. 13.

[26]Ndisi, J. W. *A Study in the Economic and Social Life of the Luo of Kenya.* Uppsala, 1974, p. 30.

[27]Godia, G. "Sport in Kenya." In, *Sport in Asia and Africa: A Comparative Handbook.* Westport, CT: Greenwood Press, 1989, p. 267.

[28]Ocholla, A. *The Luo Culture.* Wiesbaden, 1980, p. 122.

[29]Kenyatta, J. *Facing Mount Kenya.* Secker & Warberg, 1938, p. 101.

[30]Nteere, J. S. & Hardman, K. "Physical Education in Primary and Secondary Schools in Kenya," In K. Hardman (Ed.) *P. E. and Sport in Africa.* ISCPES Monograph, No. 1, Manchester, 1988, p. 69.

[31]D'Souza, H. "External Influences on the Development of Educational Policy in British Tropical Africa from 1923-1939." *African Studies Review* 18: 2. (1975), p. 38.

[32]Scriven, F. B. *Sports Facilities for Schools in Developing Countries.* Paris: UNESCO, 1973, pp. 15-16.

[33]Hardman, K. et al. "The Structure and Organization of Sport in Kenya and Malawi," In, *Sport for All Into the 90's.* ISCPES, Vol. 7. Aachen: Meyer & Meyer Verlag, 1991, p. 253.

[34]Monnington 1986, p.153; Nteere, J. S. "A Comparative Assessment of the Central Organizations for Amateur Sport in England and Kenya." Unpublished Ph.D. thesis, University of Manchester, 1990, p. 121.

[35]Godia; and Nteere, 1990.

[36]Hall, S. O. "The Role of P. E. & Sport in the Nation Building Process in Kenya." Unpublished. Ph.D. thesis, Ohio State University, 1973.

[37]Hardman et al. 1991, p. 254.

[38]Government Committee Nairobi, 1987, p. 2.

[39]Habte, A. "Education. Africa's Unfinished Business." *Journal of Health, Physical Education & Recreation,* XXXVI, (November-December, 1965).

[40]Krotee, M. L. et al. "The Role of Physical Education and Sport in the Nation of Kenya," In K. Hardman (Ed.) *P. E. & Sport in Africa.* ISCPES Monograph, No. 1. Manchester, 1988, pp. 57-64.

Chapter 30

Hong Kong and Macau: A Comparative Study of Women in Sport

Kitty O'Brien

The islands of Hong Kong and Macau occupy little space in today's world. Macau is a Portuguese territory consisting of a peninsula extending from the southeast coast of China, and two small islands. Its people live in a total land mass of 16 square kilometers (6 miles), and it lies approximately 64 kilometers (40 miles) from Hong Kong. Hong Kong has been under British jurisdiction since the First Opium War. The population fits very tightly into the 420 square kilometers (402 square miles) of land.

Both countries are affected by the imposing presence of China and have large populations of Chinese people. In 1997, the Chinese will assume control of Hong Kong from the British. In 1999, control of Macau will change from Portugal to China. While each colony can reveal some consternation over their impending takeover, there will be benefits to China's close proximity. Macau buys food and drinking water from China, while Hong Kong's residents have been allowed easy passage to and from China through Guangzhou (Canton). Transportation between Hong Kong and Macau is frequent as hydrofoils traverse the Guangzhou River estuary several times daily. Hong Kong's duty free status makes shopping there very attractive, and many of their successful businesses have found that there is a place for them in Macau's main street where gamblers are tempted by well established casinos, and can shop as well.

The population of both territories is estimated at 98% Chinese, but one cannot assume that this makes them similar in lifestyles. The 5,800.600 people in Hong Kong (1989 Census estimate) enjoy the second highest standard of living in East Asia and a GDP of $6,557 per capita, while Macau's 452,300 (1989 Census estimate) include over 135,000 Portuguese, with a GDP of $2,568 per capita. Both peoples recognize Chinese (Cantonese) as the official tongue, with English understood and spoken, and Portuguese used as a language of administration in Macau. In international sport, little would be known or heard from the athletes who represent these people. Hong Kong competes regularly in the Asian Games (1989). Macau will send representatives to the Paralympics section of the 1992 Olympic Festival, which is only their second appearance there.

This chapter examines how women are coping with sport in these two Southeast Asian colonies. It represents a descriptive study incorporating interviews with several women involved in sport in Hong Kong, and with sports authorities in Macau. The interview questionnaire on women in sport in the Pacific Rim countries was originally designed for postal correspondence. Topics for the interviews included the areas of participation, facilities, coaching, and the administration of sport. The study could not have been completed without the special assistance of Mrs. Mee-Lee Ng of the Hong Kong Polytechnic Institute, and Mr. Steve Chen, my interpreter in Macau, and I acknowledge my debt to them.

Participation

Some opportunities in sport for girls and women are present in both countries in the schools and in the community. Schools present the best occasions for Macau schoolgirls to learn physical activities as there has been little or no recreational activity for post-school ages, and the schooling years are short. Approximately 38% of girls finish high school. It is only in the past five years that 26 sport clubs, or organizations, have been established allowing for female participation. The most popular activities are table tennis, swimming, basketball, badminton, judo, rowing, and martial arts or Kung Fu.[1] In 1983, in Hong Kong, Pedro Ng conducted a survey of secondary school pupils and found that only 15.2% of females would choose physical activities as their most frequent leisure activity.[2] Speak's 1990 questionnaire that was given to incoming university students identified female pursuits in schools as badminton, basketball, athletics, volleyball, table tennis, dance, swimming, handball, softball, cycling, aerobic dance, hockey, and trampoline, in that order. He notes, with interest, that the preferred activities at the university chosen by females would be mainly those individual sports of squash, badminton, swimming, cycling, dance, and aerobic dance. Commercial urban or regional centers could have been providing the impetus for these trendy activities. While a very small percentage of Hong Kong's population goes on to university less than 2% were offered university places in 1984. Speak points out that commercial urban and regional centers are available to the general population groups as well. For the purposes of this chapter, one must accept that the sample lacks some generalizability to the overall population. By way of contrast, however, there is a resounding lack of available commercial facilities for fitness in Macau.

Facilities

The one swimming pool central to Macau residents is heavily booked on a regular basis. A new pool opened in 1989, on the island of Faipa, but it is not central to the population, most of whom must travel by foot or bicycle. Of the 23 pools listed in the *Atlas Desportivo de Macau* (Directory of sports facilities), four are small wading pools, five are located at private colleges, and 10 are owned by separate organizations such as hotels.[3] The city of Hong Kong boasts the largest number of swimming pools to teach swimming. By regulation, Hong Kong guarantees school facilities which include one outdoor playground and one indoor facility as big as a basketball court. A visiting Chinese educator claimed that, despite the fact that these facilities are guaranteed in this land-deprived society, the playground allocations are not as good as exists in mainland China.[4] Speak[5] also states that school facilities are not growing as fast as those in the community and private sectors. The report on *Sports in Education*[6] lists reasons for unsatisfactory teaching conditions in primary schools as: lack of facilities, lack of adequate extracurricular competition and appropriately qualified personnel, and the inability to recognize those children with higher levels of talent in sport. The report also provides reasons for problems in secondary schools as being similar to those for primary schools, with the additional difficulty of the sharing of facilities by morning and afternoon schools, a practice which limits extracurricular activities. Both countries have sport institutes operating where the best facilities are housed. Macau's Instituto Dos Desportos consists of four outdoor court spaces, one hockey field, one track/soccer stadium, one 25-meter and one 15-meter pool, two medium-sized multipurpose halls, and one small hall.[7] The badminton courts are covered with mats when the judo squad arrives, then taken away when basketball is played. The one hockey field was covered with artificial turf in 1989. These facilities lie in stark contrast to the Jubilee Sports Centre in Hong Kong, home of the Hong Kong Sports Institute. It houses the largest indoor sports hall in Asia as part of a complex covering 41 acres. It caters particularly to athletes in badminton, tennis, table tennis, fencing, gymnastics, rowing, soccer, squash, and swimming but a velodrome, basketball court, track and field area, and a baseball diamond are also available. Support facilities on site include a sports science department, sports resources library, lecture and function rooms, a restaurant, sports shop, and a recently opened (in 1990) Hall of Residence. The Institute's administration is now spreading its program to other sites around Hong Kong.

International Women's Participation

An interport schools sports exchange takes place between Hong Kong, Macau and Guangdong, China. These three cities take turns in running competitions in swimming, athletics, table tennis, hockey, soccer, basketball, volleyball, and badminton. This could broadly be considered as international competition, but it is simply neighborly and not at the elite level. The first ladies' tournament outside Macau occurred in the late 1950s at a table tennis tournament in Peking.[8] Only recently have they made their first entry into the Asian Games (in 1989). Bronze medals in martial arts were won by a female and a male. Macau sent one female and six males to the Seoul Paralympics, and only two males to Barcelona's Paralympics.

Female participation in the Asian and Olympic Games is a part of Hong Kong's sport history. Two female swimmers were part of the first ever contingent to the Olympics at Helsinki in 1952, and their women athletes entered the first Asian Games in Manila in 1954. The first gold medal awarded a female from Hong Kong was in the Asian Games in Bangkok of 1978, for tenpin bowling.[9] No medals have been recorded for their female Olympians, but a part of their largest medal accumulation of seven in the 1990 Asian Games included women gaining bronze medals for judo, wushu, women's all-around gymnastics, table tennis, and a silver in windsurfing. Athletic scholarships at the Jubilee Sports Centre in Hong Kong have been awarded to female participants in badminton, gymnastics, rowing, squash, swimming, table tennis, track and field, and the triathlon. Hong Kong's first medal ever, a bronze, in Asian Championship rowing, was won by Ho Kim Fai in the lightweight women's singles.[10] Therefore, when women compete, they do well.

Macau's governmental subsidies for females occur only when traveling to represent the country. Due to the unavailability of facilities, some girls have managed to obtain training funds when they are able to use a court at one of the four schools so outfitted. According to Leong[11] those girls who have been designated for higher level training have been said to be unfit, unwilling to sweat, and interested mainly in social participation. Those who are students are subject to great parental pressure to do well academically above all else.

Coaching

In 1986 and 1987, the Macau government made its initial attempts to subsidize sport. It chose 20 sports and hired several foreign coaches. All were from Beijing, China, with the exception of the judo coach from Japan. Only one, who coached swimming, was female. In 1989, when a training scheme for Macau coaches was started, no females were invited to attend. At the present time there is a female badminton coach, a sport which has already been seen as popular for women. This sport, however, was denied representation to the Asian Games by the Sport Council in 1989, due to the claim that the players were not up to standard. The coach managed to take 26 members of badminton clubs, mainly students, to Australia in 1991. Food and accommodation were offered by the Australian hosts, and one-half of the air fares were paid by the government. This is a far cry from the funds allotted for the favored judo coach, who earned three times the salary of the Chinese coaches, and who also received accommodation.[12]

Of the nine coaches employed by the Hong Kong Sports Institute for sports involving women or girls, there are only two women and they are coaching badminton and tennis. The female National Badminton coach has senior and junior squads with 20 members each. As a top sport that is well run by an association with over 80 clubs, this sport generates favorable funding, particularly through the Hong Kong Open held during non-Olympic years. Grade A players train at the Jubilee Sport Centre.[13]

Another sport which often attracts more interest among female competitors than in males is gymnastics. Hong Kong girls have been sent to the World Championships, the qualifying tournament for the Olympics, while males have not. The Sport Institute employs two male coaches to coach all scholarship gymnasts. Additionally, within Hong Kong, there are three artistic gymnastics coaches and five rhythmic gymnastics coaches. All are female and are available for international duty. At the lower levels, males often coach girls in religious schools, but more female than male coaches work in community recreation situations. Gymnastic clubs total 230 with approximately two-thirds of the 20,000 participants being female.[14]

Administration

In 1989, Portuguese administrators were sent to the Macau government to form a council to organize sport. Of the 26 sports that were active, 20 were under the control of the government as to their standards for Olympic participation. The $10 million that was allocated to sports was policed by the council, which had no competitive experience. The only female administrator, Dr. Pou Hong Leong, became interested in the fortunes of girls' and women's sports during the early days of the council. She voiced her opinions, gave of her own time and expense, and was elected to the Olympic Committee.[15] Several sports clubs for girls have been organized and the standard of play has improved, but more female administrators need to be encouraged. Of the 57 representatives on the Hong Kong Olympic Committee, four are women. They represent the Post-Secondary College Athletics Association, Gymnastics, Ten-Pin Bowling, and Ladies' Soccer.[16] Several sports employ female directors of their associations. It is accepted that the women work long hours with less pay than their male counterparts. It has also been stated succinctly, that "women are good administrators.[17] Tables 1 and 2 below show, that in the 1988 Olympic Games, 16.9% of Hong Kong's competitors and officials were females and were represented in 5 of 11 sports. In the 1990 Asian Games, that percentage was 25.5%, although women's participation increased to 16 of 21 sports.

Table 1—Hong Kong Team at the 1988 Olympic Games in Seoul.[18]

Sport	Competitors		Officials		Total
	Male	Female	Male	Female	
Archery	2	1		1	4
Athletics	1	2	1	.	4
Canoe	2		1		3
Cycling	5		3		8
Fencing	6	1	3		10
Judo	5		2		7
Swimming	6	4	2	1	13
Diving	2		1		3
Shooting	1		1		2
Table Tennis	4	2	2		8
Yachting	6		3		9
TOTAL	40	10	19	2	71

Table 2—Hong Kong Team at the 1990 Asian Games in Beijing.[19]

Sport	Competitors		Officials		Total
	Male	Female	Male	Female	
Archery	3	3	2		8
Athletics	3	2	2		7
Badminton	6	2	1	1	10
Basketball	12		2		14
Canoeing	6	2	2		10
Cycling	6		3		9

(Continued on next page)

Sport	Competitors		Officials		Total
	Male	Female	Male	Female	
Fencing	9	1	3		13
Football	18	18	5	2	43
Gymnastics	6	2	3		11
Handball		13	2		15
Hockey	16		3		19
Judo	2	4	2		8
Rowing	6	1	3		10
Shooting	10	1	3		14
Swimming	7	8	3		18
Water Polo	13		2		15
Table Tennis	5	3	2	1	11
Tennis		1	1		2
Volleyball	12		2		14
Wushu	5	4	3		12
Yachting	7	1	3		11
TOTALS	152	66	52	4	274

Summary

Limited participation opportunities, a predominance of male coaches and administrators, and restricted selection in international competitions are not new problems to girls and women in sport. The interesting factor here is that they are still quite evident in two countries which have had a later start in sport than many other larger or stronger nations. Participation opportunities are greatest in the school situations of Macau and Hong Kong, although they are far from ideal. Hong Kong's young women can achieve more physical and recreation education if they attend college. The women of both countries appear to enjoy badminton, table tennis, basketball, and swimming when they have the opportunity. The sports of field hockey and tennis, which have very limited facilities, show some popularity in Hong Kong, which may have taken the place of traditional Chinese sports. The sports institutes of both countries cater to some girls' and women's sports. Although scholarships are not yet available to Macau girls, their Institute of Sport has improved greatly on its facilities since 1987. These improvements, along with the expansion of the Hong Kong Sports Institute, will undoubtedly increase the chances of girls and women from these two countries to participate in more and larger competitions in the future, therefore providing some models for increased recreational participation as well.

Notes

[1]Leong, Pou Hong. Vice-President, Macau Badminton Association and Olympic council member. Personal interview. Macau.(1990).

[2]Speak, Michael. "University entrants: Participation in and attitudes expressed towards sport and physical recreation". Unpublished paper, Chinese University of Hong Kong, Hong Kong, 1990.

[3]*Atlas Desportivo de Macau* (Directory of sport facilities).Macau: Institute dos desportivos de Macau, 1990.

[4]Yixian, L. "On the characteristics, strong points, and shortcomings of education in Hong Kong," In G. A. Postiglione, (Ed.). *Education and society in Hong Kong: Toward one country and two systems.* Armonk, N.Y.: M. E. Sharpe, Inc., 1991, pp. 253-263.

[5]Speak.

[6]Council for Recreation and Sport. *Sports in education: A report (1988). Hong Kong.*

[7]Atlas.

[8]Leong.

[9]Sales, A. de O. Hong Kong Olympic Council President. Personal interview. Hong Kong. (1990)

[10]*Annual Report. Jubilee Sports Centre* . Hong Kong . (1989-90).

[11]Leong.

[12]Leong.

[13]Cheung Yick, Joseph. Honorary Deputy Secretary, Hong Kong Badminton Association. Personal interview. (1990).

[14]Ho, Winnie. Executive council member, Hong Kong Gymnastics Association. Personal interview. Hong Kong. (1990).

[15]Leong.

[16]Sales.

[17]Ho.

[18]Official Records, Hong Kong Olympic Committee

[19]Official Records, Hong Kong Olympic Committee.

Chapter 31

Cross-Cultural Impacts on Effectiveness in Sport

Jean Craven

In the 1990s, as more and more sports operate international formats, cross-cultural situations are occurring with ever-increasing frequency. Amateur and professional athletes move across national and cultural borders to train and work in foreign environments. They go to gain experience (and rewards) not available in their homelands, and to compete. They spend weeks, months, or years abroad. Many clubs, associations, and national teams bring in foreign master coaches[1] to work with their elite athletes. Less established sports employ coaches from countries where the sport is prestigious to stimulate grassroots growth, and higher levels. Research from several fields, governmental foreign aid, education, multinational business, and sport, has shown that cross-cultural factors exert a strong influence on the success of such undertakings.

Many in sport are cross-culturally involved, including:

1. sport administrators.
2. members of selection boards/panels.
3. club executives.
4. coaches away from their homelands.
5. coaches considering posts abroad.
6. athletes training/playing in their homeland for a foreign coach.
7. athletes planning to train/play aboard.
8. officials and others who are involved in the sports scene.
9. people involved in large scale sports events (e.g., Olympic Games); and
10. people hosting a foreigner.

Tens of thousands of dollars can be lost if a cross-cultural undertaking is not successful or is incomplete. The costs of moving personnel, and maybe their families, to say nothing of possible contract and other compensation costs, loss of good will, and ongoing trauma to both traveler(s) and recipient(s), can produce losses of many kinds for years after an unsatisfactory or failed undertaking. The misuse or wastage of expertise and effort occur all too frequently. Small difficulties multiply and escalate into problems; benefits shrink and even become nonexistent. Good intentions are not enough; knowledgeable preparation of the groundwork and personnel; thorough and appropriate planning; and sensitive and competent execution must all occur if golden rewards are to be reaped.

The "Overseas Type"

Surveys were conducted in Canada in 1987 and 1988 among the foreign coaches, Canadian coaches, athletes, administrators, and other host nationals associated with 15 national and 23 provincial sports. Responses showed that, in particular, those who display respect, who are nonjudgmental, who are peopleoriented, and who are flexible, tend to be the most highly successful in a foreign environment. These and other characteristics found among the most successful foreigners are shown in Figure 1.

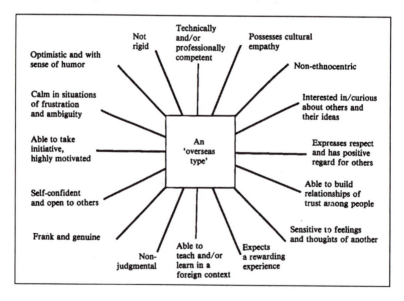

Figure 1—Characteristics of an 'Overseas Type.'

The closer a person comes to this "type," the greater is his or her potential for achieving highly abroad. Administrators, employers, and others who select need to be aware that:

1. experts/high performers at home may *not* do as well abroad (since they may be *so* finely tuned that they need their own homeland environment and norms in order to achieve so highly).

2. internationalists, competent at home, may very well excel abroad (because they are not so dependent on homeland norms and can easily draw on more than one societal base in order to achieve highly).

3. cultural compatibility is *vital* (a person successful in country A may not be so in country B), and a person's potential and tendencies in this regard *must* be assessed *before* any final decisions are made, or travel takes place.

4. the determinants of cross-cultural effectiveness must *all* be considered in the search, short-list, interview, and selection/appointment process; and

5. the cross-cultural adjustment process varies from person to person and with the "cultural distance" between home-land and host nation.

Survey respondents gave the aspects shown in Table 1 as being ones which most influenced the success of their cross-cultural involvement.

Table 1—Factors Leading to Success Abroad
(from 1987 and 1988 Canadian Surveys)

As Identified by Foreign Coaches	As Identified by Canadian Colleagues	As Identified by Other Host Nationals
Work-related aspects	Work-related skills	Adaptability of foreigner
Athletes' cooperation	Adaptability of foreigner	Work-related skills
Welcome & Support received	Language ability	Friendliness of foreigner
Personal Gains obtained	Understanding of host	Language ability
Interpersonal Skills	Nation lifestyle/customs/ people by foreigner	Enthusiasm/common sense/ open-mindedness shown

Such undertakings are challenging and are frequently stressful to almost everyone. Those considering a foreign experience should first assess why. It should matter *greatly* that the undertaking actually occur; it should be devastating if it did not. It should be viewed as an eminently worthwhile and rewarding experience, a positive and highly beneficial event.

Determinants of Cross-cultural Effectiveness

Administrators, coaches, and athletes often think that because they can function at a high level at home, similar achievements are just as easily possible aboard. They often acknowledge that it will be "different," but they do not consider that it will be any "harder." Overlooked, all too frequently, are the *extra* stresses and strains inherent in all cross-cultural situations. Most of those who select, and many of those who travel, only consider their professional qualifications, ignoring or dismissing other criteria. Research indicates that *four* main criteria should be considered and these are shown, numbered in priority order, in Figure 2.

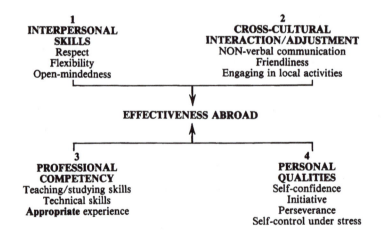

Figure 2—The major determinants of cross-cultural effectiveness (in priority order).

When references are being taken up, and when short-listed candidates with equal coaching competency and/or athletic potential and achievement are being interviewed or assessed, then their interpersonal skills and their cross-cultural interaction tendencies are the criteria on which the final choices should be determined. Past research has shown that effectiveness abroad comes from:

1. *cordial* interaction with host nationals.
2. cross-cultural knowledge, interest and involvement.
3. job and communication competency.
4. psychological adaptability and adjustment; and
5. certain personal qualities (e.g., open-mindedness, tolerance, sense of humor).

A coach or athlete thinking of going abroad, or an administrator considering hiring a foreigner, should check for:

1. strong interpersonal skills.
2. an internationalist attitude.
3. flexibility and open-mindedness.
4. people-oriented/democratic/group-centered way of working.
5. cultural compatibility.
6. a real *"want"* to be abroad.
7. communication competency.
8. teaching/studying skills.
9. a conviction that the experience will be positive/enjoyable/beneficial.
10. a positive self-image.
11. self-confidence strong enough to help weather the shocks, stresses and strains of the foreign experience; and
12. a *good match* of foreigner's qualifications/experience/needs/expectations with employer/host nation's requirements/needs/expectations.

The aim of the selection process is to identify those people who show the potential of being able to live, work, and perform effectively in a foreign environment, and whose conduct will strike a balance between the demands of self, home, and host nation (see Figure 3).

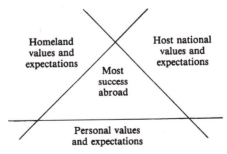

Figure 3—The overlapping of the groups of components that lead to success abroad.

Shocks Commonly Encountered Abroad

Certain *impacts* exerted by a foreign environment can *so* affect people that they perform well below their norms and the levels required of them. The most frequent "shocks" that result are:

1. Culture shock.
2. Language shock.
3. Shock of self-discovery; and
4. Role shock.

As a coach on a seasonal or longer contract, or as an athlete training/playing in your homeland with a foreign coach, or abroad on a scholarship, employed or sponsored, adjustment and adaptation to the ways of another culture will occur as the months go by. The typical adjustment path followed by most people is shown in Figure 4.[2]

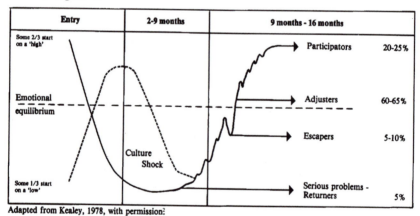

Adapted from Kealey, 1978, with permission.

Figure 4—The typical U-curve path of cross-cultural adjustment.

Whether an individual starts on a "high" or a "low," it is virtually certain that a marked negative phase will be encountered as adjustment proceeds. This is known as *"culture shock,"* and it is made up of the total of the stresses and strains that come from trying to function effectively in a foreign environment where the cultural norms and cues are different from those at home. The occurrence of culture shock, its duration, and intensity, vary from person to person and place to place. Generally, it is more severe in unprepared people and where the "cultural distance" between home and host nations is great. Culture-shocked people feel torn apart as homeland factors pull out and host nation factors press in. These are illustrated in Figure 5.

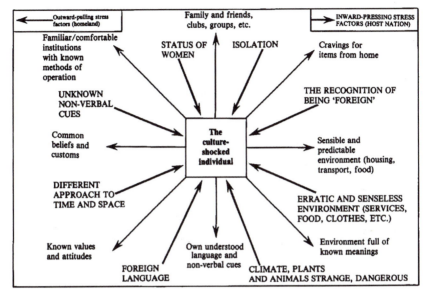

Figure 5—Forces acting on a culture-shocked individual.

Some of the more common manifestations of culture shock are given in Table 2. The effectiveness of the foreigners suffers, as does their performance. The respondents in the Canadian surveys most frequently gave the factors listed in Table 3 as being the ones that affected them adversely.

Language was a problem identified by all those surveyed. If one cannot understand the language at all, it is very hard to convey one's intelligence and knowledge. Frustrations can build. Even resentment at having to learn a foreign language, at having to re-learn how to communicate, as though a child again, can cause "language shock." Problems arise that are over and above the technical ones of coaching and learning. There are many strains involved in working with an interpreter. Double the time is needed, time which may not be available, so short cuts occur; therefore not as much is covered. Nuances present at all levels of coaching, and especially at the elite levels, frequently are not conveyed. It is hard to find interpreters who are capable *colloquially*, and even harder to find ones with the necessary *sport terminology* and *jargon* at their command. Administrators need to seek out such people ahead of the situation if maximum benefits are to accrue. Frequently overlooked are the stresses and strains imposed when the language base is the *same*. In some ways, it is less of a strain on a person to hear a noise that makes no sense, when *not* expecting to understand, than to hear a noise which *is* understood, immediately comprehended and

Table 2—Common Manifestations of Culture Shock

Feelings	*Behavior*
Fluctuate widely/wildly	Lack of control
Helplessness	Unusual actions.
Confusion	Excessive concerns about food, health, safety, cleanliness
Anxiety	Increased eating/smoking
Irritability	Loss of appetite
Frightening thoughts	Insomnia/over-sleeping
Preoccupation	Withdrawal ('flight')
Moodiness	Aggressive manner ('fight')
Fear of failure	Aping nationals ('going native')
Feel a failure	Avoid people/physical contact
Homesickness	Given to absent-minded 'far-away' staring
Cravings (for items from home)	Dependence on own expatriate nationals
Hostility	Write lots of letters home
Anger	Lodge complaints frequently
Negativity	CANNOT be detached observer
Isolation	
Loss of own identity	
Feel misunderstood	
Exhaustion	
Guilt (about hostility, etc.)	

reacted to, only to find that the "known" is the unknown, that the meaning has "changed," or that the reaction required is different. *Constant* vocabulary adjustments are very wearing on people, taking away energy needed elsewhere.

A large number of travelers abroad experience the "shock of *self*-discovery." In addition to all the new things they are seeing, finding, and experiencing, they start to see themselves anew. Sometimes this rediscovery is stimulated by the reactions to them of host nationals. Sometimes it occurs as travelers try to weld together the homeland "old" and the host nation "new." They may find that they are not the people that they thought they were; they may discover biases in themselves; they may find that they had pre-judged, wrongly or that they are not as broadminded, or tolerant, or flexible, as they thought they were. They may be expected to change, even *want* to change, and find it is not in them to do so. Such conflicts can easily lead to poor performance, and even to early return.

The most critical "shock" in relation to the success of cross-cultural undertakings of more than a few weeks in duration, particularly on the part of coaches or of athletes playing abroad, is "role shock ". Unlike culture shock, role shock

Table 3—Problem Areas Inhibiting Success Abroad
(from 1987 and 1988 Canadian Surveys)

As Identified by Foreign Coaches	As Identified by Canadian Colleagues	As Identified by Other Host Nationals
Language–especially colloquial vocabulary Work-related–lack of clear objectives and commitment from others Canadian - remoteness/ large distances/ isolation/climate's severity leisure activities educational standards Interpersonal/cultural differences Asian-Canadian Germanic-Canadian Nordic-Canadian	Language–Colloquial –sport jargon Bias E-W philosophies Lack of knowledge of/ interest in Canada Failure to know/understand motivations of Canadian (North American) athletes	Ignorance of Canada Work-related e.g., sport system/ job aspects language–colloquial English/ French sport vocabulary Personal qualities– screen out bias/ arrogance, ensure cooperative and pro-Canadian

peaks about the midpoint of the foreign stay. It is very focused in nature, it is severe, and it seldom goes away. It forms, arguably, the most common cause of the failure of cross-cultural endeavors. However, by the use of appropriate, more perceptive selection and appointment procedures, the likelihood of role shock occurring can be greatly reduced, even virtually eliminated. Role shock results from differences between the expected and actual role(s) aboard. A changed destination; a rural/urban location switch; a grassroots job, not an elite one; unexpected demands (of a non-coaching/playing nature) at work or in free time; co-coaching instead of solo work; development/paperwork/publicity involvement when not skilled in administration or public relations; and similar unexpected and distressful alterations can almost always be avoided by advanced planning. Role shock can be virtually prevented by the use of appropriate search, short-list, and interview procedures. The provision of detailed and precise *written* job descriptions, prior to the interview *and* for signature upon selection/appointment, is vital. This does not mean that the unexpected will never arise; it will. What it does mean is that many *avoidable* traumas are prevented if good communication takes place at all stages of the undertaking. Those surveyed in Canada specified the cross-cultural factors that they found contributed to role shock, and which detracted from the overall benefits of the foreign endeavor in general, relating each to the four major determinants of effectiveness abroad. These factors are presented diagrammatically in Figure 6.

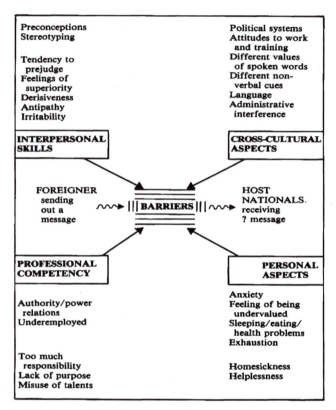

Figure 6—Barriers to effective cross-cultural communication in relation to the four major determinants of cross-cultural effectiveness.

The Value of Cross-Cultural Preparation

The traveler, the foreigner, is a point of contact between two cultures and is a bringer of change. If the traveler is a coach, that person may be a source of influence, an adviser, an assistant, a teacher of equals, a teacher of students, or any or all of these. Certainly the traveler, whether coach or athlete, is a medium for a flow of exchange in *all* fields, not just the technical one. Making contact is the first step for an individual towards success abroad, and those who cannot adjust their behavioral patterns to accommodate "very different" others and their ways are at a serious disadvantage immediately. Interaction with local people is needed to appreciate their perspectives, needs, attitudes, and beliefs in order to transfer or acquire skills successfully. Those who have worked abroad state that the communication of ideas is more important than the performance of specific tasks, and that to communicate across cultural barriers requires both verbal and nonverbal competencies. The traveler must learn what to say, and how to say it in terms of the expectations and predispositions of those listening; that is, how the recipient host nationals need to hear it. To do this, training is *vital.* Interpersonal skills; cross-cultural interaction/adjustment and culture shock; professional and communication competencies; problem areas and barriers; and personal qualities and other considerations are all topics that should be included in the pre-departure and post-arrival training. The value of such preparation is indicated below in Figure 7.[3]

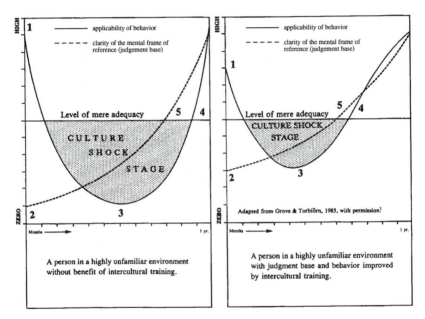

Figure 7—The value of cross-cultural training in relation to the reduction of culture shock and the acceleration of adjustment.

The graph on the left shows the typical adjustment paths for appropriateness of behavior and accuracy of the judgment base followed by a foreigner who has had no cross-cultural preparation. Typically, the culture shock period is severe, deep, and of long duration, lasting six months or more. The graph on the right shows the adjustment paths most commonly followed by foreigners who have received cross-cultural training before going abroad. The intensity and length of the culture shock period are markedly reduced. Other benefits occur, and from a comparison of points 1-5 on the two graphs these can be discerned.

1. Advance preparation reduces the total dependence of the
    travelers on their own societal norms as the base on
    which they make judgments by partially putting in place
    the norms of the host nation(s) so that the travelers are
    both *aware* of other bases and can, to some extent, *use*
    these to make judgments that are more accurate when
    abroad.

2. Immediately, the travelers' behavior is more appropriate,
    better suiting that needed in the host nation(s).

3. Such pre-departure training, and *ongoing* post-arrival
    training, helps to reduce the severity of the negative cul-
    ture shock phase; the dip is much shallower.

4. Training also brings about an earlier restructuring of the
    travelers' "functional base" and increased confidence
    results. The foreigners feel that they can operate correct-
    ly, almost normally, abroad and so the duration of culture
    shock is shortened. Increased effectiveness is seen sever-
    al months earlier; and

5. Linked to the mental restructuring, new cues are learned
    more quickly and the foreigners become "in-tune" with
    the host environment and its nuances more quickly;
    behavior, like thought, becomes comfortably accurate.

Advance preparation makes both thought processes and actions less "home-
tuned" and brings them closer to the comfortable level of adequacy required
abroad *upon arrival*. Post-arrival training supports and strengthens rapid adjustment. Pre-departure and post-arrival training means that a comfortable level of
adequate functioning is achieved and exceeded far earlier in the prepared person
than in the unprepared person, leading to greater benefits for all.

Much of the preparation for a cross-cultural experience can be incorporated into
the ongoing mental training of athletes. A session specifically on cross-cultural
aspects should be given approximately one month before departure for the new
undertaking or competition. For those going to coach, work, train, or compete
for periods of several months or years, general facts about the host nation and
more specific ones about its sport system should be acquired from books, films,
lectures, contacts who have personal experience of tne host nation, and through

attendance at workshops. Table 4 gives the topics on which foreign coaches in Canada wished to have pre-departure and post-arrival training. Wherever and whenever possible, this training should brief *both* the travelers *and* the recipient host nationals.

Table 4—Topic Areas for which Cross-Cultural Preparation and Training Were Specifically Requested (from 1987 and 1988 Canadian Surveys)

As identified by
Foreign Coaches

As identified by Candian Colleagues
and Other Host Nationals

Knowledge about host nation
sport environment, all aspects
and especially athletes
Knowlege about host country, climate,
way of life, vocabulary, customs
+ Immediate post-arrival support
mechanisms

Knowledge about host country, climate,
way of life, people, attitudes,
colloquial language
Work-related knowledge about athletes,
motivations, working conditions, the
sport environment
+ Personal qualities of foreign coach
+ Knowledge about culture shock

Requested by Foreign Coaches
In Homeland Before Departure

Requested by Foreign Coaches
In Canada After Arrival

Need	*Number of* *Times Mentioned*	Need	*Number of* *Times Mentioned*
Knowledge about Canada	15	Support and cooperation	11
COMPRISING		COMPRISING	
Sport environment		Help to settle	
Levels		Find apartment	
Administration	9	Finance	6
Organization		Car	
General needs		Travel (be shown around)	
Detailed needs		Keeping of advance promises	5
Motivations		Better organization	
Physical science		Briefing on Canadian way	8
Knowledge		of life especially re	
Sport terminology		sport i.e.,	
Canadian environment		Sport levels	
Language (English)		Competition levels	
Vocabulary	6	Athlete attitudes	
History		Athlete cultural and	
Climate		educational levels	
Honest answers from		*Coach* cultural and	
Canadians abroad		educational levels	
about Canada		Work opportunities	

During the Time Aboard

Very important is the post-arrival training. For athletes involved in major competition, a short session of perhaps one hour, given about a week to ten days
after arrival, or approximately halfway into the acclimatization period, can be
most beneficial. Some cross-cultural situations will have been experienced. Any
queries can be answered, difficulties solved while still small, problems fore-
stalled, and discussions held. The energy-sapping distractions that can spoil the
fine-tuning process can be eliminated well before the start of the competition.
For those abroad for longer stays, more benefit is obtained from a series of
cross-cultural training sessions in the first three months, with host nationals
teaching about actual experiences encountered in sport and society. Post-arrival
training should involve the foreigner *and* host nationals *throughout* the stay,
using a mixture of formal and informal settings. *Active, ongoing support* should
be provided throughout the foreigners' stay, as different needs arise in different
people at different times (see Figure 4.). In general, such preparation and support should address everyday needs first. An early working knowledge of types
of accommodation, food supply, money values, bank locations, postal system,
post office and telephone locations, shopping areas, doctor, and utilities enables
the foreigner to function with a semblance of independence. Next, work-related
aspects should receive attention, as work forms the initial contact and adjustment base. An ideal way of providing support at work is to establish a "buddy"
for the foreigner, not just for a few days, as sometimes happens, but for a period
of several months, or even for the whole duration of the stay (at least until the
foreigner has built up an individual circle of friends). As days become weeks
and months, the emphasis in training should switch more to societal and general
topics, and sessions should become increasingly informal, at lunch, during an
outing, or in the host's home. This progression reflects the typical "need"
sequence of the foreigner.

Byrnes[4] put it succinctly in 1966, saying that "the probability of successful
accomplishment is greatest when a friendly, secure individual, not distressed by
the possibility of change, is operating in a well-structured situation about which
he (she) has been given adequate information before-hand." Foreign coaches in
1987 and 1988, and the athletes with whom they worked, indicated that the following conditions are the ones that have most bearing on their effectiveness and
success:

  1. Preciseness of the role definition.
  2. Accuracy of the advance information.
  3. Realism and compatibility of objectives.

4. A good match of personnel and situations.
5. Absence of open conflict.
6. Narrowing of the cultural gap (through knowledge and acceptance).
7. Receptivity of host nationals, especially colleagues.
8. Logistic support that is active and ongoing.
9. Individual qualities/motivation/training.
10. High level interpersonal skills; and
11. High level cultural sensitivity.[5]

Conclusion

There has been found to be a strong relationship between the level of *cordiality* established with host nationals and the degree of effectiveness that is achieved by foreigners abroad. Travelers must remember that, when they are abroad, *they* are the "foreigners." Each must try to "see themselves as others see them"; each must try to put themselves "in the shoes" of their hosts and see things "their way." Travel with curiosity, interest, sincerity and joy. Travel expectantly, and as an ambassador of goodwill. Assume people are nice, they usually are! Take as luggage an openmind, a flexible attitude, a sense of humor, a willingness to learn, and an observant nature. Leave behind bias toward homeland ways, bias against "things foreign," and one's homeland cocoon. Leave behind also any thoughts that " different " means wrong or inferior. People are much the same everywhere. Differences of shape, sound, color, dress, dwellings, food, speech, and customs are really superficial, of great *interest* but *not* of great significance.[6] Cross-cultural endeavors undertaken in this manner will almost certainly be worthwhile and successful, producing "golden rewards" for all those involved.

Notes

[1]Coaches may be male or female. Cross-cultural movements may be made equally by women and men. The coaching may be given just as much to female as to male athletes. For ease of expression and for the quality of the written English, all usage of the term "coach" includes both men and women equally.
[2]Kealey, Daniel J. "Adaptation to new environments," paper from the Briefing Program of the *Canadian International Development Agency*, Ottawa, 1978.
[3]Grove, C. L., and I. Torbiörn. "A new conceptualization of intercultural adjustment and the goals of training," *International Journal of Intercultural Relations*. 9: 2 (1985), pp. 205-233.

[4]Byrnes, Frances C. " Role shock: An occupational hazard of American technical assistants abroad," *The Annals of the American Academy of Political and
Social Science,* 368 (1966), pp. 95-108.

[5]Craven, Jean. "Culture Shock and coaching effectiveness in Canadian sport: An
exploratory account of the cross-cultural experience." Unpublished M.A. thesis, University of Alberta, Canada, 1988.

[6]Craven, Jean. "Enhancing the cross-cultural sport experience." Series of book-
lets. Windermere, U.K.: Sport Consulting, 1988-90.

Chapter 32

The Development of Sporting Excellence in England and Germany: An Historical Comparison

Ken Hardman and Roland Naul

Organized competitive sport has become a significant component of modern society with highly visible world contests attracting global attention. Major international sporting events have become forums for measuring the degree of sport development in various countries. In contrast with nineteenth-century English private schools' athletic traditions and belief in character development, social accomplishments, moral and ethical codes etc., which inspired de Coubertin's ideal of participation outranking winning, there has been an almost inexorable trend in the second half of the twentieth century towards emphasis on winning first and playing for fun second, culminating in some instances in "winning at all costs" attitudes. In some regions of the world, competition has become a tainted term because it is seen largely as winners and losers, obsession with successful outcome and a demonstration of the superiority of one ideology over another. There have been increasing demands and pressures placed especially on young people in the pursuit of excellence born out of selfish motives and goals or state ends.

Following a recently completed multinational study concerned with youths' attitudes towards interscholastic sport competition,[1] the pursuit of excellence has become the subject of a research project on the provision for, and promotion of, young talented athletes, initially in England and Germany. For these two countries,[2] represented in the previous study, various and different activity patterns and structured aspects of competition were largely embedded in historico-sociocultural antecedents. Some divergences and convergences in attitudes suggested the influence of several interrelated factors, of which ideological, socio-cultural

449

and educational determinants predominated. The interplay of those forces within a historical-cultural dimension provided a context in which present features
could be viewed.[3] Such a context is important in comparative study to facilitate
a clearer understanding of meanings of present day similarities, differences and
variations. Therefore, this chapter focuses on historical approaches in the two
countries to provide that context as a preliminary stage in the research project,
with a view to highlighting respective ideological and socio-cultural bases
which reveal variations in principle and practice particularly in the former divided Germany.

In England sporting activity was engaged in, watched and paid for in the late
eighteenth century, with some activities in an advanced state of organization.[4]
However, it was in the private boarding schools of the nineteenth century that
the enduring foundations were laid down. Initially sporting activity was encouraged to structure boys' leisure as an antidote to ill-discipline, immorality, and
general antisocial conduct. Thus organized sport was used as a form of social
control. With the initiatives and support of several variously motivated
Headmasters, 'athleticism' came to be associated with a range of psycho-social
qualities embraced by character-building and with the belief that important
expressive and instrumental traits could be promoted through competitive sport.
As such, these forms of activity received 'official' recognition when the
Clarendon Commission (in 1864) gave its seal of approval that games formed
some of the most valuable social qualities and manly virtues. Significantly,
however, boys were embued with team spirit striving together for a common
aim—the boys' self was sublimated to a team: concentration was on the team
and not individual excellence!

As attitudes to the concept of the female body image changed, so competitive
sport began to feature in Girls Schools' curricular and extra-curricular activities.
Echoing the rationale espoused by her male counterparts, Headmistress
Lawrence (1898) at Roedean regarded the pleasurable healthy exercise of games
as second to none in bringing benefits and as the best arena for the "subordination of self to the good of the side,"[5] stimulation of 'esprit de corps,' and school
prestige.

In the emerging state sector, the spread of universal education facilitated the
extension of the scope of school sport. From early informally arranged 'sides'
games in school playgrounds, competition in a range of sports developed
through local town/district, county, regional to national levels administered by
hierarchically structured associations. The first Elementary Schools Association
(for football), formed in 1885, was soon followed, in the wake of their senior

'adult' associations, by national bodies: the English Schools F.A. (1904), and English Schools Athletic Association (1925). There was no systematic attempt to develop individual talent; rather it emerged incidentally through the structured network of competition. The pattern was one of progression from an individual school (students trained at midday lunch recess or after school, and played on Saturday mornings under the supervision of teachers acting in a voluntary, unpaid capacity for the well-being of the pupils), through selection in turn at town or district, county or regional, and finally to national representation.

The values attributed to sport in Public Schools came to pervade the whole education system, and were enshrined in the Government's Board of Education publications: the 1919 "Syllabus of Physical Training" emphasized the team and not the individual; competition fostered 'team spirit' with children taught to "play up, play the game, and play for the side"[6]; the Board's 1933 syllabus alluded to promotion of health, molding of character, development of team spirit and loyalty.[7] The legacy of the nineteenth-century Public Schools' 'athleticism' was potent and the residual culture has largely held fast. Generally sport was acceptable for its intrinsic (participative), and instrumental (subsummation of the individual in the team and cultivation of character-building traits) values as long as it was not taken too seriously. Young sporting talent has typically been identified through the structured network of competition or by an individual or outside agency in/out of school on an 'ad hoc' basis. Winds of change, however, were signaled in a government 'White Paper'[8] which considered "looking into means of diverting resources to those who are gifted in sport." It was a precursor to a change in philosophy, in a call for a better coordinated system of performance sport to enable young people to develop fully their potential.[9] Some governing bodies of sport (e.g., All England Netball Association, Rugby Football Union inter alia) have introduced development programs and, in the case of Soccer and Tennis, Schools of Excellence have been established. At the Football Association (FA) General Motors sponsored scheme centered at Lilleshall National Sports Center and a local Comprehensive school, 30 selected boys, aged 14-16, follow a normal school program and spend time on training (evenings/weekends) and playing (weekends) under the guidance of F.A. staff and coaches. The Lawn Tennis Association (LTA) founded a tennis school in 1983 with young talented players in residence at the Bisham Abbey National Center and enrolled at nearby schools. The 13 youngsters aged 12-13 receive coaching after school from L.T.A. qualified staff. These, largely voluntary, sector initiatives, plus those in some private Boarding Schools such as Millfield and Kelly College, which offer a limited number of bursaries to very talented youngsters, provide an integrated environment of normal education and opportunity to develop sporting excellence.

The British government is intent on promoting higher standards of performance and excellence both at home and in international competitions.[10] To this end, the Sports Council (1992), in a Consultation Document entitled "Young People and Sport," has identified a four phase development continuum—Foundation, Participation, Performance, and Excellence—a pyramidal corporate approach involving public (schools/local education and government authorities/national, regional and local sports councils), voluntary (governing bodies of sport), and private sectors, in partnership schemes, a number of which are already under way. This comprehensive, coherent progression from participation to performance designed to promote excellence "which the British public clearly wishes to see...,"[11] is somewhat removed from the Wolfenden Committee's Report's (1960) recommendation that national prestige should be kept within reasonable bounds,[12] and a far cry from the nineteenth-century antecedents of healthy, pleasurable exercise pursued for its 'manly' benefits and efficacy in social cohesion and control.

Late-eighteenth-century German bourgeois schools absorbed the Guts Muths' (1793) model of physical education which embraced the spirit of competition and the aim of increasing individual skills in accordance with the general educational philosophy of the period. The 'outdoor' orientation of Guts Muths' 'natural' movement activities was also a feature of the gymnastic exercises embodied within F.L. Jahn's "Turner" system of the early nineteenth century,[13] adopted by several German States' governments (especially Prussia) as part of their reforms in education. A subsequent, politically motivated, ban on "Turnen" (1820-1842) paved the way for developments in indoor gymnastics, in which the emphasis was on discipline and obedience through drill, free-standing exercises, and exercises on horizontal and parallel bars. Criticism returned attention to the ideas and exercises promoted by Jahn. Concurrently, the influence of the English sport movement was being felt. University philologues visited Public Schools, where they were exposed to sport and games activities, the outcome of which was the appearance of football (1874) and cricket (1876) in Brunswick schools. Subsequently. in the latter part of the century, British businessmen, tourists, and students brought a range of 'English' sports into Germany including pedestrianism and athletics, rowing, lawn tennis, and football. Football began its career as a youth sport and physical education activity at Grammar Schools in the 1870s; rowing spread earlier but was only incorporated into the school physical education curriculum in the 1880s; athletics followed in the same period; and even lawn tennis featured as a part of the so called "Games Afternoon" in the 1890s. The first German National Sports Associations founded were those of rowing, in 1883, and swimming in 1886. The German Football Association was established in 1900, and the Lawn Tennis Association in 1902.

Meanwhile, some other sports federations were founded in the 1890s. German Grammar Schools started to incorporate British sports into their physical education curriculum[14] towards the end of the century, but there was no impact on creating interschool sport competition. Instead, schools began to promote German 'Turnen' with a consequent reduction in influence of British games after the turn of the century. At the same time, the newly established German Sport Associations with their club system, extended their sphere of influence. Football, for example, became a popular youth sport but most of the Grammar Schools were reluctant to take up the game. Indeed, in many schools, football was banned from afternoon physical activity sessions and pupils were forbidden from becoming members of a sport club. It is notable that neither the new developing youth sport departments in the club system nor the school system paid any attention to gifted/talented young people up to World War I. The spirit of competition was not an ideal of school physical education, which was still dominated by the spirit of the Turners. British sports were assimilated 'physically' and not 'mentally' in terms of education.

The first steps towards selection of gifted athletes were taken in 1913 when Carl Diem, the new Secretary General for the designated Berlin Olympics in 1916, established a general school fitness badge award with track and field disciplines for grammar school boys, and when physical fitness measurements in the Army were introduced to select athletes.[15] The intervention of war halted these developments. In the early 1920s, Diem reestablished the award scheme as the "Reich Youth Competition" in athletics, and other kinds of sports. Competitive sports and games were organized by the schools as mass-intramurals during their compulsory "Games Afternoon" but there was no attempt or obligation to identify or select gifted students in sports. Every boy and girl was encouraged to participate in physical education as many times each week as possible. Those boys and girls who preferred more exercise, and wanted to compete in sport, joined a sports club where youth sport teams competed in interclub competitions for local, district, and regional championships.

Under Nazi rule, all sports clubs and their federations lost their status of independence and came under the strict political control of the government. Physical education lessons were extended to five hours a week in 1937, but promotion of gifted performers was not a main ambition of the Nazi philosophy of body culture, contrary to the impact of the Berlin Olympics in 1936. In the 1950s, and early 1960s, many efforts were made by the German Sport Association (DSB) to promote physical education, to raise its status in schools, and to rebuild the links between physical activity in the school system and the club system. Once again, Carl Diem had a hand in reinstating the former Weimar athletic award badge, now renamed the "Federal Youth Games." Any gifted student identified by a physical education teacher was directed to a local sport club where, at that time, many physical education teachers still worked as volunteer coaches in the youth departments. Thus, many physical education teachers trained gifted students in the afternoon in the clubs in which they were involved.

In the middle of the 1960s, there was wide debate on the issues of establishment of comprehensive schools and new types of upper forms in the Grammar Schools. Meanwhile, elite sport had become a part of the so called "Battle of the Systems" between the East and the West (just before the 1972 Olympic Games were awarded to Munich in 1966). One year later (in 1967), the well-known weekly journal *Der Stern,* initiated a new competition to improve competitive sports at school. The German Sport Association (DSB) introduced a special program to improve competitive sport at schools in the same year. The increasing success of the GDR sport system was studied with special interest in "Youth Sport Schools," where nearly all the GDR medalists were educated and trained. Therefore, it was not surprising that some sport politicians and sport association officials now demanded special classes and upper forms for talented students in reformed grammar schools. New syllabi were advocated to increase time for training and competition. Some State Ministries of Education started programs for selected "Sport Grammar Schools" in the late 1960s, which were converted into the general curriculum reform of the upper stage of the Grammar Schools in 1972. Now every student of a Grammar School, in grade 11, could select four main subjects for three years to attain the "Abitur" as a general certificate to enter university. Sport received the status of one of two special subjects, each given six hours per week, on which students could focus in their learning (four hours exercises, a two-hour course in one kind of sport, and another two-hour course of theoretical instruction in areas of sports science).

However, prior to 1972, some Federal Sport Federations (e.g., Nordic Skiing, Swimming, Gymnastics, Track and Field) established their own federal boarding schools where the young talented students resided and were trained by top coaches. The sports associations ran full-day or half-day boarding schools and signed contracts with local grammar schools or secondary technical schools where their students were educated. Later, in the 1970s when social and dropout problems increased, some boarding schools were closed. Some others changed to a new model, including types of schools with special classes for their young athletes.

More popular and effective is the model which has been promoted for several years by the State Ministries of Education in conjunction with some State Sport

Associations, and sometimes with the "Olympic Headquarters" which were founded between 1985 and 1989. A school with excellent sport facilities is selected in a city. This school is a local base which offers training time, coaches, and social services (e.g., for homework), for all talented students who join the training group in the afternoons. All children live with their families in the city, except those who come from other cities to attend this special type of school. There is a team of schoolteachers, highly qualified coaches of local elite clubs, and social workers who assist the group, more or less sponsored by a local donor or a company. The Ministry of Education has reduced the number of lessons the teachers have to give if they are involved in the local "swimming," "rowing" or "track and field" project. At present there is a system of decentralization because the regional sports associations cooperate with well-known local clubs, and the Ministry of Education cooperates with selected city schools.

Concluding Comments

Whereas a comprehensive hierarchical structure of interscholastic sports competition evolved to play a deeply significant role in English curricular and extracurricular programs, in Germany such activity developed outside the school system in youth sections of sports clubs. The mid-nineteenth-century 'Corinthian' values laid down in England determined the path of attitudes to sporting activity. The value system accorded with popular and state ideology whilst the nature of the prevailing educational philosophy prescribed the minimal, if any, commitment to achieving excellence in performance. Similar features were apparent in Germany. The outdoor 'Turnen' activities created by Guts Muths and Jahn, together with 'imported' forms of English sports, were seen to foster qualities such as courage, resolution and reliability. Just as in England the 'self' was subordinated to the team and 'the game' was more important than the outcome.

Such antecedents underpinned the attitudes of individuals and institutions to the development of excellence until the medal-winning achievements of communist countries.[16] These achievements were grounded in sophisticated networks of systematic identification, selection, screening, and development of young talented athletes in specialist training centers and sports schools with ancillary medical and other support services. They stood in sharp contrast with the traditional, 'ad hoc,' and decentralized, fragmented approaches which were mainly school or club based. Here talent detection was haphazard, more often than not dependent on the initiative of individual child, parent, teacher, or local coach.

The dominance of East German athletes in the German teams of the 1960s was a cause for West German concern, a situation which was exacerbated by the fear of East German collection of medals in the West German-constructed Olympic facilities, in Munich, in 1972. The solution was a concerted effort and shift in practice towards improved structures for competition, and identification and promotion of young gifted athletes through school sport. A number of action program measures were introduced which served to transform the delivery system of the pursuit of excellence.

Meanwhile, in England, the philosophy of the participation of the many, overriding the importance of the excellence of the few, was undergoing modification. This modification was flagged by the Minister of Sport's Working Party's consideration of the development of sporting talent in boys and girls of school age. With the premise that the development of talent should be commensurate with educational needs and future career, the Working Party pronounced against Sports Schools (they were "educationally undesirable"), preferring partnership schemes where promotion of talent could be pursued out of school. Interestingly, the 1976 Education Act made it illegal for local education authorities to open secondary schools with a selective entry (except for music and dance), thereby effectively placing sporting excellence in the domain of voluntary and private sectors. In 1977, the Sports Council began experimental schemes in regional centers of excellence to help young athletes optimize their sporting potential without compromising their career opportunities. Increasingly, central government has altered its historically laissez faire position to one of 'programmed intervention.' A primary objective is to help sports participants achieve higher performance standards and enable those with the potential to excel to do so,[17] in the belief that a high standard of school sport is an essential prerequisite for success at national and international levels.[18]

Thus, in both England and Germany, there has been a reorientation of attitudes, especially in government and sports institutional circles, witnessed in the introduction of new programs. Their respective traditional school- or school/club-based approaches have been deemed inadequate to meet the demands of present day top-class sport. This review of historico-socio-cultural antecedents reveals changes in the ideologies within the two countries. The former ideals of Public Schools/Guts Muths and Jahn value systems, which determined differences in practice, have been gradually eroded (sacrificed) for the optimization of individual achievement and, some would argue, in the greater pursuit of national well-being and international prestige. Increasingly, convergence and variation, rather than divergence and difference, are being evidenced.

Notes

[1]See Blair, P. F., et al., "A Cross-Cultural Study of Youths' Attitudes Concerning the Role of Sport in the Educational Process," *Journal of Comparative Physical Education and Sport.* XIV: 1 (1992), pp. 4-15.

[2]Specifically the Federal Republic of Germany prior to unification in 1990.

[3]Refer to Hardman, K. and R. Naul, "Interschool Sports Competition: Historical-Cultural Antecedents in England and Germany" *Journal of Comparative Physical Education and Sport.* XIV: 1.(1992), pp. 15-30.

[4]Brailsford, D., "1787: An Eighteenth Century Sporting Year," *Research Quarterly for Exercise and Sport.* 55: 3.(1984), p. 225.

[5]Lawrence, P., "Games and Athletics in Secondary School for Girls," *Education Department, Special Reports on Educational Subjects.* Vol. 2. London: H.M.S.O., 1898, p. 149.

[6]Board of Education, *Syllabus of Physical Education for Schools 1919* London: H.M.S.O., 1919, p. 216.

[7]Board of Education, *Syllabus of Physical Education for Schools 1933.* London: H.M.S.O., 1933, pp. 30-37.

[8]A "White Paper" is a government statement of policy. Department of the Environment, *Sport and Recreation.* Cmnd. 6200. London: H.M.S.O., 1975, p. 19.

[9]Sports Council, *Young People and Sport. A Consultation Document.* London: Sports Council, 1992, p. 18.

[10]Department of Education & Science, *Government's Response to the Education, Science and Arts Committee Report on Sport in Schools.* London: D.E.S., 1991; Department of Education & Science, *Sport and Active Recreation.* London: D.E.S., 1991, p. 3.

[11]Department of Education & Science 1991, p. 3

[12]Wolfenden, Sir J., *Sport and the Community. The Report of the Wolfenden Committee.* London: C.C.P.R., 1960, p. 73.

[13]Jahn, F. L. & E. Eiselen, *Die Deutsche Turnkunst*, Berlin, 1816; and, Guts Muths, F., *Gymnastik für die Jugend.* Schnepfenthal, 1793.

[14]Naul, R., "The Development of Physical Education During the Period of the Industrial Revolution, 1870-1915," In Mueller, N. & J. K. Ruehl *Sport History.* Schors. Niedernhausen, 1985.

[15]Buschmann, G. & K. Lennartz, *75 Jahre Deutsches Sportabzeichen.* Frankfurt: D.S.B., 1988.

[16]The term "communist" represents the western view of the form of government adopted (grounded in Marx-Leninist doctrine). It is acknowledged that "socialist state" did have wide application in such countries.

[17]Department of Education & Science, 1991, p. 7.
[18]Department of Education & Science 1991, p. 3.

Chapter 33

The Selection and Development of Sports Talent at Provincial Level: A Comparison of Sport in Sichuan, People's Republic of China, and Leicestershire, England

Robin Jones

There are two broad questions upon which this chapter is grounded. First, "How does a particular sports system produce winners at the highest level?," and second, "How does a talented individual progress within that system?" Some possible answers to these questions are explored in relation to China and Britain, at the provincial level, using swimming as the example. Swimming is an interesting point of comparison between the two countries because in each case, while it is a popular sport, they have only a modest record of success at Olympic and international levels. That, of course, says nothing about any potential for success!

Lemons and apples may not taste the same, but they can certainly be compared. Sichuan and Leicestershire are lemons and apples in many respects and, in order to help in the understanding of sport in the respective regions, the social and cultural setting in which sport takes place will be fully explored. Sichuan Province in central, southwest China has the largest provincial population in the country, 100 million people in an area roughly the size of the state of Texas. This would rank Sichuan alone among the 20 largest countries of the world and would make it, by far, the biggest country in Europe, and much greater than the population of California. By contrast, Leicestershire is one of England's smallest counties with a population of 850,000, in an area of about 50 miles by 30 miles. However, both Sichuan and Leicestershire comprise large rural areas involved in agriculture and food production. Leicestershire, additionally, has a diverse range of industrial companies in light engineering, hosiery, and footwear, while industrial production includes engineering, aeronautics, electronics and chemicals. The range and diversity of Leicestershire's economy, notwithstanding the current recession in Britain, has traditionally provided its people a buffer against difficult times and, indeed, its image is one of relative wealth when measured against the deprivations more usually associated with the northwest and northeast regions of the country. Sichuan Province is considered as the bread basket, or rice bowl of China, providing its citizens with a sense of self-reliance that would be less typical of provinces not endowed with good natural resources and an equitable climate. On the face of it, therefore, Sichuan and Leicestershire have something in common with regard to their own local identity, but it would be wrong to press that commonalty to the point where they are considered as simply large and small versions of the same thing. They are most certainly not. The differences are rooted both in tradition, which embraces all the complexities of cultural values, and in the practicalities of their socio-economic-political reality.

Locating sport in the broad social context, thus, demands considerable care especially when crossing the boundaries from one's own culture to an entirely different one. Ancient China was influenced by three major themes, Buddhism, Taoism, and Confucianism which deal, respectively, with the future world, the natural world, and the secular world. The latter two in particular, are significant in that Taoism lies behind the traditional martial arts of China that are still practiced today, while Confucianism represents the intellectualism of their early system and the barriers to sport that followed. Modern China, under Mao Zedong, challenged many of these traditional values and customs but did not, and could not, eradicate them all. Thus, there is an amalgam of old and new in Chinese sport that can be puzzling when first encountered.[1]

The rigors and realities of everyday life in contemporary China are quite different from any British example. 800,000,000 people live in the countryside of rural China following a lifestyle that is still largely untouched by the trappings of consumerism and twentieth-century technology. Sichuan Province is fortunate in being a major food producer, and there are many small towns and village communities where rural life is dominated by the seasons, the crop cycles, the harvest, and the labor-intensive routines of their agriculture. In this setting, the Sichuan Provincial Physical Culture and Sport Commission is responsible for the whole sports network of its 100 million people. This clearly is a totally different scale of operation than the county level in Leicestershire, England, but each in its own system represents an important "staging post" for the talented swimmer to progress to national level.

Sichuan invests considerable effort in the search for, and identification of, talented swimmers and any success of China's national team at the international level is sufficient justification for that effort to continue. The Province is divided into 217 counties, eight of which have been given enhanced sports facilities (i.e., for sport in general), and about 40 counties have a swimming program in their schools. There are five levels in the swimming program: 1). school, 2). county, 3). city, 4). provincial, and 5). provincial/professional. Thus, access to swimming pools is reasonable in the towns and cities and Chengdu, the Provincial capital, has about 20 pools. Children's programs for nonswimmers and beginners are arranged at some of these pools during after school and holiday periods when youngsters may learn the rudiments of swimming. Coaches at the pools have the chance to encourage the better swimmers to attend training sessions as one part in the process of sifting through the potential talent. The process of selecting talent also takes place in schools, where children are measured and tested in a battery of water-based tests. Sports scientists supervise the physiological side while the water tests are administered by the coaches. The purpose of these trials is to bring together three groups of people, swimmers, coaches, and sports scientists in the highest level of training at the special sports schools. The testing and measuring that first started in the normal schools continue in the sports school with detailed records maintained.[2] All swimmers here are tested twice a year. From these schools will emerge the Provincial swimming team that can then train full-time for regional and national championships.

Rewritten from research by Ye Guo Shi and He Zhong Tao,[3] the physiological tests include 30 morphological measurements, three functional tests, one index of physical development, 10 tests of general physical ability, three of special abilities, three psychological, and one of competitive competence for a total of 74 indices. Each swimmer's physiological profile is recorded and comparison is made between the predictive power of the tests and the actual results achieved by the swimmers in competition over a period of time (currently about three years). In the city of Le Shan, in August 1991, 300 young swimmers between the ages of 10 and 15 gathered for the trials. Also in attendance were 30 or 40 coaches, sports scientists, and officials.

The young swimmers displayed all the exuberance of being on a fun outing, laughing, chattering, and running around but there was clearly work to be done. In the 50-meter outdoor pool, they were timed in a variety of stroke tests, for example, 50 meters, legs-only butterfly. Observing these tests, it was evident that there was a wide range of ability, from the able and accomplished, to those who (in some tests at least) had difficulty breathing or who struggled to reach the end of the pool. However, no child retired or was withdrawn without finishing, even though there was a big gap between first and last positions. The process of selection was based on several factors, only one of which was the recorded time of the water trial. The coaches, at the trials, were watching for signs of potential based on their own intuitive assessment, but they were also in receipt of the objective test results from the sports scientists who gave their judgment on individuals who might be worthy of special consideration. Ultimately it was the coaches who made the final decision as to which swimmers were to be selected for further training but, from that group of 300, it was expected that perhaps five or six would be suitable.

Once a talented swimmer has been identified, he/she could become a pupil at one of the top sports schools in the Province from which the best would become full members of the Provincial swimming team. This would be the final stage at the Provincial level, any move beyond this being to the National squad in the capital, Beijing. Membership of the Provincial swimming team means being professional and training on a full-time basis at the premier facility in Chengdu, which is housed in its own building and includes a 50-meter competition pool, a training pool, and a 10-meter diving pool. Every aspect of the swimmer's life is thus dedicated towards the aim of improving performance and the Province provides a remarkably comprehensive package to achieve these ends. First, schooling and accommodation are provided 'on site,' with conventional lessons taking place on a half-day arrangement and shared dormitory-type rooms provided for living (four to six persons in a small room). A six-day week is standard for schooling but this may be adjusted according to the demands of the competitive season. Swimming training (land- and water-based), is conducted adjacent to the student dormitories and occupies the major part of their lives, perhaps as much as 42 hours per week. Training is fully monitored by coaches and there is medical supervision of the program by on-site doctors. Nutritional aspects of performance are also balanced according to results in training and competition, and the net effect is that the young swimmers have very little control over their own lives. For their endeavors, they receive a monthly allowance of about 100 to 120 yuan (a school teacher's salary is about 130 to 150 yuan per month), together with the chance to win prize money which, at the highest level, can be measured in thousands of yuan. Medical treatment, hospitalization, or injury rehabilitation is taken care of by the sports school and any special equipment or sports clothing is provided free of charge. All this provision is, of course, subject to the swimmer's continued progress and development. The inducements, the rewards, the attractions of a professional sporting career are thus fairly clear and explicit.

There is, however, another aspect that is less obvious but which is, nevertheless, relevant. Chinese citizens do not, in the normal course of events, have the right to live in any part of the country they choose. To be classed as a 'town person' or a 'country person' (hu kou) dictates where one lives and, with regard to work, it is not simply a matter of deciding to relocate to a city for the opportunity of a better job. Having the status of "country" or "town" person may mean the difference between a culture with some choice and one with uncertainty. The individual cannot choose. However, success in sports, besides the rewards just mentioned, also allows a change of status from country to town (because the sports school is in the town), and for some, this is a greater reward than the sport itself. Country life is the lot of 80% of the people and, while the villages are not so overcrowded as the towns, there is less opportunity for full employment and fewer services and facilities available. Sport represents a significant opportunity even if one is not all that keen on sport. The young swimmer is thus part of an extensive network of full-time, paid professionals all working towards the end of competitive success.

Provision for swimming in Leicestershire, in common with most parts of England, centers on public pools provided by the local councils of the towns and cities. Leicestershire has about 25 such public pools, including six in the city of Leicester itself. There are no 50-meter pools in the county, and the climate dictates that all the pools are indoor and heated. The provision of swimming pools by local councils is part of their overall provision of sports facilities as a public amenity for recreation and leisure. As a public amenity, therefore, the reservation of water time for the exclusive use of competitive swimmers in training is invariably a bone of contention, with clubs having to negotiate with the management of the pool for a limited amount of exclusive pool time, perhaps four or five hours per week, and for which the club will have to pay.

In addition, 60 schools (out of 600 in the county) have their own swimming pools, some of which may also be open to the public after school hours. Schools with their own pools obviously have a better chance of being able to secure exclusive water time to provide competitive training for their able swimmers but much will depend on the special interests and strengths of the physical education teachers at the school. Swimming coaching at the school pool takes place outside of formal instructional hours and the teacher receives no extra payment for this work. There is no fixed pattern to the way school pools are utilized as training grounds for the talented swimmer, but in Leicestershire they are not a major factor in the development of such talent.

To understand how the talented swimmer emerges in Leicestershire, it is necessary to appreciate that swimming clubs, as with all sporting clubs in Britain, are essentially groups of individuals who have decided to promote their own particular interests in sport. Those who become 'officials' of the club do so on a voluntary basis, and different clubs may have different aims and objectives. While some clubs include sections for nonswimmers, some may be keen to promote the health and fitness aspect of swimming along with the enjoyment factor, all of them are involved with competitive swimming. The more successful clubs (i.e., competitively successful) may be able to pay the expenses of a part-time coach which will help to continue to attract the better swimmers and thus enable them to enter the higher level competitions. Smaller, less successful clubs will have to make arrangements for club coaching from within their own voluntary ranks but all clubs have to address the financial problem of payment for use of pool facilities, the costs of affiliation to national governing bodies, competition costs, traveling costs, administrative costs, and the like. These costs are borne by the fees charged to members by the club committee. Transfer by an individual to a better club, in order to get improved training, coaching, and competition will almost certainly involve increased costs and increased traveling time but this is up to the individual to arrange. Clubs may be able to negotiate modest sponsorship deals with equipment or sportswear manufacturers for a few dozen costumes, but such deals are unlikely to have any significant effect on club finances. Cash deals are extremely rare. Thus, being a member of a swimming club in Leicestershire is rather more involved, than just turning up to swim at the appropriate time. It involves, first, the decision by the individual to seek and join a club. A young person may do this with the encouragement and support of parents, or with the advice of a local pool, or just through self-interest. Second, there is the ongoing commitment by the club member (or parent/guardian) to meet the financial dues of membership. Third, there is the evaluation by the member that what he or she is doing is worthwhile in terms of the personal motivation involved. Finally, and related to motivation, is the ability of the member to schedule the swimming alongside the other commitments of school study, or work, along with any other leisure or social activity that may occupy the swimmer's life. Obviously, individuals bring different backgrounds, interests, and motivations with them into the club situation.

Membership of the club, however, is based largely on interest rather than ability, and it is up to the individual to follow the training program of the club (under the guidance of the club coach) to make any improvement in times. Up to the age of 12 or 13 years, swimming clubs in Leicestershire attract roughly equal numbers of boys and girls. Thereafter, there is a decline in female membership.

Throughout Leicestershire, there are 20 swimming clubs (plus a further two for synchronized swimming, and one for diving) with a combined membership in excess of 4,000. For six months of the year, the clubs take part in a network of local swimming leagues catering for the under-nines to senior level, together with a series of club and district championships, thus giving the opportunity for virtual year-round competition. For the best swimmers from each club, an elite club has been formed, membership of which does depend on times in the various strokes. The qualifying times for age groups are set by the coach of the elite club who, incidentally, is the only full- time swimming coach in the county. This club competes in the larger regional league and also in championships up to the national level. This provides a competitive target which improving club swimmers can aim for, although there is no compulsion that they must join this elite club as their performances improve. Responsibility for coaching is left to the club coach, and much will depend on this person's knowledge of coaching techniques, the amount of time he or she has available (it's a voluntary position for the vast majority), the additional voluntary help that other club members may be persuaded to give, and access to back-up resources such as coaching clinics and information from the Amateur Swimming Association's national officers. All this leaves scope for a wide variation in the standard of club coaching. The better clubs operate a swimming development program aimed at improving the abilities of all members, and they plan the training schedules for their swimmers with some care, urging club members to be regular and hard-working in their training "if they are to get the best from it," thus emphasizing the swimmer's individual commitment.

To be "adopted" by the sporting leaders in China is to open the door to considerable security and opportunity. The Chinese government is a great "provider" and the uncontentious nature of sport, coupled with its inherent qualities of personal challenge and intrinsic reward, make it an ideal model, within the context of their political system, for State investment. The sport system provides an opportunity for employment in their overcrowded society and focuses public attention on their national success. In this respect, sport is both bread and circuses. The high commitment to swimming success in China is but part of their overall sporting plan, which in turn, and this is easy to overlook, is part of government planning and the 'open door' policy started in the late 1970s. The modernization of China, insofar as it is successful, will depend not only on investment and industrial development but also on image-building and a continuing belief by the people that the government is leading them forward. Sport fits this mold. Thus, young swimmers with the potential to go on to greater things find themselves in an incredibly supportive yet highly pressurized system. Failure to maintain progress within the system may ultimately result in the swimmer being returned to his or her home town and having to readjust to a normal school environment or taking employment in the locality. Other options for those who have achieved some measure of success may include coaching, university/institute study, or administration. Such decisions obviously could have important consequences for the swimmer's future. The system of extrinsic rewards that is an integral part of the successful swimmer's lifestyle, even at Provincial level, would seem likely to be a dominant feature of the individual's motivation to continue to strive for success in competition.

There is not quite the same sense of urgency in the English system for success at the elite level, although England does produce world champions in most sports, including swimming. It is almost certainly the case that for many elite performers in this country the financial costs of competing outweigh any financial returns that may accrue, except for a very small number who win at the international level and who attract commercial endorsements and appearance money. Swimming does not find itself in the 'glamorous' league in this respect. Any commitment to swimming success in Leicestershire rests with the clubs and their members. The Amateur Swimming Association is certainly active from the national level to the local level in promoting the sport, but this is not part of any broad national sporting plan, much less any government one. Support for the talented young swimmer comes from parents and families and, although there is plenty of opportunity to swim competitively and receive a modest amount of coaching help, there is little certainty that the potential of any one individual is fully explored by the system. However, what does seem certain is that those who do progress to the higher echelons of competition are likely to demonstrate enormous personal commitment to the rigors and pressures of training and to value the sport for its intrinsic rewards.

The stark conclusion of the opening question of this chapter, "How does a talented individual progress within the system?," is that, in Leicestershire, it occurs in spite of the system that the talent develops whereas, in Sichuan, it is a direct outcome of the system. Projecting this to national level, it perhaps offers some explanation why England remains out of the top 20 ranking and why China is beginning to emerge as a global swimming power.

Notes

---

[1]Jones, Robin, "Sport in China," *China Now*. 141 (Summer 1992).

[2]As well as recording data from the 74 index test, the record booklet also notes competition results, written comments of the swimmer, estimate of bone age (from x-ray of hand), and the swimmer's parents' height.

[3]Ye Guo Zhi & He Zhong Tao. "Research on multiple index evaluation criteria for the selection of juvenile swimmers," *Journal of China Sports Science Society*. XI (1991).

Chapter 34

A Six-Nation Study Concerning Attitudes and Participation Patterns of Youth Toward Competitive Sport[1]

**March L. Krotee, Paul F. Blair, Roland Naul, H. Neuhaus,
Ken Hardman, H. Komuku, K. Matsumura,
P. Numminen, and C. Jwo**

In an ever-changing and dynamic interdependent global village, it is requisite that we systematically investigate the forces and environs that shape our programs as well as our societies. The roots of such systematic cross-cultural inquiry were conceived in the epoch of the 1800s when scholars began to delve into the origins, meaning, differences, and social control of games, and texts such as Strutt's *Sports and Pastimes of the English People* and Smith's United States sequel of *Festivals, Games, and Amusements* were introduced to the popular literature.[2] Concomitant with growth and development of games and sport literature was the formation of conceptual frameworks elucidated by Mallinson, Bereday, Anthony, Jones, Lauwerys, and Hanafy and Krotee,[3] that for the most part followed a sociogenic approach espoused by Huizinga[4] and Roberts and Sutton-Smith[5] who believed that play, games, and sport did not originate in various other aspects of culture by chance, but were a wellspring of many cultural forms, and possessed many cultural correlates. Indeed the integral role of comparative physical education and sport across the physical and sport continuum[6] is just now beginning to be fully realized.[7] The influence that competitive sport might play in the educational process is also coming into focus.[8]

Answering the challenge

In the past, social scientists such as Bennett,[9] Broadfoot,[10] and King[11] have pointed out the value of comparative physical education and sport. The need for internationally uniform and reliable data to assist in analyzing change and examining current development, trends, issues, problems and other sociogenic phenomenon is also noted by these prominent researchers. This project provides a research paradigm delving into attitudes of youth toward interscholastic sport across cultures and national boundaries.

Specifically addressed in the study were questions relating to differences in youth's attitudes toward participation patterns in competitive sport. Research focused on differences between the countries, between males and females, and between sport participants and non-participants.

Methods

A total of 1,824 students from Finland, Germany, Japan, England, the Republic of China (ROC), and the United States served as subjects. The students ranged from 13-15 years of age and were members of physical education classes in schools located proximate to the urban areas of Jyväskylä, Finland; Essen, Germany; Tsukuba, Japan; Manchester, England; Taipei, ROC; and Minneapolis-St. Paul, USA. Subjects were asked to volunteer to complete a questionnaire that was administered in accordance with the standard guidelines of each respective university and country. Figure 1 provides a classification of the subjects by country, gender and participatory status:

Finland		Germany		Japan		England		ROC		USA		
M	F	M	F	M	F	M	F	M	F	M	F	
56	31	61	32	128	97	48	30	30	41	119	116	Participants
87	59	103	91	34	61	102	106	158	154	35	41	Non-participants

Figure 1—Subjects classified by country, gender, and participatory status.

The Instrument

The instrument employed in this study was designed by Krotee, Naul, and Hardman in 1990, and consisted of two parts. The first section included demographic considerations and identified participatory status. The second section contained 19 additional statements that pertained to competitive sports activity in each school environment. Students were asked to respond to each statement utilizing a five-point Likert-type scale of strongly agree, agree, not sure, disagree, and strongly disagree. The English-language questionnaire was translated into Finnish, German, Japanese, and Chinese and back translated in order to establish the acceptability of the instrument. Idiosyncratic differences in English word usage between England and the US were addressed. Pilot studies were conducted in order to ensure that the questionnaires were meaningful and suitable for the targeted populations.

Throughout this study the labels "sex" and "play" are used for references to gender and interscholastic or school team participatory status. The term "subject-group" identifies one of the 24 'Country x Sex play' groups, such as "US male non participants."

Analysis of Data

The subjects were grouped by country, gender, and participatory status establishing 24 cells of data that were designed as a 6 x 2 x 2 analysis of variance. Descriptive data including means, standard deviations, and frequency distributions were examined. The data were then statistically treated by use of an SPSSx package for three-way analysis of variance and follow-up t-tests (Fisher's LSD) were employed to provide further analysis of significant comparisons.

Results

Examination of the demographic data revealed a total of 1,820 respondents of which 12.8% (n=233) were from Finland, 15.8% (n=287) from Germany, 17.6% (n=320) from Japan, 15.7% (n=286) from England, and 17.1% (n=311) from the USA. Males accounted for 52.8% (n=961), while females represented 47.2% (n=859). The participatory status breakdown indicated that 43.4% (n=789) participated in interscholastic sport, while 56.6% (n=1,031) were found to be non-participants. Non-respondents to the question included .002% (n=4) of the sample. Figure 2 depicts the overall means for each additional statement:

Statement	Fin $\overline{X}$	Ger $\overline{X}$	Jap $\overline{X}$	Eng $\overline{X}$	ROC $\overline{X}$	US $\overline{X}$	Overall $\overline{X}$
1. The main reason for participating in interscholastic sport is to gain prestige for the school							
	2.57	2.30	2.47	2.63	2.33	3.39	2.79
2. One can meet new friends by participating in interscholastic sport							
	2.04	1.91	2.43	2.17	1.90	1.73	2.01
3. A school is often judged by the success of its sports teams							
	2.77	2.95	2.47	2.75	4.20	2.35	3.00
4. Taking part in interscholastic competition makes other students respect you more							
	2.73	3.75	2.51	3.17	3.45	2.66	3.06
5. The main reason for participating in interscholastic sport is to improve physical fitness							
	2.49	2.22	2.32	2.14	1.86	2.38	2.22
6. I am proud when my school wins a championship, even if I have not taken part							
	1.83	2.13	2.29	1.88	1.92	1.55	1.94
7. It is not necessarily the best players who are chosen to represent the school in competition							
	3.27	3.23	2.68	2.94	2.50	2.87	2.89
8. The only point of playing interscholastic contests is to win							
	3.78	2.74	2.97	3.63	3.77	3.81	3.46
9. Members of school teams enjoy being praised in school pep rallies and assemblies							
	2.37	2.41	2.41	2.40	1.98	1.97	2.22
10. Interscholastic sport competitions are not a very important part of school life							
	2.80	3.00	3.83	3.47	3.18	3.76	3.37
11. My parents would be delighted if I were selected to play on an interscholastic sport team							
	2.25	2.40	2.26	1.98	2.66	2.00	2.27
12. Members of interscholastic sport teams have extra opportunities to improve their physical skills							
	2.04	2.25	2.08	2.05	1.80	1.76	1.99
13. Teachers think more highly of you if you play on an interscholastic sport team							
	2.49	4.02	2.50	3.22	3.53	3.60	3.25
14. If chosen at the last minute to represent one of my school's interscholastic sport teams, I would cancel another engagement rather than let the team down							
	2.37	2.52	2.64	2.70	2.86	2.65	2.65
15. When championships are won for the school, it enhances school prestige							
	2.15	2.28	2.10	2.30	1.98	1.92	2.12
16. There are other school activities which are more important than interscholastic sport competitions							
	3.19	2.63	3.24	2.95	2.28	3.08	2.86
17. I would be proud to represent my school in interscholastic sport competitions							
	2.22	2.45	2.20	1.86	1.73	1.72	2.01
18. I am not interested in taking part in interscholastic sport competitions							
	3.62	3.90	4.07	4.03	3.53	4.25	3.89
19. I like to watch my interscholastic sports team play							
	2.09	2.46	2.42	2.46	2.07	1.94	2.24

Figure 2—Additional statements with Finnish, German, Japanese, English, ROC, USA, and overall means.

Statistical significance was found for many of the main effects (i.e., Country, Sex, Play), and interactions (e.g. Country x Sex, Country x Play, Sex x Play, etc.) of the 19 attitudinal statements. Follow-up analysis further identified specific areas of statistical significance between countries, males and females, and sport participants and non-participants. However, due to manuscript page restrictions, it is not feasible to present the complete findings for all 19 attitudinal statements investigated in the study. Therefore the probabilities for the F-ratios calculated on all of the main effects and interactions for each of the 19 statements are provided in Figure 3, while the authors isolate five attitudinal statements which are addressed in this paper:

Statement	Country	Sex	Play	Country x Sex	Country x Play	Sex x Play	Country x Sex x Play
1.	.000	.181	.962	.059	.000	.143	.628
2.	.000	.001	.403	.002	.000	.945	.274
3.	.000	.538	.052	.018	.278	.173	.797
4.	.000	.128	.000	.001	.350	.246	.706
5.	.000	.844	.051	.032	.122	.907	.596
6.	.000	.000	.008	.022	.019	.727	.893
7.	.000	.336	.917	.000	.050	.556	.308
8.	.000	.000	.089	.107	.000	.892	.009
9.	.000	.581	.211	.002	.003	.011	.273
10.	.000	.616	.000	.003	.110	.071	.643
11.	.000	.149	.000	.024	.307	.650	.204
12.	.000	.987	.000	.403	.874	.859	.735
13.	.000	.154	.391	.540	.123	.152	.323
14.	.000	.021	.000	.000	.002	.214	.411
15.	.000	.534	.002	.076	.140	.204	.592
16.	.000	.004	.000	.030	.004	.643	.390
17.	.000	.079	.000	.000	.006	.125	.009
18.	.000	.522	.000	.000	.002	.133	.751
19.	.000	.000	.001	.001	.007	.724	.603

Figure 3—Three-way ANOVA F-ratio p-values on attitudinal statements.

The five attitudinal statements selected for further scrutiny include statement numbers 6, 10, 11, 17, and 18. These highly correlated (significant at .01 level) items assess the interest that students expressed for participating in interscholastic competitions (#18), the pride they reveal for school sport competitions (#17), and sport championships (#6), the students' perceptions of their parents' pride in regard to the students' sport involvement (#11), and the importance that students ascribe to interscholastic sport in school settings (#10). The means for the students in each country revealed most of them to be in agreement on all five statements.

On statement #6, the means for all countries revealed agreement with the statement. Females were more likely to agree ($\bar{X}$=1.81) than males ($\bar{X}$=2.04), except for the students in England where males were slightly more in agreement ($\bar{X}$=1.87) than females ($\bar{X}$=1.88). Sport participants in Japan, Finland, England, and the US were more in agreement with #6 than the non-participants. Sport participants from Germany and the ROC were less likely to agree than their non-participating classmates.

For statement #10, means for the countries showed the Finnish students to be slightly in agreement ($\bar{X}$=2.80), Germany undecided ($\bar{X}$=3.00), while the ROC ($\bar{X}$=3.18), English ($\bar{X}$=3.37), US ($\bar{X}$=3.76), and Japanese ($\bar{X}$=3.83) students registered disagreement. Overall, students who participated in sport indicated stronger disagreement ($\bar{X}$=3.66) than those who did not participate ($\bar{X}$=3.14). Within the German sample, the mean for male students was in slight disagreement ($\bar{X}$=3.06), while the female students' mean indicated general agreement ($\bar{X}$=2.92).

Country means for #11, were all in agreement ranging from a mean of 2.66 for the ROC to 1.98 for English students. Females expressed more agreement ($\bar{X}$=2.25) than males ($\bar{X}$=2.30). Students who participated in sport were stronger in support ($\bar{X}$=2.09) than non-participants ($\bar{X}$=2.42).

In regard to #17, the means for all six countries showed the students in agreement ranging from the U.S. ($\bar{X}$=1.72) to Germany ($\bar{X}$=2.45). Means by sex revealed more agreement among females ($\bar{X}$=1.97) than males ($\bar{X}$=2.04). Additionally, participants were more likely to support school representation ($\bar{X}$=1.82) than were non-participants ($\bar{X}$=2.15).

Finally, for statement #18, the means for all students in all countries showed them to disagree with the statement. Males ($\bar{X}$=3.94), and females ($\bar{X}$=3.86) were not widely separated on attitudinal statement. Sport and non-participants both expressed disagreement.

Discussion

The five attitudinal statements (6, 10, 11, 17, & 18) are highly correlated items which focus on basic aspects of interscholastic sport: desire to participate, pride in interscholastic sport championships and in representing one's school in sport, perceived parental pride in student's participation, and perceptions of the importance of interscholastic sport. While the levels of agreement and disagreement vary for means by country, sex, and participation, there tended to be general agreement or disagreement by the students for each individual statement. Based on statement #18, it appears that many students who, for one reason or another, are not currently participating in interscholastic sport would be interested in an opportunity to be actively engaged in interscholastic sport.

The results for #10, revealed disagreement from all countries except Germany, which was undecided on the topic, and Finland, which tended to agree ($\bar{X}$=2.80). These may be due to the sport club delivery systems within these countries.

Statement #11, students perceptions on parental attitudes resulted in the perception that students' parents would be pleased if their children were selected on a team. In all countries, this belief was stronger among participants ($\bar{X}$=2.09) than non-participants, however even non-participants expressed the belief that their parents would be delighted if they participated ($\bar{X}$=2.42). Students in the samples from England ($\bar{X}$=1.98) and the U.S. ($\bar{X}$=2.00) indicated higher perceptions of parental satisfaction regarding sport involvement than students in other countries. Students of the ROC ($\bar{X}$=2.66), and Germany ($\bar{X}$=2.40), were less strong in their support of the statement. Statements #6 and #17 found agreement concerning pride, and representing one's school in sport competition across all countries. Female students expressed higher levels of agreement in #6 ($\bar{X}$=1.81) than did male respondents ($\bar{X}$=2.04). The participation breakdown showed that even non-participants took pride in school championships ($\bar{X}$=1.99), although not at the same level as those who participated ($\bar{X}$=1.86).

Additionally for #17, the means for each country once again found the students to be in agreement ranging from 1.72 for the U.S. sample, to 2.45 for the German students. Females were stronger in support ($\bar{X}$=1.97) than the males ($\bar{X}$=2.04). Students who participated in sport were found to be more supportive of the item ($\bar{X}$=1.82) than were those who do not take part in sporting activity ($\bar{X}$=2.04).

Conclusions

This study of youth's attitudes and participation patterns in the international arena identified differences between the students from country to country, between males and females, and between participants and non-participants. The focus remains on five highly correlated attitudinal statements with evident similarities between the students sampled across countries. The authors note a common thread that runs throughout the five statements isolated in the study. It is the thread that weaves together overall student expressions that they value interscholastic sport opportunities, that they and their parents take pride in the students' involvement in school sport, and that students are interested in taking part in interscholastic sport competitions, including both students who already participate and those who do not.

The imminent merging of myriad educational and sport processes will undoubtedly impact upon the delivery systems that shape the world of the future. It is a requisite that delivery systems are responsive to the changing needs of the citizens. The complex world presents professional educators and sport practitioners with opportunities and challenges to cooperatively design, implement, and conduct dynamic inclusive programs which will contribute to international peace and understanding and improve worldwide quality of life.

Notes

[1]This is the final report of an ISCPES sponsored research project.

[2]Avedon, E. M., and B. Sutton-Smith. *The study of games.* New York: John Wiley & Son. 1971.

[3]Anthony, D. W. "Comparative physical education." *Physical Education.* 58 (1966); Bereday, G. Z. F. *Comparative methodology in education.* New York: Holt, Rinehart, and Winston. 1964; Hanafy, E. H., and M. L. Krotee. "A model for international education comparison: Middle East perspective". In, M. Krotee and E. Jaeger (eds). *Proceedings of the International Society of Comparative Physical Education and Sport.* Champaign, IL: Human Kinetics, 1986, pp. 253-266; Lauwerys, J. "What is comparative education?" In, Lauwerys & Taylor (eds.). *Education at home and abroad.* Boston: Routledge & Kegan Paul, 1973, pp. 11-13; Mallinson, V. *An introduction to the study of comparative education and sport.* New York: Macmillan, 1973; Jones, P. *Comparative education: Purposes and method.* St. Lucia: University of Queensland Press, 1971.

[4]Huizinga, J. *Homo ludens: A study of the play element in culture.* Boston: Beacon Press, 1950.

[5]Roberts, J. M. and B. Sutton-Smith. "Child training and game involvement." *Ethnology.* 1 (1962), pp. 166-185.

[6]Krotee, M. L., I. H. Chien., and J. F. Alexander. "The role of psychological study in physical activities and sport." *Asian Journal of Physical Education.* 3

(1980), pp. 83-89.

[7]Grüpe, O. "A theoretical framework for comparative physical education and sport." H. Haag, D. Kayser, and B. L. Bennett (eds.). *Proceedings of the International Society of Comparative Physical Education and Sport.* Champaign, IL: Human Kinetics. 1987, pp. 3-8.; Hardman, K. "Comparative physical education and sport: Respect or neglect?" In, J. Standeven, K. Hardman and D. Fisher (eds.). *Comparative Physical Education and Sport: Sport for All in the 90's* . Aachen, Germany: Meyer & Meyer Verlag. 1991, pp. 88-96; Krotee, M. L., and P. F. Blair. "International dimensions of HPERD, sport, and aging." *Journal of Physical Education, Recreation and Dance.* 62: 5 (1991), pp. 49-50.; Krotee, M. L. *The dimensions of sport sociology.* West Point, New York: Leisure Press. 1979; Krotee, M. L. "The saliency of the study of international and comparative physical education and sport." *Proceedings of the International Society of Comparative Physical Education and Sport.* 8 (1981), pp. 23-27.

[8]Hardman, K., M. L. Krotee. and A. Chrissanthopoulos. "A comparative study of international competition in England, Greece and the United States." In, E. Broom et. al. (eds.), *Proceedings of the International Society of Comparative Physical Education and Sport.* Champaign, IL: Human Kinetics. 1988, pp. 91-102; Hardman K., D. Bean, A. Chrissanthopoulos, N. Kahn, M. Krotee, and J. Piccoli. "Students' and teachers' attitudes toward interscholastic sport competition: A transnational comparison." *Proceedings of the International Society for Comparative Physical Education and Sport.* Hong Kong: The Chinese University of Hong Kong. 1989, pp. 183-192.; Ichimura, S. and R. Naul. "Cross-cultural assessments and attributions to female soccer: Japan and West Germany." In, J. Standeven, K. Hardman and D. Fisher (eds.). *Comparative Physical Education and Sport: Sport for All in the 90's.* Aachen, Germany: Meyer & Meyer Verlag, 1991, pp. 212-220; Krotee, M. L., C. Y. Huang, and R. Naul. "A cross-cultural study of the socialization process of female soccer athletes". In, J. Standeven, K. Hardman, and D. Fisher (eds.), *Proceedings of the International Society of Comparative Physical Education and Sport: Sport for All in the 90's.* Aachen, Germany: Meyer & Meyer Verlag. 1991, pp. 242-248.

[9]Bennett, B. L. "What's new around the world in comparative physical education and sport?" In, M. L. Krotee and E. M. Jaeger (eds.). *Proceedings of the International Society of Comparative Physical Education and Sport.* Champaign, IL.: Human Kinetics, 1986, pp. 91-96.

[10]Broadfoot, P. "The comparative contribution—A research perspective," *Comparative Education.* 13 (1977), pp. 133-138.

[11]King, E. J. *Other schools and ours.* London: Holt, Rinehart and Winston, 1979.

Chapter 35

Daily Physical Activities and Motor Performance of West German and Czechoslovakian Schoolchildren[1]

Roland Naul, Werner Neuhaus, and Antonin Rychtecky

This study represents a three-year longitudinal survey consisting of two parts. Data collection of the first part began, in June 1987, on boys and girls from grade 6 in general physical education classes in Prague, Czechoslovakia, and was completed with grade 8 measurements in 1989. When research collaboration between the Physical Education Department of the Charles University, in Prague, and Essen University in Germany was agreed upon in 1989, the German part of this project started in 1989 and was completed in July 1991.

In order to ensure the compatibility for comparison with the Czechoslovakian studies the West German research group followed the same research design, methods, and procedures. Problems of adaptation, translation, and validation led to the exclusion of one motor test (Ruffier Test), and a psychological questionnaire on achievement motivation. This project was previously reported on at the last 7th ISCPES Conference at Bisham Abbey in 1990, when results from the first Czechoslovakian (1987) and first German (1989) measurements of the study were presented and compared.[2] The final report will focus on selected findings of the longitudinal study to underpin convergencies and divergences from a comparative perspective.

There were no serious methodological problems in adapting the tests, as the collaborators in Prague had chosen tests used internationally for measuring motor performance and physical metabolism ranges of activities. However, some problems arose in assigning an identical and comparable strain index to the different motor leisure activities of the students, which were recorded in a daily regime for one week. No students from Prague, for example, indicated skateboarding as a leisure activity, and no students in Essen spent the weekend with their parents working in the garden of their datscha in the country. Although the different qualitative aspects of the motor activity culture in the two countries were interesting and noteworthy, the respective national peculiarities had to be classified in a rating process according to a general strain index in order to ensure quantifiability and comparability of the activities.

Subjects and Design

Table 1 presents the Czechoslovakian and German test groups of the study:

Table 1—The Sample

		1987	1988	1989	1990	1991
	Grade:	6	7	8		
CSFR	Number:	126	126	126		
	Age:	12.4	13.3	14.3		

	Grade:			6	7	8
FRG	Number:			92	102	113
	Age:			12.5	13.5	14.5

As mentioned before, the CSFR study had already started in 1987 and was completed in 1989; the German part of the project did not start until 1989 and was finished in 1991. Four different physical education classes, from grade 6 in Prague and Essen respectively, were examined every year in June/July for three years up to grade 8. The daily physical regime was completed over one week (7 days) during these periods of measurement. Both samples in the CSFR and the FRG consisted of an identical age group and a comparable group of the students with respect to the demographic data.

There are indeed some differences between the West German and the Czechoslovakian boys regarding height and weight after the 3-year period. Measurements of the German boys began with the lowest value in body height and body weight but, during the two years of development, they surpassed all other groups. There are fewer gender-related differences in the development of German girls and Czechoslovakian boys, but some important differences between their Czechoslovakian counterparts.

Tables 2/3—Height and Weight

Increasing of Height

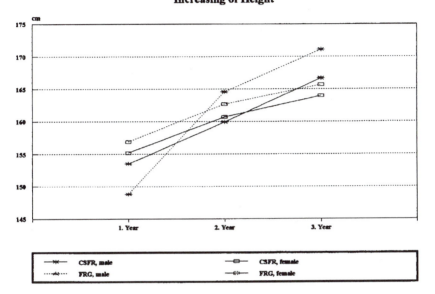

	CSFR, male	CSFR, female
FRG, male		FRG, female

Increasing of Weight

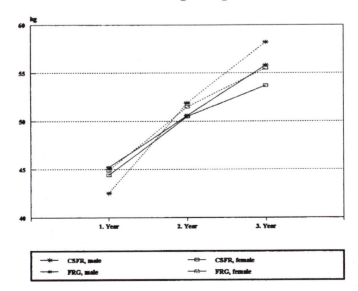

	CSFR, male	CSFR, female
FRG, male		FRG, female

The test methods and the most important items and classifications are given in Table 4:

Table 4—Test Methods

Motor Performance			Daily Regime		Ruffier Test	Motivation Test
Run	**Jump**	**Throw**	**Categories**	**BMR**		
50m-dash	standing broad jump	standing throw	K1 sleeping	110%		
	long jump with run	flying throw	K2 relaxing	120%		
			K3 learning	150%		
Power	**Flexibility**	**Endurance**	K4 walking	300%		
flexed arm hang	exercise with stick	shuttle test cooper test	K5 playing	500%		
sit-ups	complete motor test		K6 exercising	800%		
	ball throwing and catching					

Four test batteries were used in the design. A complex motor performance test was employed for measuring six different performance indicators (running, jumping, throwing, as well as power, flexibility, and endurance). The measurement items are listed in Table 4. As a third test component the students were asked to record their daily regimen over one week (7 days), together with the time spent on the respective activities. The motor tests were conducted on two different days prior to this week. Each morning, at the beginning of class, the records of the previous day were checked to ensure that the complete 24-hour rhythm was recorded. If there were time gaps the respective students were interviewed in order to determine the activities and fill in the missing data. All activities reported by the students were classified according to the strain index (K1-K6) and added up as minutes per week. For each level a relative metabolic value was defined, which allowed the calculation of a metabolic value for each student based on his/her average daily activity. If a student, for example, were to sleep for 24 hours a day his/her metabolic value would be set at 110%; if, on the other hand, he/she were to do physical exercises and training for 24 hours a day the value would be 800%. The average daily rhythm as a basic metabolic range (BMR %) was calculated for each student from the minute volume of the respective strain level on the basis of the relevant metabolic percent value.

Motor Performance

The results of selected motor performances are compiled in Table 5:

Table 5—Motor Performance/50m dash and standing broad jump

50 m Dash		1. Year		2. Year		3. Year	
		male	female	male	female	male	female
CSFR	Seconds:	9.28	9.41	8.63	8.96	8.50	9.15
	Stdev:	0.67	0.73	0.68	0.75	0.69	0.70
FRG	Seconds:	8.73	8.81	8.35	8.69	7.86	8.42
	Stdev:	0.71	0.58	0.63	0.54	0.72	0.60

Standing Broad Jump		1. Year		2. Year		3. Year	
		male	female	male	female	male	female
CSFR	cm:	171	170	178	168	193	170
	Stdev:	23.8	20.6	23.6	16.9	26.7	22.4
FRG	cm:	181	178	203	188	216	182
	Stdev:	15.8	21.9	18.9	19.1	23.7	15.9

In grade 6, German boys and girls are about half a second faster than their Prague counterparts and they stabilized their superiority over the three years. A clearly superior performance to the Czechoslovakian students exists in standing broad jump as well. There were no significant sex differences within both national groups at the grade 6 level. However, sex differences developed over the three years in both national groups and between the German and Czechoslovakian girls and boys, respectively.

In the standing throw, the Czechoslovakian female students dominated their German counterparts. For the German girls there is only a very low range of development which is regressive in the last year. The German boys developed their performance only slightly better than the Prague male students. A similar level of performance was achieved by all boys and all girls in the flexed arm hang. However, the Czechoslovakian male and female students performed much better than the German students did in grade 6.

Table 6—Motor Performance/standing throw and flexed arm hang

Standing Throw		1. Year		2. Year		3. Year	
		male	female	male	female	male	female
CSFR	m:	27.8	20.3	31.1	21.9	33.6	24.1
	Stdev:	6.1	4.8	6.0	5.1	7.1	5.0
FRG	m:	27.9	18.7	31.3	19.9	35.3	19.0
	Stdev:	6.0	4.6	6.2	5.8	8.4	6.1

Flexed Arm-Hang		1. Year		2. Year		3. Year	
		male	female	male	female	male	female
CSFR	Seconds:	35	23	34	22	45	29
	Stdev:	22	17	23	13	23	15
FRG	Seconds:	20	17	34	29	44	30
	Stdev:	14	11	17	16	19	14

A similar trend was found for endurance performance measured using the Cooper Test. The Prague students showed better endurance capacity than their German counterparts in grade 6, but German boys and girls developed their endurance better in the following two years. In grade 8, Essen boys surpassed the Czechoslovakian students and the German girls reached the same level as their Prague counterparts.

Table 7—Motor Performance/endurance

Cooper-Test		1. Year		2. Year		3. Year	
		male	female	male	female	male	female
CSFR	m:	2185	2071	2280	2096	2296	2140
	Stdev:	400	397	524	422	414	204
FRG	m:	2019	1870	2302	2027	2403	2159
	Stdev:	435	347	303	276	462	474

Summarizing the development of the selected motor performances, one can say that the German group developed better in speed and leg power while the Czechoslovakian group was superior in arm power and endurance in grade 6. However, the German boys dominated after two years and the German girls reached nearly the same level as the Prague girls except in the standing throw.

It is likely that the Prague students are trained more in gymnastics than the German students who were better trained in track and field when the project started. In general, the motor performances of boys in both national groups developed continuously, whereas some motor performances of girls seemed to be somewhat regressive in both national groups between the 2nd and 3rd year of measurement (Czechoslovakian girls in 50m dash and German girls in standing broad jump and standing throw).

Daily Regime

The evaluation of the daily regime revealed some interesting differences between the German and the Czechoslovakian students, as shown in Table 8:

Table 8—BMR range

BMR		1. Year		2. Year		3. Year	
		male	female	male	female	male	female
CSFR	%:	177	175	185	183		
	Stdev:	16	13	20	19		
FRG	%:	202	196	215	192	220	194
	Stdev:	30	31	40	24	43	23

On average, the Czechoslovakian students have a lower percentage of basic metabolism than the German students. Unfortunately, it is not possible to compare the final stage of the 3rd year because the Prague medical doctor passed away in 1989 and his position was not filled. Nevertheless, there seems to be a trend of fewer sex differences in the Czechoslovakian sample within the calculated basic metabolism range of motor activities. The German girls have a higher BMR percentage than the Czechoslovakian boys. However, the German girls did not increase their total range of motor activities within the three years; instead a slight regressive trend can be seen from grade 6 onwards. There seem to be two different physical youth cultures with varying sex profiles in each national group as it was reported for the strain indexes two years ago.

A statistical evaluation of significant correlations between the results of the motor performance tests, and the reported data of categories of the daily regime, could only be conducted for the German test group, since the respective data from Czechoslovakia necessary for this comparison has not been available over the last two years of the study. For the German students, such a significant relationship between motor performance and daily physical activity range was only established for some motor performance items, but not generally over the three years.

Tables 9/10 show the correlation indices for the different motor performance items over the three years:

Tables 9/10—Influence of Activity Profile on Motor Performance

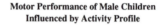

**Motor Performance of Male Children
Influenced by Activity Profile**

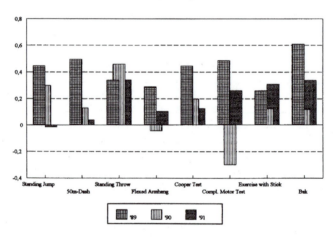

**Motor Performance of Female Children
Influenced by Activity Profile**

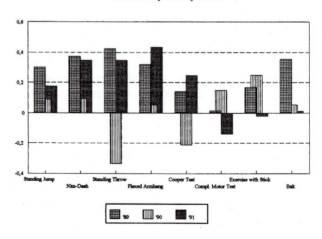

Good motor performances are not generally influenced by high basic metabolism values; that means, by the time spent doing exercises. For the boys significantly more convergences were found than for the girls in 1989. For both sexes a significant correlation between high metabolism range and good motor performance existed only for really basic motor activities like running and jumping, except for the endurance run for girls (Cooper Test). Yet over the three years the influence of metabolism on motor performance continuously decreased. An increase of physical activities has no influence on the development of power and flexibility as measured by items like standing throw, flexed arm hang, complete motor test and exercise with stick. It is likely that the different time of reaching sexual maturity for boys and girls, and the more qualitative range of upcoming special training of different kinds of sport, are more important factors for these kinds of motor skills. The consequences of high maturity for motor skill development, which is in grade 7, influenced the different and somewhat confusing correlation scales for boys and girls between the 1st and 2nd time of measurement. The later special training of different kinds of sport in grade 8, may be an important reason for more similarities between a high BMR range and motor performances in running and jumping than there were in grade 6.

Conclusion

The fact that German students have to attend one hour per week more of physical education at school, than the Czechoslovakian students, cannot explain the differences measured between both groups. The German girls practice organized sports almost three times as much as the Prague girls in the first year, which is probably due to the degree of organization combined with the large membership in sports clubs. Only slightly more than 20% of the Prague students are organized in a sport group outside of school, or are active members of a sport club, while the comparable value for the German students is 50% in the 1st year of the study. However, more and more girls reduce their exercise time in the second and third year, whereas the Czechoslovakian girls did increase their range of physical activities up to the second year. Other German studies have indicated that, particularly, the girls leave sport clubs between the ages of 12 and 14.[3] In summary the findings verify that medical measurements of daily physical activities are often not valuable to investigate predictors of motor performances. So many contextual, sex, motor, and social related factors of development have to be reflected in this special age group between 12 and 14, that in subsequent cross-cultural projects this type of test will be rejected. Motor and medical tests were utilized in the belief that they are better to use for cross-cultural comparison than other tests because they are neutral and therefore more valid to identify cross-cultural divergences and convergences. In fact, significant differences in the sex profile of physical activities and development of motor performances in Czechoslovakian and German students were found; however these important cross-cultural differences exist more in a truly cultural context than in the quantitative measurements of performances and activity ranges. That is the main outcome of this study and, of course, that traditional medical and motor tests are not necessarily valid across cultures, since elements specific to a certain culture play a significant role for various aspects of a test, for example in its construction. Nevertheless the authors have learned much more about what must be changed in cross-cultural research design than about practical information that can be positively recommended.

Notes

---

[1]This is the final report of an ISCPES sponsored research project.
[2]Naul, R., Paur, M. & Rychtecky, A. "Daily Physical Activities and Motor Performance of West-German and Czechoslovakian School Children." In K. Hardman, R. Fisher, & J. Standeven, *Sport for All in the 90s*. Aachen: Meyer & Meyer, 1991, pp. 204-211.
[3]Brettschneider, W. D,. & M. Braeutigam. *Sport in der Alltagswelt von Jugendlichen*. Frechen: Ritterbach, 1990.

Part 8: Theoretical and Methodological Considerations in the Cross-Cultural Study of Sport

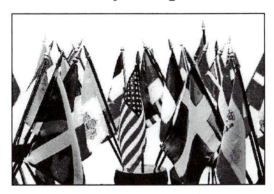

Part 8: Theoretical and Methodological Considerations in the Cross-Cultural Study of Sport

As with a number of the humanities and social science sub-disciplines of sport, cross-cultural and comparative studies have a short history. Huizinga[1] in 1950 and Caillois[2] in 1961 stand out as writers who recognized the importance of play and games in our understanding of cultures; Roberts and Sutton-Smith broadened their forerunners' perspective on the place of play in disparate cultures. It was not until sometime later (1970), that Luschen edited a series of papers on the cross-cultural analysis of sport and games. In 1983, Harris and Park[3] edited more papers on play. games and sport. However, apart from individual papers from a variety of sources, it was not until the late 1970s that comparative research in sport, based on cross-national and cross-cultural data, became more formalized.

A significant event which highlighted this was a conference organized by Simri, in Israel during 1978, which brought together 60 interested scholars who, collectively, helped to establish a society whose main focus was the sharing of ideas with special interest in comparative research. Every two years thereafter, a group of comparativists have met to share knowledge of the phenomenon of sport in disparate cultures, together with a section to examine theories and methods most appropriate for this endeavor.

A persistent and logical section of each conference has been devoted to methods and theories, as well it should! All areas of study must seek to find appropriate theoretical and methodological approaches to assist those undertaking research as well as those using research findings to arrive at the most appropriate conclusions. Discussions about methods and changes which might be made to programs and materials must be based on valid research approaches. Consequently, there is a continuous need to explore new theories, test existing ones and keep trying new methods of data collection, treatment and translation. Each biennial conference has included a theoretical and methodological section to stimulate new ideas and re-evaluate former ones.

The three papers in this section, not surprisingly, use different approaches and focus upon different themes. In Chapter 36, DePauw, Goc Karp and Smith address the issue of internationalizing the curriculum in physical education. This coincides with a change in the International Society's perspective which very recently has included international as well as comparative issues in sport and physical education in its journal and has expanded the papers given at conferences to include both foci. Undoubtedly in cross-national or cross-cultural studies of sport, 'international' contributions are a first step; that is, these comparisons can only be made when data have been collected from unique societies or cultures. One must have a data base on a culture or country before these (data) can be compared with others.

A second reason why internationalism can be justified is in order that students can be introduced to different sports, methods of teaching them as well as the form sport takes in different cultures and countries. We need to have a much more global perspective in order to appreciate our own. The authors argue that although efforts have already been made at the university level to allow some individuals (both students and faculty) to expand their horizons—both literally and figuratively—through exchange programs and international visits both to and from other countries, a more sustained and expanded program is necessary to benefit all Americans. That is, the curriculum itself must make a concerted effort to overcome and more generously provide a more global inclusion of knowledge.

Furthermore, they argue for an 'infusion' of knowledge, that is, one in which "international perspectives become(s) more of an integral part of the curriculum." They further expand on how this may develop and be implemented. An infusion model is offered to show how this may occur; examples are explained.

The intent of Haag's chapter is to determine how triangulation, a new concept to many, may be usefully employed as a way to improve comparative research in, what Haag refers to as, sport sciences. Triangulation is combining several research methodologies when studying the same phenomenon. Several advantages are enumerated and a 'Kiel Model' is further explained—which is a specific application of the concept. The overriding justification is the improvement of comparative research.

The final chapter is devoted to the past, present and future of comparative research written as a collective enterprise by three former presidents of the International Society for Comparative Physical Education and Sport. Notable events and publications are identified, themes are explained and further directions offered.

Further developments will occur in both theoretical and methodological considerations in cross-national and cross-cultural studies of sport. They must if the field is to remain healthy and grow in stature. To use a cliché, the world is becoming ever smaller; we must learn from each other and our work must have a defensible research base to give it credibility.

John C. Pooley

Notes

---

[1]Huizinga, J. *Homo Ludens: A Study of the Play Element in Culture.* Boston: Beacon, 1961

[2]Caillois, Roger. *Men. Play, and Games.* New York: The Free Press, 1961.

[3]Harris, Janet C., and Roberta J. Park. *Play, Games and Sport in Cultural Contexts.* Champaign, IL: Human Kinetics, 1983.

Chapter 36

Internationalizing the Physical Education Curriculum: A Model for the Infusion of Knowledge

Karen P. DePauw, Grace Goc Karp, and Barbara A. Smith

For nearly as long as they have been in existence, United States colleges and universities have participated in and sponsored international activities such as foreign study, exchange programs, visiting scholars, overseas student teaching opportunities, intensive language study, and other international research or study projects.[1] As academic units in the higher education setting, physical education and sport programs have participated in many of these activities which were initiated primarily during the 1970s.

A new dimension to the international activity arena has been added recently: internationalization of the university.[2] More specifically, efforts are now being directed toward internationalizing the higher education curriculum. In a recent study by Henson,[3] 79% of United States universities were found to have already begun their internationalizing efforts. Ninety-eight percent of the respondents indicated that global issues would become increasingly more important to society and the university as well.

The university, by virtue of its very nature as well as from an historical perspective, has been devoted to the pursuit of truth and the advancement of knowledge. Inasmuch as knowledge and truth know no national boundaries, the global perspective of the university must be nurtured,."..the pursuit of knowledge and truth will lead us to internationalization and ultimately, to the globalization of the universities."[4] Thus, institutions of higher education must accept the responsibility to educate individuals to become citizens of the world.

Sport (physical activity) is highly visible throughout the world; it exists in the global village. Due to the universal nature of human movement and the fact that sport (physical education, dance, etc.) is never free of the politics of its culture,[5] physical education and sport in higher education are ideally situated to participate fully in, if not lead, internationalization efforts. Similar to other academic units in the university, physical education departments have a role to play in preparing citizens for life in the global community.

Although international activity (international scholar visits, foreign travel, overseas student teaching, international conferences) in physical education occurs with increasing frequency, systematic efforts to share this knowledge with others has tended to be limited to the few professionals who have international experiences and their students. A typical approach to "internationalizing" physical education programs in higher education has been the offering of a course in comparative physical education and sport or including international topics within selected courses. More attempts must be made to internationalize the entire curriculum.[6]

To internationalize the curriculum requires that not only a systematic approach toward internationalization be adopted but, more importantly, that an international perspective be valued by the faculty and administration. Although it is true that an international perspective can be developed or increased by exposure to, and contact with, international activities, professionals in physical education must take the responsibility for systematizing the inclusion and dissemination of and about physical activity in the global village.

Inclusion and Infusion

To date, curricular internationalization activities in departments of physical education in higher education have been conducted along inclusion lines. Inclusion in the curriculum has been most frequently implemented through (a) the development and offering of a separate course(s) on comparative (international) physical education and sport, (b) offering academic learning experiences (e.g., visiting scholar lectures, film series, conferences, readings) outside the classroom, (c) the addition of a content-specific international perspective within a selected section of required (or elective) courses, and (d) the addition of an international perspective throughout a selected course. This approach is most often isolated to individual faculty members with extensive international experiences and strong personal commitment to enhancing international awareness.

Infusion of international perspectives within (throughout) the curriculum is the next logical step toward internationalization. Whereas inclusion includes both the imparting of knowledge and the application of this knowledge, infusion additionally requires ownership of, and commitment to, an international perspective on the part of the faculty and students. When knowledge and application are interwoven throughout the curriculum, the international perspective becomes more of an integral part of the curriculum. As this knowledge becomes more integrated, faculty and students tend to see and value the interconnectedness. Once value is attached, ownership and commitment result. In this chapter, infusion is proposed as the underlying process and ultimate goal of internationalizing the physical education curriculum.

Internationalization

To internationalize the physical education curriculum successfully, three key interrelated aspects are necessary: well-defined process, appropriate resources, and logical and effective strategies. Process refers generally to a planned and systematic approach to internationalization. The process should follow a logical progression such that strength of commitment and ownership are increased gradually over the course of time. In establishing the process, emphasis should be placed on providing experiences in the cognitive, psychomotor, and affective domains as well as on acknowledgment of, and respect for, different teaching and learning styles. In the process of internationalizing, it is important that the approach be one which moves the education from teacher-centered to learner-centered throughout the course of implementation.

Appropriate resources and support for internationalization are critical. Resources on international physical activity (sport, physical education, dance, etc.) are actually plentiful. Numerous books, journals/periodicals, international conferences, and international organizations have international perspectives as their focus. Examples are shown in Table 1. From the various publications available, international bibliographies (coded by topic, country, etc.) and listings of films/videos, publications etc., can be easily developed. In addition, interviews (audio, video) with visiting scholars and foreign students about physical activity in one's country could be catalogued and available to students and faculty. (Specific questions can be pre-selected and asked systematically of all interviewees). Slide/tape presentations and/or computer-assisted learning modules could be developed on specific topics (e.g., elementary games around the world; organization and structure of sport in Scandinavia). The availability of existing programs and/or access to culturally specific locations will provide opportunities to enhance the learning experiences.

Table 1—Selected Resources for Internationalizing the Physical Education Curriculum

<u>Organizations</u> (selected, 50+):

Association Internationale des Ecoles Superieures d'Education Physique (AIESEP)
International Society on Comparative Physical Education and Sport (ISCPES)
International Federation on Adapted Physical Activity (IFAPA)
International Council on Health, Physical Education and Recreation (ICHPER)
Federation Internationale d'Educationale Physique (FIEP)
International Committee for the Sociology of Sport (ICSS)
International Association of Physical Education and Sport for Girls and Women (IAPESGW)

<u>Conferences</u> (selected):

Regularly scheduled conferences sponsored by organizations identified above and many others.

<u>Journals</u> (selected):

> *ICHPER Journal*
> *Physical Education Review*
> *ISCPES Journal*
> *International Journal of Sport Psychology*
> *Scandinavian Journal of Sport Sciences*
> *Soviet Sports Review*

<u>Books</u> (selected):

> *Comparative Physical Education and Sport (Volumes 1-7)*
> Knuttgen, Ma and Wu., *Sport in China.* Champaign, IL: Human Kinetics, 1990.
> Williams, T., L. Almond, and A. Sparkes, *Sport and Physical Activity.* London: E. and F. N. Spon, 1992.

Along with appropriate resources and a well established process, the identification and selection of logical and effective strategies are necessary for internationalizing the physical education curriculum. Among these strategies are assigned readings followed by discussion, literature reviews, research papers and/or studies, comprehensive exams, problem-solving tasks, debates, identification of trends/issues, assimilation/role playing experiences, participation in actual physical activity/games/sports from different cultures, and practicum experiences in culturally diverse settings.

Infusion Approach

The three aspects described above are central to the infusion approach to internationalizing the physical education curriculum advocated here. Inasmuch as internationalization is a gradual process, three implementation levels are proposed. These levels (additive, inclusion, infusion) are described in Table 2. As shown, each level builds upon the preceding level until infusion is achieved. Essential in the model is the gradual addition of commitment required by the professor and the students alike.

Table 2—Level and Approach to Internationalization.

Level	Approach	Content	Commitment	Learning Exp	Value Added
I	Additive	knowledge	little or none	single isolated unrelated	exposure initial awareness
II	Inclusion	knowledge application	partial	multiple related	enrichment partial understanding
III	Infusion	knowledge application synthesis	strong	integral integrated	enrichment ownership understanding

Infusion Model

As in most models, these are a number of steps that need to be taken. These steps and their interrelationships are shown in Figure 1:

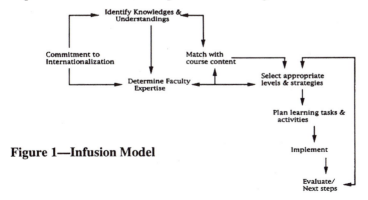

Figure 1—Infusion Model

The first step to internationalizing the curriculum is to establish a commitment to internationalizing. Internationalizing can occur with the addition of relatively few new financial resources. The commitment of time to these efforts, especially by the coordinators of such activity, is far greater than any real financial commitment. Without a commitment of time and effort on the part of all faculty, internationalizing efforts will be less than desired.

Given a commitment to internationalizing, the next step is to identify the knowledges and understandings desired of physical education majors and minors (undergraduate and graduate). These knowledges and understandings should be identified in all three domains of learning: cognitive, psychomotor, and affective.

After identifying the desired outcomes in terms of developing an international perspective among physical education students, faculty expertise needs to be determined as well as matching the specific knowledges and understandings (outcomes) with existing courses in the curriculum (e.g., understanding the role of sport in culturally diverse countries could be matched with courses on sport sociology, introduction to P.E., elementary or secondary methods). An alternative approach to matching international knowledge with courses is to examine the current content of each course and identify topics which could be "internationalized" (e.g., similarities and/or differences across countries regarding the legal aspects of sport).

Effective internationalization is dependent upon the selection of the appropriate implementation level (additive, inclusion, infusion), and identification of appropriate strategies. These are related, in part, to the extent of faculty expertise and the specific content to be infused. The specific learning tasks and experiences selected should be appropriate to the content offered in the specific courses. Implementation begins after selection of the appropriate level and strategies, and the learning tasks and activities are designed. Both formative and summative evaluation should occur within each course and across the curriculum. One of the important questions to be determined is the next step. It is anticipated that, after success at one implementation level, an effective plan can be developed for the next implementation level. Thus, the same step in the model can be traversed again for optimal implementation at a different level. The ultimate goal is to achieve the infusion of knowledge throughout the curriculum and to have this knowledge become a natural part of the course.

Examples

Internationalization can occur in all courses offered in the physical education curriculum; theory, laboratory, and activity courses. Three examples are included below: (a) adapted physical education methods course; (b) elementary physical education methods course; and, (c) college physical activity class. Please note that the examples provided are course specific but that the strategies are applicable in other situations.

Within the adapted physical education class, the following assignment could be given. Divided into groups, students would be asked to select a country and report about the country's approach to physical education and sport for individuals with disabilities. The presentation could include topics such as existing organization and structure of sport, current opportunities and approaches to integration or segregation of individuals with disabilities, educational approaches, financial support, and more. Key in the presentation would be the relationship among culture, society, and individuals with disabilities. A second assignment might be the teaching of a game selected from a specific country appropriately modified by disability and/or culture.

In an elementary methods class, a similar assignment could be given. Groups could be asked to present elementary games from a number of countries and to compare and contrast from a cultural perspective. In addition, students could incorporate the use of language cues, such as words of the day, in the language of the country from which the game was selected. Another assignment could be the use of movement activities that include the geography and regional information about countries throughout the world. For example, a bean bag toss onto a world map depicted in the gym or classroom could be used to identify the location of countries around the world. Another example could be to dribble a ball to areas identified as highly or sparsely populated. These types of activities could also be used to identify environmental issues common to many countries around the world.

The focus of internationalization shifts somewhat when infusion is applied to a physical activity class. In a racquetball class, a related game such as squash could be introduced to students as a sport similar yet different to racquetball. The historical and cultural aspects of the two sports could be compared and contrasted in a manner which educates students about different cultures but does not detract from the learning of racquetball. Little known facts (e.g. In Malaysia, the badminton finals rank equal in importance with the Super Bowl in the U.S.) could be shared periodically throughout the semester.

Concluding Comments

Internationalization of the physical education curriculum often begins from an inclusion perspective which is an important first step, but should progress toward an infusion approach. An infusion approach requires a paradigmatic shift from an additive, ethnocentric (perhaps even homogenization) approach to a more global perspective; an integrated approach in which one culture does not take precedence over another. Infusion implies a curriculum-wide systematic approach to increasing international awareness and global understanding. Inasmuch as knowledge and understanding of human movement (physical activity, physical education, sport, etc.) belong in the world university, these authors advocate an infusion model for internationalizing the physical education curriculum in colleges and universities.

Notes

[1]DePauw, 1990; Pacheco & Fernandez, 1992
[2]Henson, 1990
[3]Henson, 1990
[4]Pacheco & Fernandez, 1992
[5]DePauw,1990; Sage, 1988
[6]DePauw, 1990; Toohey, 1987

Chapter 37

Triangulation: A Strategy for Upgrading Comparative Research Methodology in Sport Science

Herbert Haag

The aim and purpose of this chapter is to examine the concept of triangulation and consider its application to comparative sport science research. The review of literature indicates that the amount of literature dealing with research methodology is characterized by the descriptive method, a status quo survey design, content analysis as a technique of data collection, and hermeneutic-oriented techniques in analyzing data coded in words. The following major issues are analyzed within this investigation:

- The concept of triangulation.
- "Kiel Model of Research Methodology" (KMRM) Position of techniques of data collection.
- Characteristics of comparative sport science research.

Furthermore, the relationship of these three aspects was carefully evaluated with the intention of upgrading research in comparative sport science.

The Concept of Triangulation

"Triangulation is the application and combination of several research methodologies in the study of the same phenomenon."[1] The need for triangulation can be summarized as follows:

a. To get more information on the real world, therefore combining naturalistic and rationalistic or qualitative and quantitative approaches.[2]

b. Because movement, play, and sport are very complex phenomena, they have to be seen in a varying social-cultural context.

c. Triangulation offers a possibility to reconcile the hermeneutic-theoretical and empirical-analytical research approaches.

Denzin[3] distinguishes four types of triangulation as part of a multiple method
approach:

I.   Data triangulation (time, space, persons).

II. Investigator triangulation (e.g., engaging multiple
     observers).

III. Theory triangulation (e.g., using more than one theoretical
     scheme in the interpretation of the phenomenon).

IV. Methodological triangulation (i.e., using more than one
     method, design, technique of data collection, technique of
     data analysis).

Multiple triangulation occurs when a researcher combines multiple sources of data,
multiple observers, more than one theoretical perspective, and several methodologies in one study. In this investigation type IV will be further analyzed, since it is
the most complex form of triangulation and indirectly related to types I and III.

Very often, triangulation is neither considered nor accepted among the different
possibilities for shaping a research process, since there are also problems connected with its application. These include:

• Locating a common subject of analysis to which multiple data,
  observers, methods and theories can be applied.

• Locating a problem that has not been investigated before, the
  issue of novelty; and

• Restriction of time and money.[4]

Some of these problems, however, seem to be problems of research in general and
therefore should not give cause to reject triangulation as a research process.

Olafson's reaction to Standeven has provided a very useful and practical concept of triangulation.[5] He proposes to see triangulation as the combination of data derived from selected quantitative and qualitative methods in order to reach an intercept of important results.[6] This means the utilization of data, coded in words and numbers (for which a variety of techniques of data collection are necessary in order to investigate complex issues). This interpretation of triangulation by Olafson[7] is fitting into the concept of research methodology (KMRM) presented subsequently to further clarify the concept of triangulation.

The "Kiel Model of Research Methodology" (KMRM). Position of Techniques of Data Collection

The KMRM is characterized by the following six steps, making up a logical process of conducting research in sport science:[8]

I. Scientific theory; this means theories of gaining knowledge (hermeneutical, empirical, phenomenological), and theories related to the politics of science (idealistic subjectivism, dialectic materialism, critical theory, critical rationalism, logical empiricism, positivism).

II. Research methods; this means approaches like descriptive, correlational, experimental.[9]

III. Research designs; this means more detailed indications on the realization of the research process (examples for research designs: historical, time-historical, survey, action research, ethnographic research).

IV. Techniques of data collection (examples include observing, questioning, and analyzing content).

V. Techniques of data analysis; this means strategies for analyzing data coded in words and/or numbers (hermeneutical and statistical strategies).

VI. Transfer of research results; this means short range, medium range, and long range measures to transfer research results to practice through, for example, conferences, workshops, journals ("practice to theory and theory to practice" paradigm).

Within these six steps of a research logic process, point IV "techniques of data collection" plays an important role, since at this stage the specificity of research related to sport science emerges. Techniques of data collection have a direct relation to triangulation due to the fact that triangulation, in many cases, means the utilization of more than one technique of data collection. In this regard it seems necessary to report, in some more detail, on the techniques of data collection.

There appear to be three distinct categories of data collection techniques:

- Formal orientation (observation, questioning, content analysis, apparatus-based techniques).

- Theory field orientation. Techniques of data collection organized according to theory fields of sport science (e.g., sport medicine, sport biomechanics, sport psychology, sport pedagogy, sport sociology, sport history, and sport philosophy).[10]

- Theme field orientation (techniques of data collection organized according to their use in regard to different central themes of sport like movement, play, and training/coaching).[11]

Thus it is apparent that many different techniques of data collection are available to the researcher. This, in turn, facilitates the application of the process of triangulation in order to arrive at better and more valid results and conclusions.

Characteristics of Comparative Sport Science Research

A closer look at the characteristics of comparative sport science is necessary in order to make final conclusions on triangulation as a strategy for upgrading comparative research methodology in sport science.[12]

Comparative sport science research can be characterized by the following traits:

- A large and diversified data base due to the fact that the total socio-cultural background has to be analyzed in order to formulate solid and valid research results in a comparative setting.

- Multiple research approaches on the level of the KMRM in order to evaluate a comprehensive understanding of the research topic.

- Balance between theoretical-hermeneutic and empirical-analytical research approaches in order to come up with holistic answers on a research question.

These characteristics prove indirectly that, in many cases, triangulation is an appropriate strategy to utilize in research on comparative sport science. The utilization and application of triangulation thus can enhance comparative research and insights into foreign developments, as well as international aspects of sport, sport education, and sport science.

Summary of Results

The results of this investigation can be summarized in the following four points:

a. Triangulation, in regard to the six aspects of the KMRM (especially to aspect IV "techniques of data collection"), is a useful strategy for comparative research in sport science.

b. Data are produced in words and/or numbers, thus often requiring a multiple approach such as triangulation. The "word and/or number" paradigm seems more logical, at least from a semantic point of view, since the qualitative versus quantitative paradigm is rather confusing and misleading.[13]

c. The discussion around triangulation has revealed, once more, that establishing the research question should remain the foremost consideration after which an appropriate research methodology is identified.

d. The utilization of triangulation in comparative sport science research can contribute to the reconciliation of the two extreme research positions like hermeneutic-theoretical and empirical-analytical. Not only one research paradigm should be considered. A paradigm in comparative research implies methodological choices. Therefore, there is a great challenge for the development and application of triangulation also within a comparative research process in sport science.

Concluding Comments

The purpose of this chapter was to analyze three aspects: the concept and strategy of triangulation; the KMRM; characteristics of comparative sport science research and the relationship to triangulation.[14] The primary conclusion is that the application of triangulation can indeed upgrade the quality of research within comparative sport science, and triangulation will become more and more important to those engaged in sport science research.[15]

Notes

[1]Denzin, "Triangulation," *Educational research, methodology, and measurement: An International Handbook.* Oxford: Pergamon, 1988, pp. 511-533.

[2]Guba, E., & Y. Lincoln, "Naturalistic and rationalistic inquiry," *Educational Research, Methodology, and Measurement.* Oxford: Pergamon, 1988, pp. 81-85.

[3]Denzin, pp. 511-533.

[4]Denzin, pp. 511-533.

[5]Olafson, G. "Triangulation in comparative research: Mixing qualitative and quantitative methods," *Sport for all: Into the 90's.* Aachen: Meyer & Meyer, 1991, pp. 39-44.; Standeven, J. "Trying triangulation: A response to Gordon Olafson and Denzin," *Journal of Comparative Physical Education and Sport Cross-Cultural and International Studies.* XIII: 2, pp. 55-61.

[6]Haag, H. "Zum paradigm qualitativ-quantitativ," *Sportpsychologisch Forschungsmethoden.* Koln: Bps, 1991, pp. 69-77.

[7]Olafson, pp. 39-44.

[8]Bauersfeld, K. *Forschungsmethoden in den sportmethodischen Wissenschaftsdisziplinen.* Leipzig: Zeitschrift der DHfK, 1987; Haag, H. "Forschungsmethodologie der sportwissenschaft," *Einfuhrung in das Stadium der Sportwissenschaft.* Schorndorf: Hoffman, 1991, pp. 292-306.

[9]Haag, H. "Methodenentwicklung in der Sportwissenschaft," *Sport und Wissenschaft.* Leipzig: Zeitschrift der DHfK 1991, pp. 46-67.

[10]Haag, H., B. Strauß, & S. Heinze. *Theorie und Themenfelder für Sportwissenschaft.* Schorndorf: Hofmann, 1989; Haag, H., & K. Hein. *Informationswege für Theorie und Praxis des Sports.* Schorndorf: Hofmann, 1990.

[11]Haag, Strauß & Heinze, 1989.

[12]Haag, H. "Forschungsmethodologie in der Sportwissenschaft. Grundlagen des vergleichenden Forschungsansatzes," *Beitrage zu Grundfragen des Sports und der Sportwissenschaft*. Schorndorf: Hofmann, pp. 28-40.; Haag, H. "Research methodology in sport sciences. Implications for the comparative research approach," *ISCPES Halifax 1980. Proceedings of the Second International Seminar on Comparative Physical Education and Sport*. Halifax: University of Dalhousie, 1982, pp. 89-110; Haag, H. "Comparative sport pedagogy - Comparative education. A basic intrarelationship within educational sciences," *Comparative Physical Education and Sport*. Champaign, Ill.: Human Kinetics, 1986, pp. 33-48; Haag, H. "Concerning the importance of research methodology in comparative education for sport pedagogy," *Comparative Physical Education and Sport*. Hong Kong: Chinese University of Hong Kong, 1989, pp. 253-267.

[13]Haag, pp. 69-77.

[14]Thomas, J, & J. Nelson. *Research Methods in Physical Activity*. Champaign, Ill.: Human Kinetics, 1990.

[15]Thomas & Nelson, 1990.

Chapter 38

The Past, Present, and Future of Comparative Methodology in Physical Education and Sport: Presidential Perspectives

Herbert Haag, John C. Pooley, and C. Lynn Vendien[1]

Way back in the early 1950s and early 1960s, there seemed to be an abundance of literature on the history of physical education and sport but very little in the area of comparative study or research in sport and physical education, except in news reports on international competitions and proceedings from international congresses. Most of the promotion and motivation for increasing study and research in this area of comparative came from history scholars and other dedicated leaders active in international associations. Descriptive techniques with some analysis seemed to be the most common method used.

Early Comparative Courses

Even without adequate literature, pioneer courses in comparative sport and physical education began as early as 1948 at Springfield College with Atallah Kidess, followed by Charles Speidel and John Lawther at Pennsylvania State University in 1955, and Lynn Vendien at the University of Massachusetts in 1962. By the mid-1960s, courses soon began to increase worldwide stimulating the need for further study and research.

Early Comparative Literature

This area of study had only two comparative textbooks by the 1960s. The first was by Pierre Seurin, of France. Published in 1968, *L'Éducation Physique dans le Monde* included 42 countries. In 1968, the first book in English by Vendien and Nixon, *The World Today in Health, Physical Education, and Recreation*,[2] appeared and included information on 26 countries. In both of these pioneer efforts, the contributing authors were asked to follow specific topics for comparative purposes. Although this request was not always adhered to, through these publications, dedicated scholars and graduate students were stimulated into doing further extensive comparative research projects.

Other significant literature in the 1960s included the ICHPER worldwide questionnaire study published in 1963, and revised in 1967-68; "Teacher Training for Physical Education," "Physical Education in the School," and "The Status of Teachers in Physical Education"; the seven monographs entitled, "Physical Education Around the World," and edited by William Johnson (in 1966, 1968, 1969, 1970, 1971, 1973, and 1976), which were later (in 1950) condensed into the volume, *Sport and Physical Education Around the World.*[3] Again mostly area descriptive techniques were used.

In an effort to obtain more information about comparative methodology for future research and to assist teachers in a relatively new field of study, four surveys were conducted:

I. Comparative Education.[4] Thirty nationally recognized scholars in Comparative Education were contacted and 21 responded.

II. Comparative Health, Physical Education, Recreation and Sport.[5] Thirty-one individuals offering such courses were contacted and 21 responded.

III. Comparative Sport and Physical Education.[6] Thirty national and international scholars teaching such courses were contacted and 29 responded.

IV. Comparative International Sport and Physical Education.[7] Three hundred national and international scholars teaching such courses were contacted and 190 responded.

Another textbook completed in 1975, and revised in 1983, *Comparative Physical Education and Sport,*[8] was written by Bruce Bennett, Maxwell Howell, and Uriel Simri. This book was one of the first to use specific topics for comparative analysis.

Early Comparative Studies with International Organizations

Many international organizations contributed to comparative literature, research, and study in the area of comparative sport and physical education as presented at their meetings and published in proceedings. To name a few, International Federation of Physical Education (FIEP); International Association for History of Sport and Physical Education (HISPA); International Association of Physical Education and Sport for Girls and Women (IAPES-GW); International Council for Health, Physical Education and Recreation (ICHPER); International Council on Sport and Physical Education (ICSPE); International Relations Council of the American Alliance for Health, Physical Education, Recreation, and Dance (IRC); International Society for Comparative Physical Education and Sport (ISCPES); and the United Nations Educational, Scientific and Cultural Organization (UNESCO).

To cite a few examples, beginning in the early 1960s, at the national AAH-PERD conventions in the U.S.A., IRC devotes 2-4 sessions on the topic of Comparative/International Sport and Physical Education. Another is ICHPER, whose members have made outstanding contributions to this area of study. Aside from the worldwide questionnaire reports in the 1960s, at their congresses, they began to offer a variety of SIGs (Special Interest Groups), including Comparative Sport and Physical Education. For many years their Comparative Coordinator, Lynn Vendien, was assigned the task of inviting scholars from all over the world to come and present their papers on comparative topics. The methods used for these presentations varied from simple description to a variety of comparative research techniques. In 1975, at their Congress in Rotterdam, and again in 1977 at Mexico City,[9] time was provided to examine the need for forming a comparative organization. This organization (now ISCPES) was founded in 1978, so at ICHPER in Kiel, in 1979,[10] and ICHPER in Manila, in 1981, the combined, cooperative efforts of these two organizations were evident in the variety and quality of comparative research presentations.

The Founding of ISCPES

In recognizing the role of ISCPES in developing, increasing, and improving comparative research and studies in sport and physical education, it is worthwhile to examine its formative years. During the Christmas week of 1978, the First International Seminar on Comparative Physical Education and Sport convened at the Wingate Institute in Israel, directed by Uriel Simri, and co-sponsored by ICHPER and FIEP.[11] It was a rather small group of some 60 delegates, dedicated leaders, representing 14 countries from around the world, who gath-

ered to focus on various comparative topics and techniques. The quality of presentations, the feeling of caring and belonging to a closely knit group, along with
a very special social-cultural program including tours, made this Comparative
Seminar, the first of its kind, such an outstanding success, that it was one never to
be forgotten.

On December 29, 1978, this Society was founded as an International Committee
on Comparative Physical Education and Sport (ICCPES), and elected a Steering
Committee comprising: Lynn Vendien, U.S.A., Chair; Uriel Simri, Israel,
Secretary-Treasurer; John Pooley, Canada; and Svein Stensaasen, Norway. This
Committee was asked to explore possibilities for its future and then make recom-
mendations for:

1. affiliation with another organization.
2. administrative functions.
3. Membership categories.
4. Constitution and By-laws; and
5. Plans for a Second International Seminar.

ICCPES: Suggested Purposes

1. Strengthen and promote the specialized area of comparative
   study.
2. Encourage development of programs of study.
3. Help promote, support, and exchange research information.
4. Support and cooperate with all levels of organizations with
   similar goals.
5. Sponsor meetings bringing together worldwide people on
   comparative study.
6. Issue appropriate publications (Fall, Winter, and Spring).

ICCPES Memberships

1. *Founding members* are those who attended the First International Seminar in
   Israel.
   - 21 in number.
2. *Charter members* are those who joined after the 1st Seminar and before the
   2nd Seminar.
   - 123 in number

The 2nd International Seminar

The 2nd International Seminar on Comparative Physical Education and Sport was held in September 1980 (at Dalhousie University in Halifax, Nova Scotia, Canada) under the direction of John Pooley. Some 50 delegates, representing 13 countries, provided another rich and challenging environment. A constitution was drafted, and membership categories established. At this time, including the 21 Founding Members, 123 Charter Members, and 11 new Members who came to the Seminar, the total membership was 155 representing 25 countries. During this meeting the name ICCPES was changed to the ISCPES. The Committee became a Society with a newly elected Executive Board comprising Vendien, President; Simri, Secretary-Treasurer; Pooley, Vice-President; and Stensaasen, Member.

The main purpose of this Seminar was to exchange ideas about Comparative Physical Education and Sport Research and Teaching.[12] Research methodology was especially highlighted. Papers for presentation were selected mostly on the basis of research that compared two or more countries, or topics, along with teaching methods in comparative physical education and sport.

Comparative Research in Sport and Physical Education

There is no one accepted style of teaching in a comparative classroom anymore than there is one accepted method in comparative studies or research. The one accepted fact is that there must be at least two or more well-defined topics to compare. However, Bereday, as early as 1964,[13] emphasized the need to clearly define the problem along with appropriate sampling techniques and methods of collecting the data. He then listed four distinct and commonly used steps for completing comparative research, 1. Description of data; 2. Interpretation and evaluation of data; 3. Juxtaposition, thus establishing the similarities and differences; and, 4. Comparison with hypothesis and a conclusion. Considering that any research in the area of Comparative Sport and Physical Education was a relatively new field of study, it had rather rigid guidelines for early interested scholars. Survey methodology was common in the early years and remains so today. Even still, the sampling techniques need to be scrutinized more carefully as they are so critical to the conclusions drawn. However, in those earlier days, when area descriptive technique was most often used, it did have great value in arousing interest and understanding, but without some comparative analysis, it could not be classified as comparative research. The topical approach depended upon the individual, the locale, and availability of instruments to be used. Most of all, some concept of flexibility was necessary in order to understand and utilize new approaches that could benefit a study.

Since the mid-1960s, and especially in the 1970s after ISCPES was founded, the interest in comparative sport and physical education continued to increase greatly, producing a considerable amount of literature including books, journal article, and conference proceedings. As stated before, one of the primary goals of ISCPES has always been to promote research in comparative sport and physical education, to provide assistance to those seeking to initiate studies, and to help promote programs of teaching.

At this 8th Conference of ISCPES, delegates must never forget the true value of face to face contacts at conferences, with exchange of ideas, and a much deeper understanding of and from people and programs of all cultures around the world. Acknowledging there is no one accepted method to follow, one must continue to be flexible in approaches and together help develop an exciting new future in the area of Comparative Sport and Physical Education research.

The Present Status

Today, the continuing debate on comparative methodology in physical education and sport is healthy. It began for members of ISCPES at the first seminar, in Israel fourteen years ago, when a formal structure for the field began to develop. Early scholars relied principally on colleagues in comparative education and only secondarily from others in the social sciences to provide methodological guidance. Frankly, the early methodological focus was piecemeal with a mixture of regional, national, cultural, and individual case studies, only some of which were marginally comparative, if at all. Usually, an international flavor was enough to convince some that this was the same as 'comparative' studies or that, subsequently, one could make a comparison *ex post facto*. This very quickly changed, in the minds of most.

Slowly, a growing cadre of scholars from various cultures, whose education had been nurtured in diverse university settings, joined what became a Society in 1980. Methodological practices were diverse; and so they have remained. The thrust of the criticism aimed at the embryonic field of comparative physical education and sport, in the early 1980s especially, was about the absence of comparative data rather than on its treatment. A typical plea was that some studies were accepted either for presentation at the biannual conferences (they were originally named as *seminars* and treated accordingly), or for publication in the *Journal*, which were single case studies with the comparative element absent. The comparative focus, it was argued, was the root of the Society's work and should be protected.

During very recent years, there has been a return to an acceptance of single case studies, usually, though not exclusively, in the form of single country or culture studies, as an essential step in comparative work. It can be argued that case studies alone (without a comparative component) *should* be included in the Society's publications, as well as at conferences. This author disagrees, although for years comparative education has accepted such papers as legitimate in the field. Whatever the type of data used, studies should include two or more elements of the same variables or phenomena for a comparison to be made. Alternatively, the justification of a single case (such as a country's youth sport offering or an analysis of discriminatory practices in sport as a function of gender, race, or ability) should only be accepted by the Society if a discussion section is added where comparisons are made with other cases. I draw the reader's attention to the *purpose* of the Society in emphasizing comparison as *the* focus.

Notwithstanding these remarks, since Pooley's article in 1986 entitled "The Use and Abuse of Comparative Physical Education and Sport,"[14] in which a number of suggestions were made, there has been more comparative research by individuals representing different countries who collect data (in varying forms), or who conclude with a comparison of it, pointing out similarities and differences between theirs and other cultures and countries. Moreover, more scholars have visited other cultures and countries and there would appear to be a greater likelihood of comparative research to be undertaken soon in spite of a worldwide recession.

However, many challenges made in Pooley's earlier address have not been accepted. There is much to do in the comparative domain, for the chance to learn about our world neighbors using a variety of strategies is increasingly easier than 10 or five years ago. In spite of this, we continue to practice sport in isolation and in ignorance of others. Interested scholars have a great responsibility to examine, carefully and critically, issues and programs so that we may see our system in clearer perspective and make adjustments where necessary.

For a debate about methodology, Gordon Olafson's article on "mixing quantitative and qualitative methods,"[15] together with Joy Standeven's[16] constructive criticism of it, is useful in articulating current issues. More fundamentally, Patton's[17] contemporary and comprehensive treatment of *qualitative research methods* is recommended as an excellent guide for new courses. It is assumed that most scholars have a fundamental knowledge of *quantitative* research, since university research methods courses, internationally, usually focus on this type of methodology. Overall, qualitative research is likely to be used in comparative studies much more in the future. As Siedentop[18] has indicated, it is natural, responsive, context relevant and flexible, if complex. Recognizing the element of complexity merely acknowledges that issues in physical education and sport are, by their nature, complex, especially when using 'macro' variables involving systems of sport or physical education. Complexity is heightened when dealing with cross-national and cross-cultural settings. Qualitative research is interpretive. As Locke[19] asserts, a key assumption holds that it is not possible to understand people and their actions unless they are taken within the whole context. Qualitative research sometimes is called "naturalistic" because it is not interventionist, and it involves observations of settings in their natural state. Suggestions for avoiding subject falsification include (1) being aware of the risk of making unjustifiable assumptions and not letting down one's guard; (2) remembering that most dissembling is triggered by perceived threat; (3) remembering that faking is difficult to sustain over time; and, (4) following procedures for cross-checking subject accounts.[20] Earlier, the same author[21] recognized that novices in qualitative research encounter problems which are familiar in any form of inquiry, but which often require responses different from those used in quantitative designs. His paper discussed, within the framework of research in physical education, external and internal problems and issues faced by the researcher using the qualitative design. The paper concluded with three pages of selected references for the novice.

Using a somewhat different approach, Schriewer[22] defines comparative (physical) education as an elaborate form of mediating between cross-cultural data and social scientific theories. He presents analytical possibilities for methodological analysis and socio-historical reconstruction, while West,[23] using the novel title "How not to do comparative education," urges comparative researchers to immerse themselves in a society in order to study its physical education or sport system.

Finally, although again focused on comparative education but recognizing the similarities with our field, Sheehan[24] has warned against the assumption that the values we hold as individuals are the correct ones! He has indicated that a major problem affecting the comparative field has been the way in which Western values have infected the analyses of non-Western educational systems. Researchers (especially those involved with underdevelopment) have not remained scientifically neutral, have too often played advisory and advocacy roles, and have thus helped to perpetuate dependency and exploitative relationships. Comparative education, he said, should return to the goals of its pioneers, and approach the systematic study of the educational problems and proposed solutions of other countries and cultures in terms of the difficulties diagnosed in society. The tensions in the discipline of comparative education will be resolved only if it is generally recognized that the question of what can and cannot be done in the study of foreign countries is a moral one. The same can be said of comparative physical education and sport, although the use of the term pioneers is a bit grand!

The debate about methodology will continue and so it should. A variety of approaches will be applied and so they should. Charles Ragin,[25] a comparative sociologist has produced a new view [to me] of comparative methodology which, as he says, moves beyond qualitative and quantitative strategies. From an initial, and only cursory view of his work, there would appear to be much promise in his thesis and in our future use of it.

Future Directions

Concentrating on future prospects of comparative methodology in physical education and sport, it is imperative to consider the immense changes which have taken place in recent years. These include breakdown of the East-West confrontation; development of international cooperation (see Europe); development of small state units with national identity and civil war conflicts; awareness of two basic world problems, the environment, and migration South to North as well as East to West (leading to more multicultural societies); and the installation of a humanistic form of economy, the so-called social marked economy, replacing the planned communistic economy and avoiding the extreme capitalism of a western nature.

All these developments require a solid understanding of socio-cultural diversity all around the world. Since movement, play, and sport are integral parts of culture and society, there is an increased need for true comparative research in sport and physical education in order to help the future development of mankind under a humanistic perspective. Movement, play, and sport can play an important role in this regard. Thus it is the responsibility of sport science, in its comparative dimension, to engage in this direction. Since the targets for research are very complex and multidimensional, the research methodology for comparative sport science has to be constantly refined and sophisticated.

Consequently the challenge is quite great for sport science especially in its dimension of research methodology. The following points seem to be important for the future development of sport science as a scientific field with a solid methodological basis and a grasp for investigating the urgent topics and questions of the present-day world:

- The process of finding hypotheses or assumptions for research studies has to be realized very carefully. Only in this way science, and also sport science, can meet their responsibility in an institution of society, serving its purposes.

- The question, issue, or problem at hand always has to be considered first and only then the aspects of research methodology can be decided upon.

- There has to be a balance of hermeneutic-theoretical and empirical-analytical research approaches in order to provide sound analysis of complex phenomena in comparative research.

- New and unusual aspects of research methodology, from the broader realm of academe, should be considered in sport science, in general, and in comparative sport science specifically in order to upgrade research in this field (compare triangulation, meta-analysis, objective hermeneutics, multivariate analysis).

- The transfer of knowledge gained by scientific endeavor has to be secured in order to get a maximum benefit from research. The paradigm "practice to theory and theory to practice" underscores this objective.[26]

Improved research methodology will further support the relevance and importance of cross-cultural and comparative research in physical education and sport. Finally, the primary purposes of such study remain:

- To learn more about other countries.

- To learn more about oneself through being exposed to other models (i.e., enhancing self-evaluation).

- To search for human betterment through implementing "foreign" elements into one's own system.

Notes

---

[1] As former Presidents of the International Society for Comparative Physical Education and Sport, Professors Vendien, Pooley, and Haag chose each to focus on the "past," "present," and "future" respectively.

[2] Vendien, C. Lynn & John E. Nixon, *The World Today in Health, Physical Education, and Recreation.* Englewood Cliffs: Prentice Hall Inc., 1968.

[3] Johnson, William (Ed.), *Sport and Physical Education Around the World*, Champaign, IL: Stipes Publishing, Inc., 1980.

[4] Vendien, C. Lynn, "Survey on Comparative and International Education Courses," Paper presented at IRC, 1969.

[5] Miller, Ben W. "Highlights of Facts and Opinion Survey on Courses in Comparative and/or International HPER and Sport, Paper presented at IRC, 1970.

[6] Vendien, C. Lynn, "Survey of Existing Courses in Comparative Sport and Physical Education," Paper presented at IRC, 1968.

[7] Vendien, C. Lynn & John E. Nixon, "Survey on Comparative National and International Courses in Sport and Physical Education," Paper presented at IRC, 1977.

[8] Bennett. Bruce L., Maxwell L. Howell, and Uriel Simri, *Comparative Physical Education and Sport.* Philadelphia: Lea & Febiger, 1975, 1983; also see, Howell, Reet, Maxwell L. Howell, Dale P. Toohey, and Margaret D. Toohey, *Methodology in Comparative Physical Education and Sport,* Champaign, Illinois: Stipes Publishing Co., 1979.

[9] ICHPER, *Proceedings from the World Congress.* Rotterdam, The Netherlands, 1975; and, ICHPER, *Proceedings from the World Congress,* Mexico City, Mexico, 1977.

[10] ICHPER, *Proceedings from the World Congress,* Kiel, Germany, 1979.

[11] ICCPES, Newsletters 1, 2, 3, & 4, Wingate, Israel: Wingate Institute, 1979, 1980; and ISCPES, *Proceedings from the First International Seminar on Comparative Physical Education and Sport in 1978,* Wingate, Israel: Wingate Institute, 1979.

[12] ISCPES, *Proceedings from the Second International Seminar on Comparative Physical Education and Sport in 1980,* Halifax, Nova Scotia: Dalhousie University Printing Center, 1982.

[13] Bereday, George Z. F. *Comparative Education,* New York: Holt, Rinehart &Winston, Inc., 1964.

[14] Pooley, John C. "The Use and Abuse of Comparative Physical Education and Sport." *Journal of Comparative Physical Education and Sport.* IX: 1 (1987), pp. 5-24.

[15]Olafson, Gordon, "Triangulation in Comparative Research: Mixing Qualitative and Quantitative Methods." *Journal of Comparative Physical Education and Sport*, XII: 2, (1990).

[16]Standeven, Joy, "Trying Triangulation: A Response to Gordon Olafson (and Denzin)." *Journal of Comparative Physical Education and Sport*, XIII: 2, (1991), pp. 55-61.

[17]Patton, Michael Quinn, *Qualitative Evaluation and Research Methods* (2nd Edition). Newbury Park, California: Sage Publishing, 1990.

[18]Siedentop, Darryl, "Dialogue or Exorcism? A Rejoinder to Schempp." *Journal of Teaching in Physical Education,* 6: 4 (1987), pp. 373-376.

[19]Locke, Lawrence F. "The Question of Quality in Qualitative Research." Paper presented at the Measurement and Evaluation Symposium (Baton Rouge, LA), 1986.

[20]See also Locke, Lawrence F. "Qualitative Research as a Form of Scientific Inquiry in Sport and Physical Education." *Research Quarterly for Exercise and Sport,* 60: 1 (1989), pp. 1-20.

[21]Locke, Lawrence F., "Qualitative Research in the Gymnasium: Old Problems and New Responses." Paper presented at the Seminaire International La complementarite, 1985.

[22]Schriewer, Jurgen, "The Twofold Character of Comparative Education: Cross Cultural Comparison and Externalization to World Situations." *Prospects*, 19: 3 (1989), pp. 389-406.

[23]West, Peter, "How Not To Do Comparative Education," *Comparative and International Studies and the Theory and Practice of Education.* Proceedings of the Annual Conference of the Australian Comparative and International Education Society, Hamilton, New Zealand, 1983.

[24]Sheehan, Barry A. "Comparative Education: Phoenix or Dodo?" *Comparative and International Studies and the Theory and Practice of Education.* Proceedings of the Annual Conference of the Australian Comparative and International Education Society, Hamilton, New Zealand, 1983. Also see, Smith, Nick L. "The Context of Investigations in Cross-Cultural Evaluations." *Studies in Educational Evaluation,* 17: 1 (1991), pp. 3-21; and, Speakman-Yearta, Maureen A., "Cross-Cultural Comparisons of Physical Education Purposes." *Journal of Teaching in Physical Education*, 6: 3 (1987), pp. 252-258.

[25]Ragin, Charles C. *The Comparative Method: Moving Beyond Qualitative and Quantitative Strategies.* Berkeley: University of California Press, 1987.

[26]See, Bassler, R., *Quantitative oder qualitative Sozialforschung in Sportwissenschaten.* Wien: Osterreichischer Bundesverlag, 1989; Clarke, D. H. & H. H. Clarke, *Research process in physical education. recreation and health.* Englewood: Prentice-Hall, 1970; Guba, E.G. & Y. S. Lincoln,

"Naturalistic and materialistic inquiry." In J. P. Keeves (Ed.), *Educational research methodology and measurement* Oxford: Pergamon, 1988, pp. 81-85; Haag, H. "Development and structure of a theoretical framework for sport science (Sportwissenschaft)" *Quest.* 31 (1979), pp. 25-35; Haag, H. "Quantitative methods of research on instruction in physical education and sport," In, H. Rieder & U. Hanke, *Sportlehrer und Trainer heute.* Koln: Strauss, 1987, pp. 311-335; Haag, H. "Zum paradigm qualitative - quantitative," In, R. Singer (Ed.), *Sportpsychologische Forschungsmethoden. Probleme, Anstatze.* Koln: Bps., 1991, pp. 69-77; and Haag, H., O. Grupe, & A. Kirsch (Eds.), *Sport science in Germany. An interdisciplinary anthology.* Berlin: Springer, 1992.